T0257917

Encyclopedia of Diabetes: Retinopathy and Treatment for Type 1 Diabetes

Volume 11

Encyclopedia of Diabetes: Retinopathy and Treatment for Type 1 Diabetes
Volume 11

Edited by **Rex Slavin, Windy Wise and Roy Marcus Cohn**

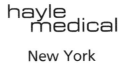

hayle
medical

New York

Published by Hayle Medical,
30 West, 37th Street, Suite 612,
New York, NY 10018, USA
www.haylemedical.com

Encyclopedia of Diabetes: Retinopathy and Treatment for Type 1 Diabetes
Volume 11
Edited by Rex Slavin, Windy Wise and Roy Marcus Cohn

© 2015 Hayle Medical

International Standard Book Number: 978-1-63241-153-2 (Hardback)

This book contains information obtained from authentic and highly regarded sources. Copyright for all individual chapters remain with the respective authors as indicated. A wide variety of references are listed. Permission and sources are indicated; for detailed attributions, please refer to the permissions page. Reasonable efforts have been made to publish reliable data and information, but the authors, editors and publisher cannot assume any responsibility for the validity of all materials or the consequences of their use.

The publisher's policy is to use permanent paper from mills that operate a sustainable forestry policy. Furthermore, the publisher ensures that the text paper and cover boards used have met acceptable environmental accreditation standards.

Trademark Notice: Registered trademark of products or corporate names are used only for explanation and identification without intent to infringe.

Printed in the United States of America.

Contents

Preface

This book contains extensive analysis regarding the pathogenesis of Type-1 Diabetes. Type-1 Diabetes is a classic autoimmune disease. Genetic factors are responsible but they cannot describe the rapid, even overwhelming extent of this disease. It is important to comprehend etiology and pathogenesis of this disease. The complexities related to Type-1 Diabetes include a number of clinical problems. Several veterans in this field have analyzed a number of topics for consideration that are appropriate for clinicians as well as researchers alike. The book gives appropriate elucidation of advanced technologies and applications in the constant search for cure and treatments for diabetes which are organized under three sections namely, Retinopathy, Treatment and Diabetes & Oral Health.

This book is a result of research of several months to collate the most relevant data in the field.

When I was approached with the idea of this book and the proposal to edit it, I was overwhelmed. It gave me an opportunity to reach out to all those who share a common interest with me in this field. I had 3 main parameters for editing this text:

1. Accuracy – The data and information provided in this book should be up-to-date and valuable to the readers.

2. Structure – The data must be presented in a structured format for easy understanding and better grasping of the readers.

3. Universal Approach – This book not only targets students but also experts and innovators in the field, thus my aim was to present topics which are of use to all.

Thus, it took me a couple of months to finish the editing of this book.

I would like to make a special mention of my publisher who considered me worthy of this opportunity and also supported me throughout the editing process. I would also like to thank the editing team at the back-end who extended their help whenever required.

Editor

Part 1

Retinopathy

Ocular Complications of Type 1 Diabetes

Daniel Rappoport, Yoel Greenwald, Ayala Pollack and Guy Kleinmann
Ophthalmology Department, Kaplan Medical Center, POB 1, Rehovot,
Israel

1. Introduction

Type 1 diabetes is a complex metabolic disease involving multiple organ systems which may cause severe visual impairment. Almost all parts of the eye may be affected including: the extra-ocular muscles, intra-ocular lens, the optic nerve, and retina.

Diabetes is the leading cause of blindness between the ages of 20 and 74 in many developed countries (Cheung et al., 2010; Powers, 2008). Individuals with diabetes are 25 times more likely to become legally blind than individuals without diabetes. Blindness is primarily the result of diabetic retinopathy that accounts for ¼ of blind registrations in the western world (Cheung et al., 2010; Powers, 2008).

Prevention of severe visual impairment in type 1 diabetes includes: optimal glycemic control, the treatment of ancillary risk factors such as hypertension, regular ophthalmic screening, and early diagnosis and treatment of ocular complications.

In the following chapter we will describe the ocular complications of diabetes and the treatments for these conditions.

2. Extra-ocular muscles

Diabetics may present with a sudden onset of diplopia (double vision). This is usually caused by the partial or complete paralysis of one of the extra-ocular muscles due to microvascular damage to the third, fourth or sixth cranial nerve (Thomas & Graham, 2008; Kline et al. 2010).

When a third cranial nerve palsy occurs, it is important to differentiate between a diabetic nerve palsy and paresis due to compression of the nerve from an aneurysm at the junction of the posterior communicating and internal carotid arteries. In diabetic nerve palsy the pupil is often spared meaning that it continues to react to light appropriately despite damage to the motor capabilities of the third cranial nerve. Typically in cranial nerve palsy due to a space occupying lesion such as an aneurysm, the pupil in the affected eye is dilated. In 20% of patients with diabetic nerve palsy there may be pupil involvement, however this is usually a mild efferent defect (Kline et al. 2010). Aneurysms are rare in children but may be present in adolescents, so ruling it out, by neuroimaging, is crucial. Pain may also be present in diabetic third nerve palsy. When there is paresis of the fourth or sixth cranial nerve, referral to a neuro-ophthalmolgist is also recommended for follow-up and to exclude other causes, such as myasthenia gravis or brain lesions.

When the oculomotor defect is due to microvascular complications of diabetes the prognosis is good.

Recovery of ocular motor function generally begins within three months of onset and recovery is usually complete. Although the diplopia can be debilitating, due to the generally limited course of these complaints, patients can usually be effectively managed conservatively with eye patching. Surgery is rarely indicated.

3. Lens: Cataract and refractive changes

Hyperglycemia can reduce lens clarity. Hyperglycemia also induces changes in the refractive index and accommodative amplitude of the lens, both of which also act to reduce visual function (Flynn & Smiddy, 2000).

3.1 Refractive and accommodative changes

One of the most frequently encountered ocular manifestations of diabetes is abrupt changes in the refractive power of the lens. When the blood glucose level is high, the glucose concentration in the aqueous humor, the fluid surrounding the lens, increases as well. This causes the glucose concentration in the lens to increase by diffusion (Flynn & Smiddy, 2000). Under normal conditions glucose is metabolized inside the lens by glycolysis. However, when the glucose level in the lens is very high, glycolysis enzymes are overridden and some glucose is reduced by the enzyme aldose reductase and converted to sorbitol (Stirban et al., 2008). Sorbitol is metabolized slowly by the lens cells and accumulates, increasing the osmotic pressure inside the lens. This increased osmotic pressure leads to an influx of water from the aqueous humor and the lens swells. This larger lens is more convex and therefore more powerful at bending incoming light which alters the focal point of the eye, causing acute nearsightedness (myopia) and blurred distance vision.

These refractive changes may be up to three to four diopters and may last for several weeks. Thus, patients with poorly controlled blood glucose levels experience transient refractive changes due to fluctuating levels of glucose in the blood. Acute blurring of vision may be the first symptom of undiagnosed or poorly controlled diabetes.

Accommodation, the ability to adjust focus for near tasks such as reading, is also affected in patients with diabetes. Studies have shown that diabetics have decreased amplitude of accommodation compared to age matched controls, and require spectacle correction for near work at a younger age than non-diabetics (Flynn & Smiddy, 2000).

3.2 Cataract

Cataract is a common cause of visual impairment in patients with diabetes. Epidemiological studies have revealed an up to five-fold increased prevalence of cataracts in diabetic patients. Individuals with type 1 diabetes manifested a greater prevalence of cataracts between the ages of 18 to 44 than age-matched controls (Obrosova et al., 2010). Duration of diabetes and quality of glycemic control are the major risk factors for early cataract development.

Potential mechanisms of diabetic cataract formation include accumulation of lenticular sorbitol, as described in the previous section (3.1). This reduces lens clarity leading to early cataract formation. It has also been postulated that recurrent high levels of glucose in the lens lead to the glycolation of lens proteins from increased non-enzymatic glycation and oxidative stress to the lens (Obrosova et al., 2010). This causes diabetic patients to develop age related lens changes similar to non-diabetic age related cataracts, except at a younger age than non-diabetics (Bobrow et al. 2010). Several studies have analyzed the effect of vitamin and anti-oxidant supplements, such as vitamin C, E and beta carotene and zinc on preventing or slowing progression of age related cataracts in diabetes without showing any statistically significant benefit with their use (AREDS report no. 9, 2001 as cited in Obrosova et al., 2010).

A rarer form of cataract in diabetics that is seldom encountered in clinical practice today is called the 'true diabetic cataract'. This is typically seen in young patients with uncontrolled diabetes. Any rapidly maturing (i.e whitening) cataract in a child or a young adult should raise awareness to the possibility of diabetes.

Cataract surgery is indicated when visual function is significantly impaired by the cataract. Surgery is also indicated if the cataract obscures the view of the retina and makes the diagnosis and treatment of diabetic retinopathy difficult. Cataract surgery is safe in diabetic patients and there is a 95% success rate in terms of improved visual acuity (Obrosova et al., 2010). Good glycemic control, fluid and electrolyte balance should be maintained perioperatively and the patient's primary care physician and anesthesiologist should be involved. It is recommended that the surgery be scheduled in the morning to minimize changes in the patient's usual schedule (Purdy et al., 2010). Some controversy exists regarding a potential association between cataract surgery and a subsequent worsening of diabetic retinopathy. Patients should be made aware of this risk pre-operatively. Cataract surgery and its effect on diabetic retinopathy will be discussed in more detail the diabetic retinopathy section (7.6.2).

4. Cornea

Structural changes to the corneal basement membrane in diabetes decrease the adhesion of corneal epithelial cells to the deeper stromal tissue. This increases the risk of recurrent corneal erosions (Reidy et al., 2010). In addition, accumulation of sorbitol in the cornea during periods of hyperglycemia leads to hypoesthesia (a loss of corneal sensation). Both hypoesthesia and epithelial adhesion dysfunction occur more frequently with increased severity and duration of diabetes. In these patients, any epithelial injury, either from trauma, during ocular surgery or from routine contact lens use, may result in prolonged healing times. This increases the risk of severe complications such as bacterial infiltration and ulceration.

5. Iris and pupil

Bilateral tonic pupils may be seen in diabetic patients (Kline et al., 2010). This manifests with sluggish, segmented pupillary reactions to light and better response to near effort, followed by slow redilation of the pupil. Tonic pupils are caused by microvascular damage to postganglionic parasympathetic pupillomotor nerve fibers. Diminished pupillary response is also seen due to glycogen infiltration of the pigment epithelium and sphincter and dilator muscles (Thomas & Graham, 2008).

Rubeosis iridis, neovascularization in the iris, is a serious complication of diabetes which occurs in patients with severe diabetic retinopathy (Thomas & Graham, 2008). Growth factors released from the ischemic retina induce the development of intertwining blood vessels on the anterior surface of the iris (figure 1). These vessels can block the normal drainage of fluid from the anterior chamber, leading to a sharp and persistent rise in intraocular pressure. This complication is known as neovascular glaucoma. This type of glaucoma is often refractory to treatment and can be associated with pain from very high ocular pressure. Topical medical therapy used commonly in other forms of glaucoma is often less effective. Treatment should include aggressive control of the underlying retinal disease with peripheral laser ablation to reduce ischemia. The treatment of proliferative diabetic retinopathy will be discussed in more detail in section 7.6.2.3.

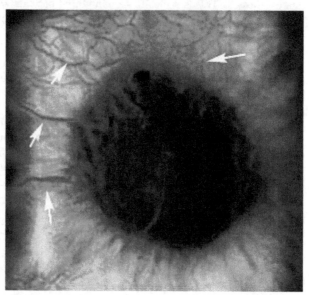

Fig. 1. Neovascularization of the Iris: These pathologic blood vessels on the iris (white arrows) are associated with retinal ischemia in proliferative diabetic retinopathy. The normal iris has no visible surface blood vessels.

6. Optic nerve

6.1 Diabetic papillopathy
In diabetic papillopathy, chronic swelling of the optic disc often associated with mild visual impairment. The suspected cause is mild reversible ischemia of the optic nerve head (Ostri et al., 2010; Kline et al., 2010). Risk factors include pronounced recent decrease in hemoglobin A_{1C} and a small cup to disc ratio of the optic nerve head. Patients often present with no visual complaints or with a mild nonspecific visual disturbance such as mild distortion or blurring. There is no pain and visual acuity is usually normal but may be slightly diminished. There is no afferent pupillary defect. An enlarged blind spot is seen on visual fields. Clinical examination reveals unilateral or bilateral hyperemic edema of the optic disc, accompanied by dilation of inner disc surface vessels, vascular leakage and axonal swelling (cotton wool spots). These enlarged vessels may be confused with neovascularization of the disc but these radially dilated vessels do not extend into the vitreous (Figure 2).

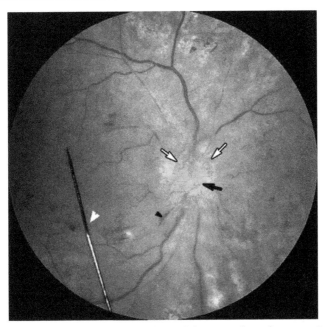

Fig. 2. Diabetic Papillopathy. A chronic swelling of the optic disc often associated with mild visual impairment. This color fundus photograph shows blurred disc margins (white arrows), flame shaped hemorrhages (black arrowhead). The dilated blood vessels on the optic disc (black arrow) may be confused with neovscularization but are radially dilated, do not enter the vitreous cavity and do not leak on fluorescein angigraphy.[marked by the white arrowhead the pointer aiding the patient's fixation during photography].

When diabetic papillopathy is suspected, it is important to perform fluorescein angiography. In diabetic papillopathy, dye leakage is limited to the disc and peripapillary retina as opposed to the intravitreal leakage seen in the case of neovascular lesions. Diabetic retinopathy is usually present at diagnosis, but in 20% of reported cases there was no clinical evidence of any diabetic retinopathy (Kline et al., 2010). If the optic disc edema is bilateral, the initial evaluation should include brain imaging and lumbar puncture to rule out intracranial space occupying lesions and elevated intracranial pressure.

The optic disc edema resolves in many cases without treatment, usually within two to ten months. Minimal optic atrophy is seen in 20% of cases. In rare cases, especially in poorly controlled patients, diabetic papillopathy may progress to non-arteritic anterior ischemic optic neuropathy (NAION) with significant optic atrophy and arcuate visual field defects. In most cases, long term visual acuity depends on the associated diabetic retinopathy. There is no proven treatment for diabetic papillopathy.

6.2 Non-arteritic anterior ischemic optic neuropathy (NAION)

Non-arteritic anterior ischemic optic neuropathy (NAION) occurs as a consequence of the interruption of blood flow to the optic nerve at the level of the optic disc. NAION is characterized by diffuse or segmental, hyperemic or pale optic disc edema. It is usually unilateral, and in contrast to diabetic papillopathy, damage to the optic nerve ganglions causes decreased visual acuity and/or visual field loss. Vision is usually not worse than 20/200 and the typical visual field defect is altitudinal. Diabetes is a risk factor for NAION and the condition may present at a younger age in diabetic patients (Kline et al., 2010).

After an episode of NAION visual acuity may be stable but can also decline slowly over weeks to months until eventual stabilization. The initial finding upon examination is optic disc swelling, but this resolves over time and is replaced by optic disc atrophy within 4-8 weeks. There is no proven treatment for this condition.

7. Diabetic retinopathy

Damage to the retinal capillaries and other small vessels is the hallmark of diabetic eye disease and is known as diabetic retinopathy. This condition is the major cause of blindness and visual disability in patients with type 1 diabetes.

7.1 Epidemiology

Diabetic retinopathy is one of the most frequent causes of blindness in working aged adults (20-74 years) (Regillo et al., 2010; Cheung et al., 2010). In the USA an estimated 86% of patients with type 1 diabetes have some degree of diabetic retinopathy. Data from the Wisconsin Epidemiologic Study of Diabetic Retinopathy (WESDR) showed that within 5 years of diagnosis of type 1 diabetes, 14% of patients developed retinopathy, with the incidence rising to 74% by 10 years (Klein et al., 2008; Varma, 2008). In people with retinopathy at the WESDR baseline examination, 64% had their retinopathy worsen, 17% progressed to proliferative diabetic retinopathy (PDR) and about 20% developed diabetic macular edema during 10 years of follow-up.

The WESDR data in type 1 diabetics showed that 25 years after diagnosis, 97% of patients developed retinopathy, 43% progressed to PDR, 29% developed diabetic macular edema and 3.6% of patients younger than 30 at diagnosis were legally blind (Klein et al., 2008). Fortunately, recent advances in glycemic control, ophthalmic treatment and patient education seem to be working. The WESDR results also showed a reduction in the yearly incidence and progression of diabetic retinopathy during the past 15 years (Varma 2008).

The course of diabetic retinal disease in children is fairly benign. Severe complications such as proliferative diabetic retinopathy are uncommon in children before puberty (Raab et al., 2010).

7.2 Risk factors

Several risk factors influence the development and progression of diabetic retinopathy. The following list contains most of the important risk factors known today.

1. Diabetes duration: The longer the duration of diabetes, the higher the risk of developing diabetic retinopathy and of having a severe manifestation of the disease. (Simon et al., 2010; Cheung et al., 2010).

2. Hyperglycemia: Good glycemic control has been shown to significantly prevent the development and progression of diabetic retinopathy. Every 1% decrease in hemoglobin A_{1C} leads to a 40% reduction in the risk of developing retinopathy, a 25%

reduction in the risk of progression to vision threatening retinopathy and a 15% reduction in the risk of blindness (Cheung et al. 2010, DCCT group, 1995).

3. Hypertension: Good blood pressure control is important in reducing the risk of retinopathy. Every 10 mmHg reduction in systolic blood pressure leads to a reduction of 35% in the risk of retinopathy progression and a reduction of 50% in the risk of visual loss (Cheung et al. 2010).

4. Hyperlipidemia: High cholesterol may also be a risk factor for diabetic retinopathy progression (Cheung et al., 2010).

5. Genetic factors: The Diabetes Control and Complications Trial (DCCT group, 1997) showed a heritable tendency for developing diabetic retinopathy, regardless of other risk factors.

6. Ethnicity: Diabetic retinopathy in America is more prevalent among African Americans, Hispanic and south Asian groups than in Caucasians with otherwise similar risk profiles (Cheung et al., 2010).

7. Pregnancy: Pregnancy is associated with worsening of diabetic retinopathy (DCCT group, 2000). All pregnant women need to be closely monitored throughout pregnancy. Pregnancy in type 1 diabetes is discussed in further detail in section 7.6.1.

7.3 Pathophysiology

The normal retina has a blood–retinal barrier (BRB) which consists of cells that are tightly joined together to prevent certain substances from entering the retinal tissue. An important part of the BRB is the non-fenestrated capillaries of the retinal circulation. In diabetic retinopathy, damage to retinal blood vessels leads to a breakdown of the BRB and the leakage of fluid, blood and protein into the retinal tissue.

Diabetic retinopathy is induced when hyperglycemia and other causal risk factors trigger a cascade of biochemical changes leading to microvascular damage in the retina. Hyperglycemia leads to rise of sorbitol concentrations via the action of aldose reductase. This process increases oxidative stress by reducing intracellular levels of reduced glutathione, an important antioxidant (Stirban et al., 2008). Intracellular hyperglycemia also increases synthesis of diacylglycerol an activating cofactor for protein kinase C (PKC). Activated PKC decreases the production of anti-artherosclerotic factors and increases production of pro-artherogenic factors, pro-adhesive and pro-inflammatory factors (Stirban et al., 2008). Hyperglycemia also leads to accumulation of advanced glycated end products which are pro-inflammatory and activate PKC (Stirban et al., 2008). Intracellular hyperglycaemia increases intracellular N-acetylglucosamine levels. This byproduct reacts with serine and threonine residues in transcription factors, resulting in pathologic changes in gene expression (Stirban et al., 2008). The final consequence of these pathological processes is increased inflammation and increased oxidative stress which cause endothelial cell dysfunction in retinal blood vessels.

Endothelial cell dysfunction induces retinal arteriolar dilatation which increases capillary bed pressure. This results in microaneurysm formation, vessel leakage and rupture (Cheung et al., 2010). Vascular permeability is also increased from loss of pericytes and increased endothelial proliferation in retinal capillaries. The breakdown of the blood-retinal barrier allows fluid to accumulate in the deep retinal layers where it damages photoreceptors and other neural tissues. This is the mechanism by which macular edema reduces visual acuity.

In some capillaries there is endothelial cell apoptosis. Vessels become acellular leading to vascular occlusion and non-perfusion of local retinal tissue (Stirban et al., 2008). The resultant retinal ischemia promotes the release of inflammatory growth factors, such as vascular endothelial growth factor (VEGF), growth hormone- insulin growth factor and erythropoietin (Cheung et al., 2010). These factors influence neovascularization, the proliferation of new capillaries, which is the hallmark of proliferative diabetic retinopathy.

7.4 Classification and clinical features

Diabetic retinopathy is classified into two stages: non-proliferative diabetic retinopathy (NPDR) and proliferative diabetic retinopathy (PDR). In NPDR the vascular changes occur within the retina and do not cross the retinal surface. The more advanced stage of PDR is marked by neovascularization wherein new blood vessels grow out from the retinal surface towards the vitreous cavity.

A major cause of vision loss in diabetic retinopathy is diabetic macular edema (DME). DME occurs when leaky capillary beds allow fluid to accumulate in the part of the retina responsible for central vision. This edema can occur in patients with any stage of underlying retinopathy from mild NPDR to severe PDR.

Visual impairment is usually related to the state of macular disease and the consequences of neovascularisation such as vitreous hemorrhage and retinal detachment. As such, the level of retinal disease does not always correlate with visual function and severe diabetic retinopathy can be present initially without significant visual loss.

7.4.1 Non-proliferative diabetic retinopathy (NPDR)

In NPDR the retinal microvascular changes occur within the retina and do not extend beyond the surface of the retina. The patient with NPDR is usually asymptomatic and visual acuity is preserved unless the macula is affected.

Clinical findings include microaneurysms (saccular enlargements of weakened capillaries), intra-retinal hemorrhages, hard exudates (lipid filled macrophages), cotton wool spots (nerve fiber layer infarcts)(figures 3-4), venous beading (focal venous dilatations and constrictions) and intra-retinal microvascular abnormalities (IRMA's, dilated pre-existing capillaries) (Regillo et al., 2010, Cheung et al., 2008).

Fluorescein angiography (FA) is an essential tool for evaluating the retinal circulation and retinopathy stage. Sodium fluorescein is injected into the systemic circulation, and an angiogram is obtained by photographing the fluorescence emitted after illumination of the retina. In NPDR, the FA shows microaneurysms as dye filled outpouchings. Hemorrhages appear as black dots as the blood obscures the fluorescence from the retina and choroid below (figure 5).

NPDR is classified as mild, moderate or severe, reflecting the risk of progression to PDR (Table 1) as determined by the Early Treatment in Diabetic Retinopathy Study (ETDRS) (ETDRS group, 1995). The diagnosis of severe NPDR is made when one of three findings is present: diffuse intra-retinal hemorrhages and microaneurysms in all 4 retinal quadrants, venous beading in 2 quadrants or one intra-retinal microvascular abnormalities anywhere. Fifteen persent of patients with severe NPDR will progress to high-risk PDR within 1 year. When any two features of severe NPDR are present, the patient is said to suffer from very severe NPDR and the one year risk of progression to high risk PDR increases to 45%.

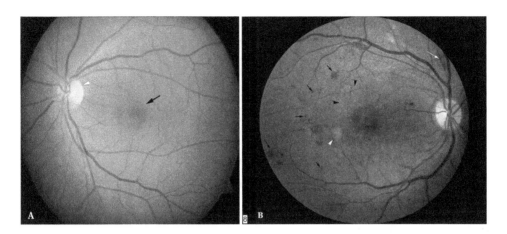

Fig. 3. A: Color photograph of normal fundus (left eye) normal optic disc (white arrow) and macula (black arrow). B: Color photograph (right eye) showing non-proliferative diabetic retinopathy and macular edema. Findings include; dot and blot hemorrhages (black arrows), flame shaped hemorrhages (white arrow), and cotton wool spot (white arrowhead) which represent nerve fiber layer infarcts. Hard exudates (black arrowheads) are lipid filled macrophages and in this photograph are radially distributed around the central macula.

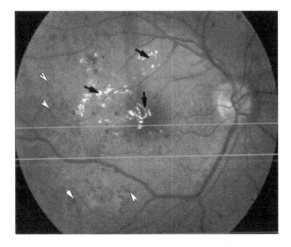

Fig. 4. Color photograph of fundus with moderate non-proliferative diabetic retinopathy with macular edema. Multiple dot and blot retinal hemorrhages are seen (white arrowheads) and hard exudates (black arrows).

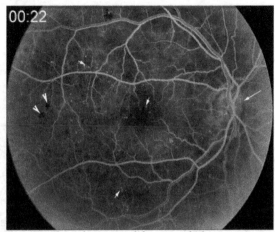

Fig. 5. Fluorescein angiography of non proliferative diabetic retinopathyof the right eye. Sodium fluorescein is injected into the systemic circulation, and an angiogram is obtained by photographing the fluorescence emitted after illumination of the retina. In NPDR the FA shows microaneurysms filled with dye (small white arrows). Hemorrhages appear as black dots because the transmission of fluorescence from below the hemorrhage is blocked (white arrowheads) . The optic disc marked with long white arrow.

Stage of NPDR	Clinical Features	Progression Risk
Mild NPDR	Few microaneurysms	5% progress to PDR within 1 year
Moderate NPDR	Microaneurysms and other microvascular lesions	12-16% progress to PDR within 1 year
Severe NPDR (Meets 1 of 3 criteria)	• Extensive intraretinal hemorrhages and microaneurysms in all four quadrants • Venous beading in two or more quadrants • One IRMA	52% progress to PDR within 1 year 15% progress to high risk PDR within 1 year
Very severe NPDR	Any two of the features of severe NPDR	45% progress to high risk PDR within 1 year

Table 1. Clinical classification of non-proliferative diabetic retinopathy

7.4.2 Proliferative diabetic retinopathy (PDR)

Diabetic retinopathy advances to the proliferative stage when new vessels (neovascularizations) are formed which grow up from the retina towards the vitreous cavity. The development of these pathological blood vessels is induced by pro-angiogenic factors released as a result of the severe retinal ischemia caused by the progression of diabetic retinal microvascular disease. Neovascularizations can be identified clinically as a jumble of disorganized, fine vessels emanating from the organized retinal vessel architecture (figure 6). Fluorescein angiography is also very effective at identifying neovascular lesions as the new vessels are porous and leak fluorescent dye into the vitreous cavity.

The new vessels in PDR evolve in three stages. Initially, the fine new vessels grow with minimal fibrous tissue. Then the new vessels increase in gauge and length with an increased fibrous component. Finally, the vessels regress and the residual fibrovascular tissue along the posterior surface of the vitreous body contracts.

Retinal neovascularizations (NV) are divided into two subtypes based on their relative risk of causing severe visual loss as demonstrated by the Diabetic Retinopathy Study (DRS). Vascular proliferations on or near the optic disc are termed NV-disc (NVD) and proliferations elsewhere are termed NV-elsewhere (NVE) (figures 6 - 8). The presence of NVD carries the higher risk of severe visual loss and requires more urgent treatment (DRS research group, 1979, 1981).

PDR is graded from early to high risk based on the risk of severe visual loss as determined by the extent of the neovascular proliferations. The DRS (DRS research group, 1979, 1981) defined high risk PDR as the presence of either: NVD with a vitreous hemorrhage, NVD larger than a quarter disc area without vitreous hemorrhage or NVE larger than half disc area with vitreous hemorrhage. Without treatment, patients with early PDR have 50% risk of developing high risk PDR in 1 year and those with high risk PDR have a 25% risk of severe visual loss within 2 years. Treatment of PDR involves extensive peripheral laser ablation of the retina and is discussed in section 7.5.2.3.

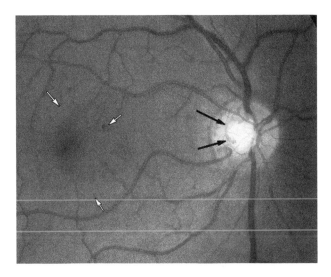

Fig. 6. Proliferative Diabetic Retinopathy with Neovascularization of the Optic Disc (NVD). Vascular proliferations on or near the optic disc are termed NV-disc (NVD).This Color photograph shows fine jumbled vessels (black arrows) typical of NVD. Multiple dot and blot retinal hemorrhages are seen (white arrows).

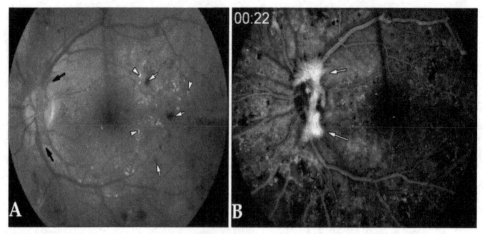

Fig. 7. High Risk Proliferative Diabetic Retinopathy with Large NVD. PDR is graded from early to high risk based on the risk of severe visual loss as determined by the extent of the neovascular proliferation. A: Color photograph showing a large neovascularization of the optic disc (black arrows) this NVD is larger than a quarter disc area therefore consistent with high risk PDR. Retinal hemorrhages (white arrows) and hard exudates (white arrowheads) are also seen. B: Fluorescein angiography in the same patient demonstrating hyper-fluorescence due to dye leakage from the disc neovascularization (white arrows).

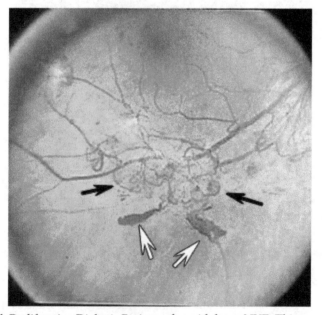

Fig. 8. High Risk Proliferative Diabetic Retinopathy with large NVE. This neovascular lesion located away from the optic disc is known as a Neovascularization-Elsewhere (NVE). This large NVE (black arrow) is associated with a small hemorrhage (white arrow).

The most frequent complication of PDR is vitreous hemorrhage (figure 9) caused by rupture in the fragile neovascular vessels. The initial complaint is often of black dots partially obscuring vision and can evolve to severe visual loss over a period of hours to days as the eye fills with blood.

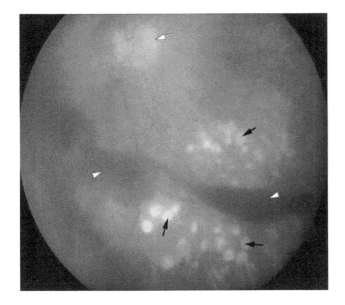

Fig. 9. Vitreous Hemorrhage. Vitreous hemorrhage is the most frequent complication of PDR. It is caused by rupture of neovascular vessels. This color figure shows partial vitreous hemorrhage causing general haze. Dense blood in the vitreous cavity is seen (white arrowheads). This hemorrhage occurred in eye after the initiation of pan-retinal photocoagulation as a treatment for PDR. Multiple white-yellow laser burns are seen (black arrows). This treatment is discussed in section 7.5.2.3. The optic disc is also seen (white arrow).

Another cause of severe vision loss in PDR is traction retinal detachment. This detachment occurs when the neovascular tissue connecting the retinal surface to the vitreous contracts causing a separation between the surface and deep retinal layers (figure 10). If this occurs in the center of the macula severe vision loss can result.

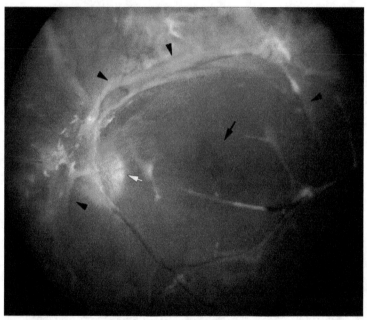

Fig. 10. Traction Retinal Detachment. This detachment is one of the serious complications in PDR and may cause severe visual loss. It occurs when the neovascular tissue connecting the retinal surface to the vitreous contracts causing a separation between the surface and deep retinal layers. This color fundus photograph shows elevated and detached retina (black arrowheads) involving the optic disc area (white arrow). The retina at the center of the macula (black arrow) is not detached.

A third serious complication of PDR occurs when proliferative and pro-angiogenic factors released from the ischemic retina induce the propagation of new vessels on the iris (figure 1). These vessels can block the normal outflow of fluid from the eye causing often severely increased ocular pressure. This complication is known as neovascular glaucoma and is discussed further previously in section 5.

Visual acuity in the absence of macular disease is often good in PDR until a complication occurs, most commonly vitreous hemorrhage. This sudden transition from good vision to near blindness can be traumatic for patients who were unaware of the severity of their diabetic eye disease.

7.4.3 Diabetic macular edema

Diabetic macular edema (DME) is responsible for most of the moderate visual loss in retinopathy patients. The vision loss is often mild at first, but without effective treatment it can progress and patients can lose the ability to perform activities of daily living such as reading and driving. Diabetic macular edema is assessed separately from the stage of retinopathy (NPDR/PDR) and it can manifest along a different and independent course.

The edema evolves when damage to the macular capillary bed causes a breakdown of the blood-retina barrier. This results in increased retinal vascular permeability and to the accumulation of fluid in the macula. Macular edema may be 'focal' and emanate from a small cluster of leaky vessels, or 'diffuse' and involve the entire macula without a clear point of origin. Clinical examination can reveal rings of hard exudates (lipid filled macrophages) which delineate the area of focal leakage (figures 3 & 4). These subtypes are often differentiated by angiography which demonstrates areas of focal leakage from specific capillary lesions and microaneurysms in focal edema. In diffuse macular edema, angiography reveals widespread leakage with no definitive point of origin from extensive breakdown of the blood-retinal barrier (Regillo et al., 2010).

Treatment decisions are based on the clinical examination in DME. Intervention is recommended only when the retinal edema involves or threatens the center of the macula. In all other cases, close follow-up alone is indicated (ETDRS group, 1995).

Optical Coherence Tomography (OCT) is a useful ancillary imaging technique in DME. Recent technological advances in OCT technology have provided ophthalmologists with high-resolution images of the retina in cross-sectional slices. Aside from demonstrating areas of retinal thickening and intra-retinal fluid (figure 11), OCT obtains quantitative measurements of central retinal thickness that are important for close monitoring and follow-up of macular edema. Serial OCT examinations are often used as a non-invasive and accurate method analyzing treatment response in DME patients (Cheung et al., 2008).

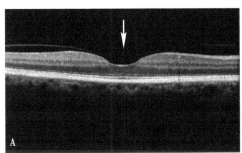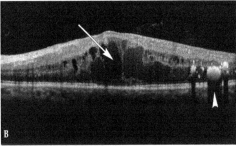

Fig. 11. Optical Coherence Tomography (OCT) of the Macula. A: OCT scan demonstrating the normal anatomic indentation in the central macula in a healthy eye (white arrow). B: Diabetic macular edema: There is loss of central macular indentation due to retinal cysts (white arrow). Hard exudates are also seen (white arrowhead).

7.4.4 Diabetic macular ischemia

Macular ischemia is a devastating complication of diabetic retinopathy. It is caused by extensive loss of retinal capillary perfusion in the macula. Clinical exam often reveals microaneurysms clustering at the margins of the non-perfused retina. Angiography can demonstrate the presence and extent of the area with capillary non-perfusion. This entity is generally associated with significantly decreased vision (Regillo et al., 2010).

7.5 Treatment and prevention of diabetic retinopathy

The main goal of treatment of diabetic retinopathy is preventing complications which can lead to vision loss. Treatment should include both ocular therapy and systemic medical intervention.

7.5.1 Medical treatment

Hyperglycemia, hypertension and hyperlipidemia are known risk factors for the development and progression of diabetic retinopathy. Treating and controlling these factors is crucial to preventing and limiting disease progression.

The Diabetes Control and Complications Trial (DCCT group, 1995) showed that intensive glycemic control reduced both the risk of developing retinopathy and the rate of progression of existing retinopathy. Intensive glycemic control reduced the risk for progression to severe NPDR and PDR, the incidence of diabetic macular edema and the need for laser treatments. Every percent reduction in hemoglobin A_{1C} lowers the risk of retinopathy development by 30-40%.

Several other systemic therapies have been investigated and found to reduce the risk of retinopathy progression including Angiotensin Converting Enzyme Inhibitors, Protein Kinase C Inhibitors and inhibitors of Advanced Glycosylation End-products formation (Cheung et al., 2008).

7.5.2 Ocular treatment

Ocular therapy in diabetic retinopathy includes panretinal or focal laser photocoagulation, intravitreal injections of either steroids or inhibitors of Vascular Endothelial Growth Factor (VEGF), surgery or a combination of the aforementioned treatments. The suitable treatment regimen must be tailored individually for each patient and is based on clinical status of the patient (ocular and systemic), previous treatments and data from several reports and ongoing studies.

7.5.2.1 NPDR

Visual acuity is not usually affected in NPDR unless there is damage to the macula in the form of macular edema or ischemia. Ocular treatment at this stage is definitively indicated only if there is evidence of macular disease. In patients with very severe NPDR who are at high risk for progression to PDR, laser treatment can be considered if the patient is not considered a suitable candidate for close follow-up. In such cases the recommended treatment is Pan- Retinal laser Photocoagulation (PRP) which will be discussed in section 7.5.2.3 (ETDRS group, 1995).

7.5.2.2 Diabetic macular edema (DME)

Treatment options for DME include focal laser photocoagulation, intravitreal injections of either steroids or anti-VEGF compounds and surgery.

7.5.2.2.1 Focal laser

The mainstay of DME treatment is focal laser photocoagulation. Focal laser treatment for DME involves the application of discrete laser burns to areas of leakage in the macula. The treatment is not painful and can be repeated up to every 4 months if edema persists. Treatment criteria are based on the ETDRS recommendations (ETDRS group, 1995) which showed that eyes with macular edema involving or threatening the central macula, defined as clinically significant macular edema (CSME), benefited from focal laser treatment. Focal laser treatment reduced the risk of moderate visual loss (loss of three lines of vision) by 50% over two years, increased the chance of improved vision and reduced central macular thickness compared to no treatment.

In eyes with macular edema that does not meet the criteria for CSME, laser treatment is not indicated. Close follow-up is recommended to determine the progression of the macular edema. Unfortunately, when the macular edema is associated with macular ischemia from a loss of macular capillary perfusion, the ETDRS showed a lesser beneficial effect for focal laser (ETDRS Group, 1995).

Side effects of focal laser photocoagulation include: paracentral visual field loss, transiently increased macular edema with decreased visual acuity and choroidal neovascularization (Regillo et al, 2010).

7.5.2.2.2 Steroid injections

Inflammatory factors play an important role in the development of diabetic retinopathy and macular edema (see section 7.3). For this reason it has long been thought that ocular steroid injections may be beneficial in DME treatment. Several trials have shown modestly improved visual acuity and central macular thickness after injection of intravitreal Triamcinolone (Grover at al., 2008; Yilmaz et al., 2009). A few recent trials on long acting steroid implants, such as Fluocinolone Acetate or Dexamethasone, have also reported short term visual acuity improvements (Grover et al., 2009).

The Diabetic Retinopathy Clinical Research Network (DRCR network, 2008) compared intravitreal injection of Triamcinolone to focal laser treatment in eyes with DME. There was no difference in visual acuity between the two groups after 1 year, and at 2 years eyes treated with laser had better vision. However, complications of intravitreal steroids, including elevated ocular pressure and increased cataract progression limit the usefulness of these drugs in DME. Intravitreal sterioid injections may be considered in patients who have previously undergone cataract surgery and in cases where the macular edema is refractory to focal laser. In these cases the injections may be given either alone or as an adjunct to laser treatment (Gillies et al., 2006; Maia et al., 2009).

7.5.2.2.3 Anti-vascular endothelial growth factor (VEGF) compounds

Vascular Endothelial Growth Factor (VEGF) is a major cause of the increased retinal vascular permeability which causes macular edema (Stirban et al., 2008). Several VEGF inhibitors have been investigated as treatments for DME with a beneficial effect on visual acuity and central macular thickness.

Injection of intravitreal Pegaptanib, a pegylated aptamer that inhibits one isoform of VEGF, was found to be better than sham injections in improving in visual acuity and decreasing the need for focal laser treatment, in the Macugen Diabetic Retinopathy Study group (Cunningham et al., 2005).

The injection of monoclonal antibodies that block all isoforms of VEGF has also been investigated as a treatment for DME. Several studies have shown a beneficial effect on visual acuity in eyes treated with Bevacizumab (trade name Avastin), a recombinant full length humanized antibody to VEGF (Nicholson & Shachat, 2010). Based on data from multiple studies (Nicholson & Shachat, 2010) repeated doses of Bevacizumab increase its average positive effect. The optimal timing for repeat dosing is unclear, but is probably between 3 to 12 weeks, with maximal effect with a 3 to 6 weeks interval between treatments.

The Bevacizumab Or Laser Treatment study (Michaelidis et al., BOLT study, 2010) compared 6-weekly bevacizumab injections to focal laser treatment in DME. One year post-randomization, eyes treated with bevacizumab had significantly better vision by over one line of acuity and less macular edema compared to eyes treated with focal laser. Bevacizumab treated eyes also had fivefold greater odds gaining at least 2 lines of vision.

Another promising drug that targets VEGF is Ranibizumab (trade name Lucentis). This a recombinant, humanized antibody fragment binds and inhibits all isoforms of VEGF. A recent study compared four treatment options; monthly injections of Ranibizumab combined with focal laser, monthly Ranibizumab alone with the option for rescue focal laser treatment, focal laser treatment alone and focal laser combined with intravitreal injections of Triamcinolone (DRCR network 2010a). After 1 year, eyes that received intravitreal injections of Ranibizumab, either combined with laser or with the option for rescue laser had better visual acuity compared with the other treatment groups. On average, eyes receiving Ranibizumab gained 1 line in visual acuity after 1 year. Half of Ranibizumab treated patients gained more than 2 lines in visual acuity, and 30% gained 3 lines or more. Two years results showed a similar positive treatment effect in DME with Ranibizumab injections.

The injection of anti-VEGF agents to the vitreous is both effective and safe. Adverse ocular effects include: cataract formation, retinal detachment, vitreous hemorrhage and infection. Potential systemic adverse effects include: hypertension, stroke, and myocardial infarction but these are very uncommon (Cheung et al., 2010; Nicholson & Shachat, 2010).

7.5.2.2.4 Surgical intervention

DME can also be treated surgically by performing a vitrectomy. This option is used sparingly because of the utility of both laser treatments and intravitreal injections in controlling the disease. Surgery is indicated in cases refractory to other treatments or when there is mechanical traction on the macula from vitreo-retinal adhesions. In such cases edema resolution can often not be obtained without resorting to intraocular surgery where the traction can be definitively released (Kaiser et al., 2001; DRCR network, 2010b).

7.5.2.3 Proliferative diabetic retinopathy (PDR) treatment

7.5.2.3.1 Panretinal photocoagulation (PRP)

The goal of treatment in PDR is to prevent complications and lower the risk of severe vision loss. The mainstay of treatment for PDR is laser ablation of the peripheral retina. In this treatment, known as panretinal photocoagulation (PRP), laser burns are placed over the entire retina, sparing only the central macula (figure 12). PRP promotes the regression and arrest of progression of retinal neovascularizations by destroying ischemic retinal tissue and reducing ischemia driven VEGF production (Cheung et al., 2010; Regillo et al., 2010).

The Diabetic Retinopathy Study (DRS) evaluated efficacy of PRP treatment in eyes with advanced NPDR or PDR (DRS Group, 1981). The DRS study recommended prompt treatment in eyes with high risk PDR (defined in section 7.4.2), because these eyes had the highest risk for severe visual loss. PRP treatment in these patients reduced the risk of severe visual loss by 50% over 5 years. The ETDRS study found that PRP treatment in eyes with early PDR reduced the risk of progression to high risk PDR by 50%, and significantly reduced the risk of severe visual loss (ETDRS Group, 1995). Based on these results, PRP treatment should be considered in eyes with any stage PDR especially if there is poor metabolic control, a non compliant patient or difficulty in maintaining close follow-up.

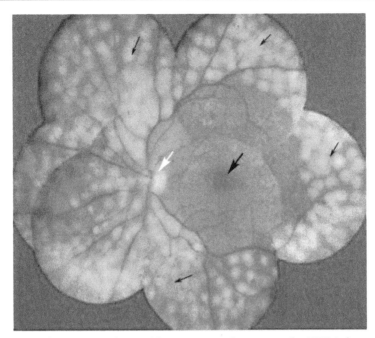

Fig. 12. Pan-Retinal Photocoagulation. The mainstay of treatment for PDR is laser ablation of the peripheral retina. In this treatment, known as panretinal photocoagulation (PRP), laser burns are placed over the entire retina (small black arrows), sparing only the central macula (large black arrow) and the optic disc (white arrow).

Full PRP treatment as recommended by the DRS and the ETDRS includes as many as 4000 laser burns. PRP can be painful and is often performed over several sessions. After the initial treatment course, additional therapy can be applied if there is persistent neovascularisation. After treatment, proliferative retinal tissue may regress and contract causing a vitreous hemorrhage or a traction retinal detachment from contracture of fibrovascular tissue. Side effects of PRP treatment also include; decreased in night vision, decreased color vision and loss of peripheral vision. These side effects can be reduced by spreading out the treatment sessions and by using less energy at each session (Regillo et al. 2010).

When PDR presents with macular edema, PRP treatment may initially increase the amount of the edema (ETDRS Group, 1991). In such case it is recommended to treat the macular edema with either focal laser or an intravitreal injection before initiating PRP (Silva et al., 2009, Mirshani et al., 2008).

7.5.2.3.2 Vitreous hemorrhage

In patients with new onset vitreous hemorrhages, laser PRP treatment is recommended if visualization of the retina is adequate. A severe, dense, non-clearing vitreous hemorrhage is an indication for vitrectomy surgery. The Diabetic Retinopathy Vitrectomy Study (DRVS Group, 1985) recommended surgery within 1 to 6 months of vitreous hemorrhage onset in type 1 diabetes patients with a non-clearing vitreous hemorrhage. Early vitrectomy improved visual acuity outcomes compared with waiting up to a year for spontaneous resolution before resorting to surgery.

Recent advances in vitreoretinal surgery, including smaller gauge instruments and the ability to perform laser ablation during surgery, have changed treatment recommendations. If a patient with a vitreous hemorrhage has not previously undergone PRP, vitrectomy is recommended when a dense vitreous hemorrhage persists beyond one to three months. Patients with vitreous hemorrhage that have preexisting complete PRP may undergo a longer observation period (Regillo et al., 2010).

Several studies have evaluated the efficacy of intravitreal anti-VEGF injections in patients with PDR (Nicholson & Shachat, 2010). Intravitreal Bevacizumab as adjunctive therapy with PRP was found to decrease leakage area from neovascularizations, improve visual acuity outcomes and reduce macular edema compared with PRP alone. In eyes with PDR and a dense vitreous hemorrhage preventing full PRP treatment, a Bevacizumab injection has been shown to aid significantly in clearing the hemorrhage (Moradian et al., 2008).

Bevacizumab has also been shown to enhance retinal surgery in patients with PDR. A single Bevacizumab injection given 1-2 weeks before vitrectomy for vitreous hemorrhage, results in decreased bleeding during surgery, decreased operating time and less post operative vitreous hemorrhage as compared to vitrectomy alone (Nicholson & Shachat, 2010; Ahmadieh et al.,2009).

7.5.2.3.3 Traction retinal detachment

Traction retinal detachment from the contraction of the neovascular tissue connecting the retinal surface to the vitreous is another serious complication of PDR. However, traction detachments which do not involve the macula can remain stable for years. Vitrectomy surgery is indicated only when the traction retinal detachment involves or threatens the central macula or if a retinal tear develops (Regillo et al. 2010).

7.5.2.3.4 Neovascular glaucoma

A third serious complication of PDR occurs when high levels of VEGF in the retina induce the development of new vessels on the iris. These vessels threaten to block the outflow of aqueous fluid from the eye and raise ocular pressure. The treatment of patients with neovascularisation of the iris involves both the minimization of retinal ischemia and the aggressive reduction of intraocular pressure if elevated. Retinal ischemia is treated with aggressive and extensive ablation of peripheral retinal tissue with PRP regardless of the stage of PDR. Injection of intravitreal anti-VEGF agents as adjunctive therapy to PRP can induce a rapid reduction or resolution of neovascularisation of the iris (Ahmadieh et al., 2009; Wasik et al., 2009). However, these injections should be seen as an adjunct to full PRP which remains the definitive treatment and not as a viable replacement.

Elevated ocular pressure in neovascular glaucoma is treated initially with topical medications. Often multiple drops are required to reduce pressure to below the target level of approximately 20 millimeters of mercury. In advanced cases, topical treatment alone may not be sufficient and systemic treatment with carbonic anhydrase inhibitors such as Acetazolamide may be considered. Common side effects of Acetazolamide include numbness and tingling in the fingers and toes, and taste alterations. Acetazolamide also increases the risk of dehydration and metabolic acidosis. Serial electrolyte and kidney function tests are recommended in all patients receiving this medication.

In refractory cases Cyclodestructive procedures are required if medical therapy fails to provide symptomatic relief. With cyclocryotherapy, the IOP-lowering effect is achieved by destroying secretory ciliary epithelium and/or reducing blood flow to the ciliary body. It is indicated as a last resort only if relief of pain is the main goal.

7.6 Special considerations
7.6.1 Diabetic retinopathy in pregnancy

In women with preexisting diabetes, pregnancy is considered an independent risk factor for the development and progression of diabetic retinopathy (Shultz et al., 2005). Gestational diabetes, in absence of preexisting diabetes does not show a similar association with diabetic retinopathy. Most of the progression of diabetic retinopathy in pregnancy occurs by the end of the second trimester. Although regression of retinopathy usually occurs postpartum, there is still an increased risk for progression during the first year postpartum (Shultz et al., 2005). Risk factors for the development and progression of diabetic retinopathy in pregnancy include longer duration of diabetes before conception, rapid normalization of hemoglobin A_{1C} at the beginning of pregnancy, poor glycemic control during pregnancy, diabetic nephropathy, high blood pressure and preeclampsia (Shultz et al., 2005; Vestgaard et al., 2010).

Severity of diabetic retinopathy before or at beginning of pregnancy is also a strong predictor of progression of retinopathy during and after pregnancy. The Diabetes in Early Pregnancy Study (Chew et al., 1995) showed that 10.3% of women without diabetic retinopathy and 18.8% with mild NPDR experienced retinopathy progression during pregnancy, and 6.3% of women with mild NPDR progressed to PDR. In women with moderate NPDR, 54.8% suffered retinopathy progression and 29% developed PDR. Overall, progression to sight threatening diabetic retinopathy, including macular edema and PDR, occurs in 6% of pregnant diabetic women (Vestgaard et al., 2010).

Progression of retinopathy during pregnancy is probably related to the hypervolemic and hyper-coagulable states in pregnancy, as well as elevated pro-inflammatory and angiogenic factor levels. This results in capillary occlusion and leakage aggravating diabetic retinopathy mechanisms (Shultz et al., 2005; Kastelan et al., 2010). Ideally, good glycemic control and full treatment of pre-existing diabetic retinopathy complications should be attained before conception.

All diabetic women who plan pregnancy should be referred by their treating physician to an ophthalmologist. The recommended follow-up of pregnant women with type 1 diabetes includes an ophthalmologic exam at the beginning of pregnancy and during the first trimester. Subsequent follow-up depends on the stage of diabetic retinopathy found on the initial examinations. In women with no retinopathy or very mild NPDR, an ophthalmologic exam is indicated when there are visual complaints. In moderate NPDR an exam should be done at least once during the second trimester and every 4-6 weeks during the third trimester. In severe NPDR and PDR, close follow-up is needed, and an exam should be done every 4-6 weeks, from the beginning of the second trimester.

Treatment of diabetic retinopathy during pregnancy includes maximal control of both glucose levels and blood pressure (Vestgaard et al., 2010). Ocular therapy such as PRP should definitely be performed for PDR and be strongly considered in cases of severe NPDR. Disease progression can be very fast in pregnancy and waiting for PDR to clearly develop may result in severe complications that necessitate invasive surgery. Ocular therapy for PDR and macular edema during pregnancy can include PRP, focal laser and intravitreal injections of Triamcinolone. Although there is not much data on the safety of intravitreal injections of anti-VEGF agents during pregnancy, the literature includes some reports on the safe and effective use of Bevacizumab (Tarantola et al., 2010).

7.6.2 Cataract surgery in patients with diabetic retinopathy

Cataract is a major factor which compromises vision in diabetic patients. While diabetics may benefit from cataract extraction, a controversy exists in the ophthalmic community as to whether cataract surgery potentiates diabetic retinopathy progression. Several studies have reported worsening of diabetic retinopathy and macular edema after surgery (Pollack et al., 1991; Hauser et al., 2004; Jaffe et al., 1992, Hayashi et al., 2009). Progression was seen during the first year after surgery and was highest in the first 3 months post-operatively. A review of several other studies, especially in the cataract surgery era using the smaller incision phacoemulsification technique, showed no significant progression of diabetic retinopathy and macular edema after surgery (Rashid & Young, 2010; Shah & Chen, 2010). Overall, diabetics with cataracts benefit from surgery, and improved visual acuity is reported in 92-94% of patients (Rashid & Young, 2010). The combined evidence suggests that in patients with low risk or absent diabetic retinopathy and no clinically significant macular edema at the time of surgery, there is little increased risk of retinopathy progression. However, in patients with severe NPDR, PDR or significant macular edema, cataract surgery carries an increased risk for retinopathy progression and a worse visual acuity outcome.

Recent studies have shown a potential benefit using intravitreal injection of Bevacizumab at the end of cataract surgery (Cheema et al., 2009; Chen et al., 2009; Nicholson & Shachat, 2010) especially in cases with poorly controlled or refractory macular edema and diabetic retinopathy before surgery. Patients who received intravitreal Bevacizumab enjoyed better outcomes in terms of visual acuity, macular thickness and retinopathy progression.

A thorough evaluation of patients with diabetes is warranted before cataract surgery. Patients who have severe NPDR or PDR should be considered for PRP treatment prior to cataract removal (Chew et al., 1999). Patients with clinically significant macular edema should undergo treatment, such as focal laser or intravitreal injection of anti- VEGF agents pre-operatively. Ideally, surgery should be delayed until stabilization of retinopathy and macular edema is achieved. In refractory cases, adjunctive therapy with an anti-VEGF agent at the end of cataract surgery should be considered. Close post-operative follow-up with an ophthalmologist is highly recommended in all patients with preexisting diabetic retinopathy.

8. Schedule for ophthalmologic examinations

Regular ocular examination can detect early ocular disease such as cataracts and glaucoma as well as retinopathy. Diabetic retinopathy in type 1 diabetes is rare during the first 5 years after diagnosis, so the baseline ophthalmologic examination could be extended to 5 years after diagnosis if blood glucose has been well controlled. In children with pre-pubertal diabetes, the baseline examination should be done at puberty (Raab et al. 2010).

The timing and frequency of follow-up ocular examinations depends on individual patient's status. In high risk patients with long term diabetes and poor systemic risk factor control annual examinations should be performed even in the absence of retinopathy. In patients with known retinopathy, the examination schedule is based on the degree of retinopathy, and on the patient's compliance and adherence to regular follow-up. In more advances stages such as PDR and when macular edema is present, more frequent and careful follow-up is suggested. (Regillo et al., 2010). Table 2 shows the recommended schedule for follow-up.

Retinopathy Stage	Follow-up Schedule
Normal or rare microaneurysms	Annually
Mild NPDR	Every 9 months
Moderate NPDR	Every 6 months
Severe NPDR	Every 2-4 months
Clinically significant macular edema	Every 2-4 months
PDR	Every 2-3 months (careful follow-up)

Table 2. Suggested time table for follow-up in diabetic retinopathy (modified from the Preferred Practice Patterns committee, retina panel, diabetic retinopathy, American Academy of Ophthalmology, 2003, as cited in Regillo et al., 2010).

9. Summary

Management of type 1 diabetes involves close cooperation between the treating primary physician and the many specialists who help manage the complications of this disease. Recent advances, including intraocular anti-VEGF injections, have added important new tools which minimize vision loss in diabetic eye disease. Proactive, interdisciplinary coordination of treatment and timely referrals can aid in the minimization of visually threatening complications, significantly enhancing patient quality of life.

10. References

Ahmadieh H.; Shoeibi N.; Entezari M.; Monshizadeh R. (2009). Intravitreal Bevacizumab for prevention of early postvitrectomy hemorrhage in diabetic patients: a randomized clinical trial. *Ophthalmology*, Vol. 116, No.10, (October 2010), pp. 1943-1948, ISSN 0161-6420

Bobrow JC.; Blecher MH.; Glasser D. et al. (Eds.) (2010). Section 11: Lens and cataract. *Basic and Clinical Science Course, 2010-2011, American Academy of Ophthalmology*. Americam Academy of Ophthalmology, ISBN 9781615251391

Bonini-Filho M.; Costa RA.; Calluci D. et al. (2009). Intravitreal Bevacizumab for diabetic macular edema associated with severe capillary loss: one year results of a pilot study. *American Journal of Ophthalmology*, Vol.147, No.6, (June 2009), pp. 1022-1020, ISSN 0002-9394

Cheema RA.; Al- Mubarak MM.; Amin YM. et al. (2009). Role of combined cataract surgery and intravitreal Bevacizumab injection in preventing progression of diabetic retinopathy; prospective randomized study. *Journal of Catarct and Refractive Surgery*, Vol.35, No.1, (January 2009), pp. 18-25, ISSN 0886-3350

Chen CH.; Liu YC.; Wu PC. (2009). The combination of intravitreal Bevacizumab and phacoemulsification surgery in patients with cataract and coexisting diabetic macular edema. *Journal of Ocular Pharmacology Therapeutics*, Vol.25, No.1, (February 2009), pp. 83-89, ISSN 1080-7683

Cheung N.; Mitchell P.; Wong TY. (2010). Diabetic Retinopathy. *The Lancet*, Vol.376, No.9735, (July 2010), pp. 124-136, ISSN 0140-6736

Chew EY.; Benson WE.; Remaley NA. et al. (1999). Results after lens extraction in patients with diabetic retinopathy; early treatment diabetic retinopathy study report number 25. *Archives of Ophthalmology*, Vol.117, No.12, (December 1999), pp. 1600-1606, ISSN 0003-9950

Chew EY.; Mills JL.; Metzger BE. et al. (1995). Metabolic control and progression of retinopathy. The Diabetic in Early Pregnancy Study. National Institute of Child Health and Human Development. Diabetes in Early Pregnancy Study. *Diabetes Care*, Vol.18, No.5, (May 1995), pp. 631-637, ISSN 0149-5992

Cunningham ET.; Adamis AP.; Altaweel M. et al. (2005). Macugen Diabetic Retinopathy Study Group. A phase II randomized double-masked trial of Pegaptanib, an anti-vascular endothelial growth factor aptamer, for diabetic macular edema. *Ophthalmology*, Vol.12, No.10, (October 2005), pp. 1747-1757, ISSN 0161-6420

DCCT 1995: Progression of retinopathy with intensive versus conventional treatment in the Diabetes Control and Complications Trial. Diabetes Control and Complications Trial Research Group. *Ophthalmology*, Vol.102, No.4, (April 1995), pp. 647-661, ISSN 0161-6420

DCCT 1997: Clustering of long term complications in families with diabetes in the diabetes control and complications trial. The Diabetes Control and Complications Trial Research Group. *Diabetes*, Vol.46, No.11, (November 1997), pp.1829-1839, ISSN 0012-1797

DCCT 2000: Effect of pregnancy on microvascular complications in the diabetes control and complications trial. The Diabetes Control and Comlications Trail Research Group. *Diabetes Care*, Vol.23, No.8, (August 2000), pp. 1084-1091, ISSN 0149-5992

DRCR network 2008: The Diabetic Retinopathy Clinical Research Network: A randomized trial comparing intravitreal Triamcinolone acetonide and focal/grid photocoagulation for diabetic macular edema. Diabetic Retinopathy Clinical Research Network. *Ophthalmology*, Vol.115, No.9, (Spetember 2008), pp. 1447-1449,e1-10, ISSN 0161-6420

DRCR network 2010a: The Diabetic Retinopathy Clinical Research Network. Randomized trial evaluating Ranibizumab plus prompt or deferred laser or Triamcinolone plus prompt laser for diabetic macular edema. *Ophthalmology*, Vol.117, No.6, (June 2010), pp. 1067-1077, ISSN 0161-6420

DRCR network 2010b: Diabetic Retinopathy Clinical Research Network writing committee on behalf of the DRCR.net. Vitrectomy outcomes in eyes with diabetic macular edema and vitreomacular traction. *Ophthalmology*, Vol.117, No.6, (June 2010), pp. 1087-1093, ISSN 0161-6420

DRS 1979: Four risk factors for severe visual loss in diabetic retinopathy. DRS report 3. Diabetic Retinopathy Study Research Group. *Archives of Ophthalmology*, Vol.97, No.4, (April 1979), pp. 654-655, ISSN 0003-9950

DRS 1981: Photocoagulation treatment of proliferative diabetic retinopathy: clinical application of Diabetic Retinopathy Study (DRS) findings. DRS report 8. Diabetic Retinopathy Study Research Group. *Ophthalmology*,Vol.88,No.7, (July 1981), pp. 583-600, ISSN 0161-6420

DRVS 1985: Early vitrectomy for severe vitreous hemorrhage in diabetic retinopathy: two-year results of a randomized trial. DRVS report 2. Diabetic Retinopathy Vitrectomy Study Research Group. *Archives of Ophthalmology*, Vol.103, No.11, (November 1985), pp. 1644-1652, ISSN 0003-9950

ETDRS 1991: Early photocoagulation for diabetic retinopathy. ETDRS report 9. Early Treatment Diabetic Retinopathy Study Research Group. *Ophthalmology*, Vol.98, No.5(suppl.), (May 1991), pp.766-785, ISSN 0161- 6420

ETDRS 1995: Focal photocoagulation treatment of diabetic macular edema: relationship of treatment effect to fluorescein angiographic and other retinal characteristics at baseline. ETDRS report 19. Early Treatment Diabetic Retinopathy Study Research Group. *Archives of Ophthalmology*, Vol.113, No.9, (September 1995), pp. 1144-1155, ISSN 0003-9950

Flynn HW & Smiddy WE. (Eds.) (2000). Diabetes and ocular disease: past, present and future therapies. In: *Ophthalmology Monograph 14*, pp. 49-53, 266, American Academy of Ophthalmology, ISBN 1560551739, San Francisco, USA.

Gillies MC.; Sutter FK.; Simpson JM. et al. (2006). Intravitreal Triamcinolone for refractory diabetic macular edema: two-year results of a double-masked, placebo-controlled, randomized clinical trial. *Ophthalmology*, Vol.113,No.9, (September 2006), pp. 1533-1538, ISSN 0161-6420

Grover D.; Li TJ.; Chong CC. (2008). Intravitreal steroids for macular edema in diabetes. *Cochrane Database Systematic Reviews*, (January 2008), CD00565.54

Hauser D.; Katz H.; Pokroy R. et al. (2004). Occurrence and progression of diabetic retinopathy after phacoemulsification cataract surgery. *Journal of Cataract and Refractive Surgery*, Vol.30, No.2, (February 2004), pp.428-432, ISSN 0886-3350

Hayashi K.; Igrarashi C.; Hirata A. et al. (2009). Changes in diabetic macular edema after phacoemulsification surgery. *Eye (London)*, Vol.23, No.2, (February 2009), pp. 386-389, ISSN 0950-222X

Jaffe GJ.; Burton TC.; Kuhn E. et al. (1992). Progression of nonproliferative diabetic retinopathy and visual outcome after extracapsular cataract extraction and intraocular lens implantation. *American Journal of Ophthalmology,* Vol.114, No.4, (October 1992), pp. 448-456, ISSN 0002-9394

Kaiser Pk.; Riemann CD.; Sears JE.; Lewis H. (2001). Macular traction detachment and diabetic macular edema associated with posterior hyaloids traction. *American Journal of Ophthalmology,* Vol.131, No.1, (January 2001), pp.44-49, ISSN 0002-9394

Kastelan S.; Tomic M.; Pavan J.; Oreskovic S. (2010). Matrenal immune system adaptation to pregnancy- a potential influence on the course of diabetic retinopathy. *Reproductive Biology and Endocrinology,* Vol.8 (October 2010), pp. 124-128, ISSN 1477-7827

Klein R.; Knudtson MD.; Lee KF. et al. (2008). The Wisconsin Epidemiologic Study of Diabetic Retinopathy: XXII the twenty-five-year progression of retinopathy in persons with type 1 diabetes. *Ophthalmology,* Vol.115, No.11, (November 2008), pp. 1859-1868, ISSN 0161-6420

Kline LB.; Tariq-Bhatti M.; Chung SM. et al. (Eds.) (2010). Section 5: Neuro-ophthalmology. *Basic and Clinical Science Course, 2010-2011, American Academy of Ophthalmology.* American Academy of Ophthalmology, ISBN 9781615251339

Maia OO, Jr.; Takahashi BS.; Costa RA. et al. (2009). Combined laser and intravitreal Triamcinolone for proliferative diabetic retinopathy and macular edema: one year results of a randomized clinical trial. *American Journal of Ophthalmology,* Vol.147, No.2, (February 2009), pp. 291-297, ISSN 0002-9394

Michaelidis M.; Kalines A.; Hamilton RD. et al. (2010). A prospective randomized trial of intravitreal Bevacizumab or laser therapy in the management of diabetic macular edema (BOLT study) 12-month data: report 2. *Ophthalmology,* Vol.117, No.6, (June 2010), pp. 1078-1086, ISSN 0161-6420

Mirshahi A.; Roohipoor R.; Lashay A. et al. (2008). Bevacizumab- augmented retinal laser photocoagulation in proliferative diabetic retinopathy: a randomized double-masked clinical trial. *European Journal of Ophthalmology,* Vol.18, No.2, (March-April 2008), pp. 263-269, ISSN 1120-6721

Moradian S.; Ahmadieh H.; Malihi M. et al. (2008). Intravitreal Bevacizumab in active progressive proliferative diabetic retinopathy. *Graefe's Archive for Clinical and Experimental Ophthalmology,* Vol.246, No.12, (December2008),pp. 1699-1705, ISSN 1435-702X

Nicholson BP. & Schachat AP. (2010). A review of clinical trials of anti-VEGF agents for diabetic retinopathy. *Graefe's Archive for Clinical and Experimental Ophthalmology,* Vol.248, No.7, (July 2010), pp. 915-930, ISSN 1435-702X

Obrosova SS.; Chung SS.; Kador PF. (2010). Diabetic cataracts: mechanisms and management. *Diabetes/Metabolism Research and Reviews,* Vol.26, No.3, (March 2010), pp. 172-180, ISSN 1262-3636

Ostri C.; Lund-Andersen H.; Sander B. et al. (2010). Bilateral diabetic papillopathy and metabolic control. *Ophthalmology,* Vol.117, No.11, (November 2010), pp.2214-2217, ISSN 0161-6420

Pollack A.; Dotan S.; Oliver M. (1991). Course of diabetic retinopathy following cataract surgery. *British Journal of Ophthalmology*, Vol.75, No.1, (January 1991), pp. 2-8, ISSN 0007-1161

Powers AC. (2008). Diabetes Mellitus. In: *Harrison's Principles of Internal Medicine*, Fauci AS., Brownwald E., Kasper DL. et al. (Eds.), Mcgraw-Hill. Retrieved from: http://www.accessmedicine.com

Purdy EP.; Bolling JP.; Di-Lorenzo AL. et al. (Eds.) (2010). Endocrine disorders. In: Section 1: Update on general medicine. *Basic and Clinical Science Course 2010-2011, American Academy of Ophthalmology*, pp. 189-205, American Academy of Ophthalmology, ISBN 9781615251292

Raab EL.; Aaby AA.; Bloom JN. et al. (Eds.) (2010). Vitreous and retinal diseases and disorders. In: section 6: Pediatric ophthalmology and strabismus. *Basic and Clinical Science Course 2010-2011, American Academy of Ophthalmology*, pp. 296-297, American Academy of Ophthalmology, ISBN 9781615251346

Rashid S. & Young LH. (2010). Progression of diabetic retinopathy and maculopathy after phacoemulsification surgery. *International Ophthalmology Clinics*, Vol.50, No.1, (Winter 2010), pp. 155-166, ISSN 0020-8167

Regillo C.; Holekamp N.; Johnson MW. et al. (Eds.) (2010). Retinal vascular disease: Diabetic retinopathy. In: Section 12, Retina and vitreous. *Basic and Clinical Science Course, 2010-2011, American Academy of Ophthalmology*, pp. 109-132, American Academy of Ophthalmology, ISBN 9781615251407

Reidy JJ.; Bouchard CS.; Florakis GJ. et al. (Eds.) (2010). Metabolic disorders with corneal changes. In: Section 8: External disease and cornea. *Basic and Clinical Science Course 2010-2011, American Academy of Ophthalmology*, pp. 307-308, American Academy of Ophthalmology, ISBN9781615251360

Shah AS. & Chen SH. (2010). Catract surgery and diabetes. *Current Opinion in Ophthalmology*, Vol.21, No.1, (January 2010), pp. 4-9, ISSN 1040-8738

Shultz KL.; Birnbaum AD.; Goldsteir DA. (2005). Ocular disease in pregnancy. *Current Opinions in Ophthalmology*, Vol.16, No.5, (October 2005), pp. 431-435, ISSN 1040-8738

Silva PS.; Sun JK.; Aiello LP. et al. (2009). Role of steroids in the management of diabetic macular edema and proliferative diabetic retinopathy. *Seminars in Ophthalmology*, Vol.24, No.2, (April 2009), pp. 93-99, ISSN 0882-0538

Stirban A.; Rosen P.; Tschoepe D. (2008). Complications of type 1 diabetes: new molecular findings. *Mount Sinai Journal of Medicine*, Vol.75, No.4, (August 2008), pp. 328-351, ISSN 1931-7581

Tarantola RM.; Folk JC.; Culver Boldt H.; Mahajan VB. (2010). Intravitreal Bevacizumab during pregnancy. *Retina*, Vol.30, No.9, (October 2010), pp. 1405-1411, ISSN 0275-004X

Thomas D. & Graham E. (2008). Ocular disorders associated with systemic disease. In: *Vaughan & Asbury's General Ophthalmology*, Riordan-Eva P. & Whitcher JP. (Eds.), Mcgraw- Hill. Retrieved from: http://www.accessmedicine.com

Varma R. (2008). From a population to patients: The Wisconsin Epidemiologic Study of Diabetic Retinopathy. *Ophtahlmology*, Vol.115, No.11, (November 2008), pp. 1857-1858, ISSN 0161-6420

Vestgaard M.; Ringholm L.; Laugesen CS. et al. (2010). Pregnancy- induced sight-threatening diabetic retinopathy in women with type 1 diabetes. *Diabetic Medicine*, Vol.27, No.4, (April 2010), pp.431-435, ISSN 1464-5491

Wasik A.; Song HF.; Grimes A.; Engelke C.; Thomas A. (2009). Bevacizumab in conjunction with panretinal photocoagulation for neovascular glaucoma. Optometry, Vol.80, No.5, (May 2009), pp. 243-248, ISSN 1529-1839

Yilmaz T.; Weaver CD.; Gallagher MJ. et al. (2009). Intravitreal Triamcinolone acetonide injection for treatment of refractory diabetic macular edema: a systematic review. *Ophthalmology*, Vol.116, No.5, (May 2009), pp. 902-911, ISSN 0161-6420

Review of the Relationship Between Renal and Retinal Microangiopathy in Type 1 Diabetes Mellitus Patients

Pedro Romero-Aroca[1] , Juan Fernández-Ballart[2], Nuria Soler[1],
Marc Baget-Bernaldiz[1] and Isabel Mendez-Marin[1]
*[1]Department of Ophthalmology, University Hospital Sant Joan, Institut de Investigació
Sanitaria Pere Virgili (IISPV), Reus,
[2]Epidemiology, Department of Basic Sciences, University Rovira i Virgili (Tarragona),
Spain*

1. Introduction

Diabetes mellitus is a group of metabolic disorders of carbohydrate metabolism in which glucose is underutilized, producing hyperglycemia. The disease is classified into several categories. The revised classification, published in 1997 (ADA, 1997; The Expert Comitee on the Diagnosis and Classification of Diabetes mellitus, 2000), defines Type 1 diabetes mellitus (formerly known as the insulin-dependent diabetes mellitus or juvenile-onset diabetes mellitus) as a disorder caused by autoimmune destruction of pancreatic h-cells, rendering the pancreas unable to synthesize and secrete insulin. In 85–90% of cases, antibodies appear against pancreatic h-cells (ICA), acting as anti-insulin (IAA), or others such as GAD, IA-2 and IA-2h (Geiss et al 1997).

The latter complications of diabetes mellitus include both microvascular complications (predominantly retinopathy, nephropathy and neuropathy) and macrovascular complications, particularly stroke and coronary artery disease. Together, these make diabetes the seventh most common cause of death in the developed world (Geiss et al 1997).

The major microvascular complications, retinopathy and nephropathy, are the more important causes of blindness and end-stage renal disease in Europe. There are few similarities in the coexistence of DR and DN being both as microvascular disease and microscopically both have capillary basement membrane thickening. However, capillary closure is apparent in the retina and kidney after sufficient exposure to disease with duration. The pathophysiology of DN and DR are more or less similar, which commence with increase in vascular permeability. The selective increase in permeability to albumin in early DN is caused by loss of polarity across the glomerular basement membrane (Myers et al, 1982) and the disease mechanism in the eye is probably a breakdown of tight junctions between cells. The onset of proteinuria and proliferative retinopathy are both related to previous poor glycemic control, duration of diabetes and hypertension.

The detection of retinopathy is easy (by the use of fundus periodical retinographies), but the diagnosis of the early stages of nephropathy needs microalbuminuria to be determined in urinalysis. Microalbuminuria has prognostic significance; thus, in 80% of people with Type 1 diabetes mellitus and microalbuminuria, urinary albumin excretion increases at a rate of 10–20% per year, with the development of clinical proteinuria within 10– 15 years. After the development of clinical grade proteinuria (>80%), patients go on to develop decreased glomerular filtration rate and, given enough time, end-stage renal disease (Geiss et al 1997). Several factors appear to influence susceptibility to the microvascular complications of diabetes mellitus, but our knowledge of the role and the importance of these genetic and environmental factors are still incomplete. The most powerful risk factor for microvascular complications was the duration of diabetes, but frequency of both retinopathy and nephropathy was impressively related to the level of plasma glucose at the time of examination.

From the recent studies, it is evident that the presence of retinopathy itself may reveal patients at risk for nephropathy (Estacio et al, 1998; El Asrar et al, 2002; Rossing et al, 2002; Villar et al, 1999). In a cross sectional study, patients with DR were 5.68, 13.39 and 3.51 times as likely to have DN among type1 and type2 diabetic patients (El-Asrar et al, 2002).

However, there is lack of evidence that determine the association of retinal-renal complications using the gold standard methods. The DR is characterized by microvascular abnormalities, proliferation of retinal vessels and increased retinal vascular permeability leading to the development of non-proliferative and proliferative DR, and macular edema (Williams et al 2004). The DN is a life threatening complication which predisposes to excess morbidity and mortality resulting from renal failure and cardiovascular disease (Ritz et al, 1999; Adler at al, 2003).

Our hypothesis was that the severity of DR correlates with the presence and severity of DN in people with type 1 diabetes. Studies in other populations documented a well-known association between advanced DR stages and overt nephropathy in type 1 diabetic patient (Looker et al, 2003; Gall et al, 1997). Similarly, our results provide further support to the close relationship between presence of DR and severity of DN in type1 diabetic patients.

It was reported that at least one fifth of the diabetic individuals are affected by multiple complications and the frequency increases with increasing age and duration of diabetes.

In the study of WESDR, there was a strong correlation between DN and severity of DR in all age groups (Klein et al, 1984; Klein et al 1984).

In the present study we determine the epidemiological risk factors that influence the appearance of diabetic retinopathy, and overt nephropathy, in a seventeen -year follow-up of a population sample of 112 patients who did not have diabetic retinopathy or microalbuminuria at the beginning of the study.

2. Methods

2.1 Sample size and study population

Since 1987 a register has been kept of any new cases of type I diabetes mellitus in Catalonia (Spain). The incidence of new cases over that period has been 11.4 cases per 100000 inhabitants (13.2 cases in men and 9.6 cases in women) (Castell et al, 1999).

Since 1990, there has been an ongoing registration of all diabetic patients (type I and 2) at St Joan Hospital, which is the only surgical ophthalmology centre in Reus (Spain), and having a dependent population of around 207,500 inhabitants. In 1999, there were 1495 patients with diabetes mellitus type I (Castell et al, 1999).

2.2 Design
The present study is prospective and was initiated in 1990 with 126 patients recruited with type I diabetes mellitus. The initial conditions included the absence of retinopathy and nephropathy (determined by the absence of microalbuminuria in three consecutive measures taken at one month intervals).

Two previous results were obtained at 5 and 10 years of the study (Romero-Aroca et al, 2000; Romero-Aroca et al, 2003). At the end of the study in 2007 only 112 patients were still being controlled (14 patients had dropped out during the follow up). At the end of the study (seventeen years of follow-up) the authors have determined the incidence of diabetic macular oedema and their risk factors, related to the appearance of renal overt nephropathy.

2.3 Diagnostic methods
Diabetic retinopathy was evaluated by retinal photographs through dilated pupils, of two 50° fields of each eye centred firstly at the temporal to the macula and secondly at the nasal to the papilla (Aldington et al, 1995). The results were then classified into four groups (Wilkinson et al 2003):

* Mild non proliferative
* Moderate non proliferative
* Severe non proliferative
* Proliferative

Macular edema was diagnosed under stereoscopic viewing of the macula with a slit lamp and Goldmann fundus contact lens, and was considered present if we found:

* retinal thickening involving or within 500 µ m of the centre of the macula
* hard exudates at or within 500 µ m of the centre of the macula, if associated with thickening of adjacent retina (but no hard exudates remaining after retinal thickening disappeared)
* a zone or zones of retinal thickening, one disc area or larger in size, any part of which is within 1 disc diameter of the centre of the macula.

The clinical classification used was the international clinical diabetic retinopathy disease severity scale, proposed by the American Academy of Ophthalmology in 2002 (Wilkinson et al 2003). In all patients with diabetic macular oedema, a fluorescein angiography was obtained, centred on macular region to determine the leakage in that area. The fluorescein angiographic findings were categorized into three types:

* focal leakage type, which was predominantly well-defined focal areas of leakage from microaneurysm or localized dilated capillaries;
* diffuse leakage type, predominantly widespread and ill-defined leakage involving the whole circumference of the fovea;
* cystoid leakage type, predominantly diffuse leakage but with pooling of dye in the cystic spaces of the macula in the late phase.

Since 2000, all patients with diabetic macular oedema have been given an optical coherence tomography OCT), repeated every 4 months as a control test. Optical coherence tomography was performed with a OCT model TOPCON TRC NW 7SF. The retinal map algorithm uses measurements along 6 radial lines, 6 mm in length, to produce a circular plot in which the foveal zone is the central circular zone of 1.00 mm in diameter. Macular edema measured by OCT was defined as a retinal thickening of more than 216 microns, and was classified as follows, using the Otani et al patterns amplified by the two tractional forms described later (Otani et al, 1999): Sponge-like retinal thickness, defined as increased retinal thickness with reduced intra retinal reflectivity and expanded areas of lower reflectivity; cystoid macular oedema, characterized by the intra retinal cystoid spaces at the macular area; serous retinal detachment was thought to be present if the posterior surface of the retina was elevated above the outer border of the highly reflective band, regarded as the signal generated mainly by the retinal pigment epithelium. Only patients with a visible separation between the layer of photoreceptors and the pigment epithelium, was classified as serous detachment; if we observed the photoreceptor layer adjacent to pigment epithelium, we classified the case as cystoid macular oedema.

2.4 Inclusion criteria
Patients with type I diabetes mellitus (insulin dependent or young-onset diabetes mellitus)

2.5 Exclusion criteria
Presence of diabetic retinopathy at the beginning of study, presence of diabetic nephropathy at the beginning of study, presence of microalbuminuria at the beginning of study, patients with LADA diabetes (latent autoimmune adult diabetes), patients with type 2 diabetes mellitus (not insulin-dependent or older-onset diabetes mellitus), patients with type 2 diabetes mellitus appeared before 30 years of age (MODY diabetes mellitus)

2.6 Definition of variables
Visual acuity in each eye was measured on the Snellen chart and recorded as a decimal value, with best refraction for distance. All data manipulations were performed on visual acuities expressed in log MAR form. The legal blind subject was defined as corrected visual acuity less than or equal to 0.1 in the better eye; reduced visual acuity as less than or equal to 0.4 and greater than 0.1 in the better eye.
The epidemiological risk factors included in the study were:
• Gender and current age.
• Duration of diabetes mellitus, classified in the statistical study in two groups: below 20 years of duration and equal to or more than 20 years duration.
• Type of diabetic retinopathy classified into two groups: first with a diabetic retinopathy lower than severe pattern, and the second with patients with severe or proliferative pattern, patients who need scattered photocoagulation were classified in tis second group.
• Arterial hypertension, which indicates a systolic measurement above or equal to 140 mm Hg and the diastolic measurement above or equal to 90 mm Hg, or when the patient is taking anti-hypertensive medications.
• Levels of glycated haemoglobin (HbA1c) as recommended i by the American Diabetes Association (ADA, 1997) as the major component of HbA1c (accounting for 80% of HbA1c), was measured every 3 months. The control of glycaemia was considered in concordance with the European Diabetes Policy Group, into two groups of patients i.e. over or under 7.0% (European Diabetes Policy Group, 1999). The value included in the statistical analysis was the mean of all values obtained over the 15 years.
• Presence of microalbuminuria, defined as increased albumin excretion (30-300 mg of albumin/24 h or 20-200 μg/min of creatinine) on two of three tests repeated at intervals of 3-6 months as well as exclusion of conditions that invalidate the test (Geiss et al,

1997). The test was performed annually. After microalbuminuria was diagnosed, repeated testing was made within a period of 3-4 months.

- Presence of diabetic nephropathy, defined as clinical albuminuria or overt nephropathy by the American Diabetes Association, corresponding to protein excretion >300 mg/24h (>200 µg/min or >300 µg/mg of albumin: creatinine ratio). Measurement of creatinine clearance as an index of glomerular filtration rate was performed on the same urine collection (Geiss et al, 1997).

- Patients were classified as having macro vascular disease if one or more of the following were present: symptoms of angina pectoris, history of myocardial infarction, coronary artery by pass grafting, percutaneous tranluminal coronary angioplasty, symptoms of or operation for intermittent claudication, history of amputation, transient ischemic attack, stroke.

- Levels of triglycerides and fractions of cholesterol (HDL-cholesterol and LDL-chorlesterol). In the statistical analysis, we classified the patient into normal or higher values, according to the ADA categories as patients with high risk if LDL-cholesterol 3.35 mmol/L (130 mg/dl), HDL-cholesterol 0.90 mmol/L for men and >1.15 mmol/L for women (35 mg/dL for men and 45 mg/dL for women), and triglycerides 1.5 mmol/dL (400 mg/dL), (Expert Panel on Detection, Evaluation, And Treatment of high Blood Cholesterol in Adults, 2001).

2.7 Statistical methods

All statistical analyses were carried out using the SPSS software package (version 18.0), results are expressed as mean±standard error, a P-value of less than 0.05 was considered to indicate statistical significance.

Differences between those included in analyses were examined using the two sample Student T-tests or one-way ANOVA, for continuous or quantitative data, as visual acuity or current age. For the qualitative or categorical data we used the Chi-square test in the univariate phase of study, with determination of Odds ratio for each variable.

The Kruskal-Wallis test and the least significant difference test using ranks for multiple comparisons were carried out to evaluate the correlation between best-corrected visual acuity an OCT findings.

In the multivariate phase of analysis the relationship of diabetic retinopathy, microalbuminuria and overt nephropathy, to various demographic and other risk factors were examined using logistic regression analysis; the full model was built including gender and age a priori.

3. Results

Demographic variables of the patients

Gender: 54 patients were men (48.2%) and 58 were women (51.8%)

The mean of age was 39.94 ± 10.53 years old (24 – 61 years), the mean of diabetes mellitus type I duration was 23.42 ± 7.57 years (12 – 45 years). The arterial hypertension was present in 44 patients (39.3%).

The means of the different quantitative data were:

- Glycosylated haemoglobin A_{1c}: 7.69% ± 1.24 (4.50% – 11.40%)
- LDL-Cholesterol: 3.50 ± 0,57 mmol/l (3.00 – 4.00)

- HDL-Cholesterol: 1.12 ± 0.42 mmol/l $(0.70 - 2.02)$
- Triglycerides: 1.47 ± 0.76 mmol/l $(0.90 - 3.00)$

Visual acuity study

Mean visual acuity after 17 years was 0.77 ± 0.34 ($0.02 - 1$) in the Snellen chart test; and $+0.37 \pm +0.72$ (+ 1.7 - + 0) in the Log MAR test.
Low vision (defined as vision in the best eye >0,1 and < 0.4 in the Snellen chart) was detected in 13 patients (11.6%) and blindness (AV < 0.1 in Snellen chart) in 14 patients (12.5%).

Incidence of diabetic retinopathy (Table 1)

After 17 years there were 62 patients (55.4%) with different types of diabetic retinopathy. The Rate of progression was 8.30 person-year.
- Mild diabetic retinopathy in31 patients (27.7%)
- Moderate diabetic retinopathy in 7 patients (6.3%)
- Severe diabetic retinopathy in 5 patients (4.5%)
- Proliferative diabetic retinopathy in 18 patients (16.1%)

There were 23 patients (20.5%) with diabetic macular edema after 17 years, the Rate of progression was 3.08 person-year. The mild or moderate form of diabetic macular edema was present in 13 patients (11.6%) and the severe form of macular edema in 10 patients (8.9%).
In the 62 patients with diabetic retinopathy 17 (27.42%) developed overt nephropathy, with a rate of progression 4.11 person-year. In patients with proliferative form of diabetic retinopathy (23 patients) 11 developed microalbuminuria (47.82%), the rate of progression was 7.17 person-year.

Statistical study of diabetic retinopathy

Univariate study with the application of chi squared test (Table 1).
The factors significant in the appearance of diabetic retinopathy were as follows: duration of diabetic retinopathy p<0.001, presence of arterial hypertension p<0.001, levels of glycated haemoglobin (HbA_{1c}) > 7.5% p<0.001, high levels of LDL-cholesterol p<0.001, high levels of tryglicerides p=0.003 and presence of overt nephropathy p= 0.001.

Logistic regression of diabetic retinopathy (Table 2).

The followings factors studied were significant in the appearance of diabetic retinopathy: Duration of diabetes mellitus more than 20 years p< 0.001, presence of arterial hypertension p<0.001, high levels of HbA_{1c} p< 0.001, high levels of tryglicerides p=0.004, high levels of LDL-Cholesterol p= 0.002, and overt nephropathy p=0.021.

Statistical study of diabetic nephropathy

Univariate analysis with the application of chi squared test(Table 1).
The factors significant in the apparition of overt nephropathy were: presence of arterial hypertension p<0.001, high levels of HbA_{1c} p<0.001, high levels of LDL-Cholesterol p=0.010, high levels of triglycerides p=0.003, and presence of diabetic retinopathy p=0.021. When we introduced the presence of proliferative diabetic retinopathy against the presence of any retinopathy, the chi squared test had a result of p<0.001, and for proliferative diabetic retinopathy p< 0.001.

Logistic regression of diabetic nephropathy (Table 2).

The significant factors were: the presence of arterial hypertension $p<0.001$, and high levels of HbA_{1c} $p<0.001$, high levels of LDL-Cholesterol $p=0.002$, high levels of triglycerides $p=0.009$,. Also the presence of diabetic retinopathy was significant $p=0,021$. When we introduced the presence of proliferative diabetic retinopathy against the presence of any retinopathy, the chi squared test had a result of $p<0.001$

Risk factor	Diabetic retinopathy				Overt Nephropathy			
	Chi square		Logistic regression		Chi square		Logistic regression	
	Signifi-cance (p)	Odds ratio	Signifi cance (p)	Odds ratio	Signifi-cance (p)	Odds ratio	Signifi-cance (p)	Odds ratio
Gender	0.237	1.397	0.829	0.881	0.743	0.107	0.870	0.910
Glycated haemoglobin (HbA_{1c} >8%)	<0.001	11.011	<0.001	5.575	<0.001	55.687	<0.001	38.360
Arterial hypertension	<0.001	28.193	0.007	6.579	<0.001	12.777	0.023	10.271
Duration of diabetes mellitus (20 years)	<0.001	33.623	<0001	12.096	0.913	0.012	0.170	0.394
HDL-Cholesterol	0.828	0.047	0.813	0.837	0.019	5.201	0.061	0.195
LDL-Cholesterol	<0001	18984	0.002	10.304	0.010	2.715	0.002	3.555
Triglycerides	0.003	8.442	0.004	1.528	0.003	3.513	0.009	2.912
Overt Nephropathy	0.001	6.097	0.021	3.498				
Retinopathy					0.021	6.097	0.021	2.153
Proliferative diabetic retinopathy					<0.001	14.814	<0.001	4.306

Table 1. Chi squared and logistic regression analysis for diabetic retinopathy and microalbuminuria.

Patients only with retinopathy	Patients only with overt nephropathy	Patients with retinopathy and overt nephropathy
Duration of diabetes mellitus (4.679)*	High levels of HbA1c (7.250)*	High levels of HbA1c (6.471)*
High levels of HbA1c (2.250)*	High levels of triglycerides (1.713)*	High levels of triglycerides (2.810)*
Arterial hypertension (2.668)*	Duration of diabetes mellitus (1.029)*	Arterial hypertension (2.657)*
High levels of LDL-cholesterol (1.277)*	Arterial hypertension (0.742)*	Duration of diabetes mellitus (2.269)*
High levels of triglycerides (1.254)*	High levels of LDL-cholesterol (-1.360)*	High levels of LDL-cholesterol (1.232)*

* = Function of classification coefficients.

Table 2. Fisher's classification coefficient.

Statistical application of discriminate analysis

At the end of the study we may observe that four groups of patients had been formed:
- those without any form of microangiopathy (overt nephropathy or retinopathy) 45 patients (group A).
- those with only retinopathy (45 patients) (group B).
- those with only overt nephropathy (5 patients) (group C).
- those with both overt nephropathy and retinopathy (17 patients) (group D).

In this case we needed to apply a discriminate analysis to evaluate the risk factors for the different groups.

Applying Fisher's coefficient indicated that (Table 2):
- for group B the risk factors were: duration of diabetes mellitus (4.679), high levels of HbA$_{1c}$ (2.250) and high levels of LDL-Cholesterol (2.268)
- for the group C only the high levels of HbA$_{1c}$ (7,250) were highly correlated
- for the group D the significant factors were: high levels of HbA$_{1c}$ (6,471), presence of arterial hypertension (2.657), high levels of triglycerides (2.810) and duration of diabetes mellitus (2.269)

4. Discussion

The diabetic retinopathy (DR) and diabetic nephropathy (DN) are the two major complications of diabetes mellitus. The proliferative diabetic retinopathy and proteinuria secondary to DN are both late complications of diabetic overt nephropathy, these usually occur 10 to 15 years after the onset of type 1 DM, and are strongly associated with each other. The epidemiology of diabetic overt nephropathy and retinopathy in type 1 DM, are different, thus for diabetic overt nephropathy increases its prevalence since 10% at ten year duration of diabetes mellitus, achieving the highest value after 40 years with a 40% of diabetic patients with nephropathy, since this point the curve levels off, and only a minority of patients develop clinically significant renal abnormalities, and patients who survive 35 years of type 1 DM without developing DN are at extremely low risk of doing so in the future. Against this curve the diabetic retinopathy succeed in a different form in type 1 diabetic patients, thus the diabetic retinopathy is rare before 10 years DM duration, and increases the prevalence, since this point to a levels upper 80% after 20 years diabetes duration, without a decreases after these 20 years of duration, as we observed in our study. The incidence of DR was 55.4%, and was lower than in other studies such as Klein et al 1998 (Klein et al, 1998), but this may be because the sample studied did not present diabetic retinopathy at the beginning and patient controls were stricter than in the rest of the patients with diabetes mellitus type I (controls every 3 months), we could concluded that the mean level of HbA_{1c} was 7.69% ± 1.24 (4.50% – 11.40%) is better than the achieved by WESDR (Klein et al, 1998). The diabetic macular edema appeared in 20.5% of patients, which was more similar to the findings in the Klein study at 14 years (26%). In the present study the incidence of diabetic macular edema is higher than the proliferative form of diabetic retinopathy in type I diabetes mellitus patients, as was observed in other studies.

With regard to nephropathy diabetes accountings for more than 19.6% of all cases of DN. The DN presents initially as intermittent microalbuminuria that progresses to persistent microalbuminuria, and is accompanied by a decline in the glomerular filtration rate. These dates were in agreement with other studies published in our country on renal failure in diabetes mellitus type I patients Smatjes et al (Esmatjes et al, 1998) found an incidence of 44.5% with some form of renal failure at 20 years in type I diabetes mellitus.

The relationship between DN and DR was well described, thus the Wisconsin Epidemiologic Study of Diabetic Retinopathy (Klein et al, 1993) associated the presence of gross-proteinuria at baseline examination with a 96% increase in the risk of progression to proliferative retinopathy. Also in the Steno study (Kofoed-Enevoldsen et al, 1987), people with type I diabetes mellitus and gross-proteinuria at baseline had an increase risk of progression to proliferative retinopathy (12% annually) compared to those without proteinuria (1%-2% annually).

At the end of our study we can see that four groups of patients had formed: those without overt nephropathy or diabetic retinopathy (45 patients), patients with only overt nephropathy (5 patients), those with only diabetic retinopathy (45 patients), and those with overt nephropathy and diabetic retinopathy (17 patients). The statistical test used for examining these data was a discriminate test, which allowed us to identify the risk factors that influence any of these groups.

In the group of patients with only DR the duration of diabetes mellitus was the more important risk factor and for the group with Dr and DN the most important risk factor is the high levels of HbA_{1c}.

We may assume then, that for the development of only retinal lesions in diabetes mellitus, the duration of the disease is the most important followed by and in a second level of importance the levels of HbA1c and arterial hypertension; and for the development of renal and retinal lesion simultaneously poor control of glycaemia measured by levels of HbA1c were more important than the duration of diabetes mellitus.

Two broader groups of patients can be assumed to have been formed in this study, the first being those patients who developed only diabetic retinopathy, and the second those with both diabetic retinopathy and renal lesion (overt nephropathy). This conclusion is consistent with previous studies as that of Lövestam-Adrian in 1998 (Lövestam-Adrian, et al, 1998), in which after a 10-year follow-up of a population of 24 patients, with proliferative diabetic retinopathy at the beginning of the study, only two developed microalbuminuria, That study concluded that there are, at least partly, different pathogenic mechanisms behind diabetic retinopathy and overt nephropathy.

5. Conclusion

Despite there being a poor relationship between overt nephropathy and diabetic retinopathy (p=0.021 in the present study), the presence of overt nephropathy correlated well with severe forms of diabetic retinopathy (as proliferative Dr p<0.001 in the present study); and in addition, at the end of study two broad group of patients had been configured, the first those who developed only diabetic retinopathy, and the second with diabetic retinopathy and renal lesion (overt nephropathy). For the first group with only DR , duration of diabetes mellitus is the most important risk factor, and for the second group (patients with DR and DN) the levels of HbA_{1c} and blood pressure are the most important.

6. References

Adler AI, Stevens RJ, Manley SE, Bilous RW, Cull CA & Holman RR (2003). UKPDS Group. Development and progression of nephropathy in type2 diabetes. The United Kingdom Prospective Diabetes Study (UKPDS 64). Kidney Int; 63:225-232. ISSN 0085-2538

Aldington SJ, Kohner EM, Meuer S, Klein R & Sjolie AK (1995). Methodology for retinal photography and assessment of diabetic retinopathy , The EURODIAB IDDM complications study. Diabetologia, 38 , 437-444 ISSN 0012-186X

American Diabetes Association (1997). Report of the Expert Committee on the diagnosis and classification of diabetes mellitus. Diabetes Care; 20:1183-1201. ISSN 0149-5992

Castell C, Tresserras R, Lloveras G, Goday A, Serra J & Salleras L (1999). Prevalence of diabetes in Catalonia, an OGTT-based population study. Diab Res Clin Prac, 43, 33-40 ISSN 0168-8227

El-Asrar AM, Al Rubeaan KA, Al-Amor SA, Moharram OA & Kangave D (2000). Retinopathy as a predictor of other diabetic complications. International Ophthalmology;24:1-11. ISSN 0161-6420

Esmatjes E, Castell C, Goday A, Montanya E, Pou JM & cols (1998). Prevalence of nephropathy in type I diabetes Med Clin (Barc). 1998 17; 110(1):6-10. ISSN 0025-7753

Estacio RO, McFarling E, Biggerstaff S, Jeffers BW, Johnson D & Schrier RW (1998). Overt albuminuria predicts diabetic retinopathy in Hispanics with NIDDM. Am J of Kidney Disease; 31:947-953. ISSN 0272-6386

European Diabetes Policy Group (1999). A Desktop guide to type I (insulin-dependent) diabetes mellitus. 1998-199. Guidelines for Diabetes care. Diabetic Med, 16, 253-266. ISSN 1464-5491

Expert Panel on Detection, Evaluation, And Treatment of high Blood Cholesterol in Adults (Adult Treatment Panel III) (2001). Executive summary of the third report of the National Cholesterol Education Program   (NCEP). JAMA, 285, 2486-2497 ISSN 0098-7484

Gall MA, Hougaard P, Borch-Johnsen K & Parving HH (1997). Risk factors for development of incipient and overt diabetic nephropathy in patients with non-insulin dependent diabetes mellitus: prospective, observational study. BMJ;314:783-789. ISSN 0959-8138

Geiss L, Engelgau M, Fraizer E & Tierney E (1997). Diabetes surveillance, 1997. Centers for Disease Control and Prevention. U.S. Departement of Health and Human Services Atlanta GA.

Klein R, Klein BEK, Moss SE & Cruickshanks KJ (1998). The 14-year incidence and progression of diabetic retinopathy an associate risk factors in type I diabetes. The Wisconsin Epidemiologic Study of Diabetic Retinopathy XVII. Ophthalmology, 105, 1801-1815. ISSN 0161-6420

Klein R, Klein BEK, Moss SE, Davis MD & DeMets DL (1984). The Wisconsin Epidemiologic Study of Diabetic Retinopathy II: prevalence and risk of diabetic retinopathy when age at diagnosis is less than 30 years. Arch Ophthalmology;102:520-526. ISSN 0093-0326

Klein R, Klein BEK, Moss SE, Davis MD & DeMets DL (1984). The Wisconsin Epidemiologic Study of Diabetic Retinopathy II: prevalence and risk of diabetic retinopathy when age at diagnosis is 30 or more years. Arch Ophthalmology;102:527-32. ISSN 0093-0326

Klein R, Moss SE & Klein BEK (1993). Is gross proteinuria a risk factor for the incidence of proliferative diabetic retinopathy?. Ophthalmology, 100: 1140-1146 ISSN0161-6420

Kofoed-Enevoldsen A, Jensen T, Borch-Johnsen K & Deckert T (1987). Incidence of retinopathy in type I (insulin-dependent) diabetes: association with clinical nephropathy. J Diabet Complications,1, 96-99. ISSN 1056-8727

Looker HC, Krakoff J, Knowler WC, Bennett PH, Klein R & Hanson RL (2003). Longitudinal studies of incidence and progression of diabetic retinopathy assessed by retinal photography in Pima Indians. Diabetes Care;26:320-326. ISSN 0149-5992

Lövestam-Adrian M, Agardh E & Agardh CD (1998). The incidence of nephropathy in type 1 diabetic patients with prol iferative retinopathy: a 10-year follow-up study. Diabetes Res Clin Pract.;39(1):11-17. ISSN 0168-8227

Myers BD, Winetz JA, Chui F, Michaels AS. Mechanism of proteinuria in diabetic nephropathy: A study of glomerular barrier functions. Kidney Int 1982;21:633-41 ISSN 1523-1755

Otani T, Kishi S & Maruyana Y (1999). Patterns of diabetic macular edema with optical coherence tomography. Am J Ophthalmol , 127, 688-693. ISSN 0002- 939

Ritz E, Orth SR. Nephropathy in patients with type2 diabetes mellitus. N Eng J Med 1999; 341:1127-33. ISSN 1533-4406

Romero-Aroca P, Espeso-Sentis O, Sarda-Aure P & del Castillo-Dejardin D (2000). Relationship between microalbuminuria and diabetic retinopathy in type I diabetes mellitus. Rev Clin Esp. 200,351-354. ISSN 0014-2565

Romero-Aroca P, Salvat-Serra M, Mendez-Marin I & Martinez-Salcedo I (2003). Is microalbuminuria a risk factor for diabetic retinopathy?. J Fr Ophtalmol, 26, 7, 680-684. ISSN 0181-5512

Rossing P, Hougaard P & Parving HH (2002). Risk factors for the development of incipient and overt diabetic nephropathy in type 1 diabetic patients: A 10 year prospective observational study. Diabetes Care 2002;25:859-864. ISSN 0149-5992

The Expert Comitee on the Diagnosis and Classification of Diabetes mellitus (2000). Report of the Expert Committee on the Diagnosis and classification of Diabetes Mellitus. Diabetes Care; 23: S4-S19 ISSN 0149-5992

Villar G, Gracia Y, Goicolea I & Barquees J (1999). Determinants of development of
     microalbuminuria in normotensive patients with type 1 and type 2 diabetes.
     Diabetes and Metabolism; 25:246-254. ISSN 1520-7560

Wilkinson CP, Ferris FL, Klein RE, Lee PP, Agardh CD, Davis M, Dills D, Kampic A,
     Pararajasegaram R & Verdaguer JT, representing the Global Diabetic Retinopathy
     Project Group (2003). Proposed international clinical diabetic retinopathy and
     diabetic macular edema disease severity scales. Ophthalmology, 110, 1677-1682
     ISSN 0161-6420

Williams R, Airey M, Baxter H, Forrester J, Kennedy-Martin T & Giarach A (2004).
     Epidemiology of diabetic retinopathy and macular edema: a systematic review.
     Eye; 18:963-983. ISSN 0950-222X

Part 2

Treatment

3

Prevention of Diabetes Complications

Nepton Soltani

Molecular Medicine Research Center, Hormozgan University of Medical Science,
Iran

1. Introduction

The constellation of abnormalities caused by insulin deficiency is called diabetes mellitus. The cause of clinical diabetes is always a deficiency of the effect of insulin at the tissue level. Type I diabetes or insulin- dependent diabetes mellitus (IDDM), is due to insulin deficiency caused by autoimmune destruction of the B cell in the pancreatic islets, and it accounts for 3-5 % of cases and usually presents in children. Type 2 diabetes, or non-insulin-dependent diabetes mellitus (NIDDM), is characterized by the dysregulation of insulin release from the B cells, along with insulin resistance in peripheral tissues such as skeletal muscle, brain, and liver. Type 2 diabetes usually presents in overweight or obese adults.

The incidence of diabetes in the human population has reached epidemic proportions worldwide and it is increasing at the rapid rate.150 million people in 2000, which is predicted to rise to 220 million in 2010.

In animals, it can be produced by pancreatectomy; by administration of alloxan, streptozocin, or other toxins that in appropriate doses cause selective destruction of the beta cells of the pancreatic islets; by administration of drugs that inhibit insulin secretion; and by administration of anti-insulin anti-bodies. Strains of mice, rats, hamsters, guinea pigs, miniature swine, and monkeys that have a high incidence of spontaneous diabetes mellitus have also been described.

Diabetes is characterized by polyuria, polydipisa, weight loss in spite of polyphagia, hyperglycemia, glycosuria, ketosis, acidosis, and coma. Widespread biochemical abnormalities are present, but the fundamental defects to which most of the abnormalities can be traced are 1) reduced entry of glucose into various peripheral tissues and 2) increased liberation of glucose into the circulation from the liver. Therefore there is an extracellular glucose excess and, in many cells, an intracellular glucose deficiency a situation that has been called starvation in the midst of plenty. Also, the entry of amino acids into muscle is decreased and lipolysis is increased.

2. Diabetes complication

Diabetic complications are divided to two parts: 1) metabolic complication and 2) vascular complication.

2.1 Metabolic complication

Obesity is increasing in incidence, and relates to the regulation of food intake and energy balance and overall nutrition. It is special relation to disordered carbohydrate metabolism and diabetes. As body weight increase, insulin resistance increase, that is, there is a decreased ability of insulin to move glucose into fat and muscle and shut off glucose release from liver. The liver takes up glucose from the bloodstream and stores it as glycogen, but because the liver contains glucose 6- phosphates it also discharges glucose into the blood-stream. Insulin facilitates glycogen synthesis and inhibits hepatic glucose output. When the plasma glucose is high, insulin secretion is normally increased and hepatic glucogenesis is decreased. This response dose not occurs in type I and II diabetes.

When plasma glucose is episodically elevated over time, small amounts of hemoglobin A are nonenzymatically glycated to from HbA1c. Careful control of the quently HbA1c level is measured clinically as an integrated index of diabetic control for the 4 to 6 weeks period before the measurement. Many studies showed that the mean HbA1c value was a good predictor of ischemic heart disease. In particular, the multivariate analysis showed that per each 1% increment in HbA1c there was a 10% increase in the risk of coronary heart disease. Some studies believed that 1% reduction in HbA1c level led to a 16% reduction in the occurrence of myocardial infarction.

Peripheral neuropathy, often expressed as hypersensitivity to painful stimuli, is among the most common complications of diabetes that develops in up to 60% of patients. It occurs in both type I and II diabetes and its incidence is linked to duration of disease. Neuropathic pain is a chronic or persistent pain characterized by alterations in pain perception, enhanced sensitivity to noxious stimuli (hyperalgesia) and abnormal pain sensitivity to previously non-painful stimuli (allodynia). Though the pathophysiology of neuropathy in diabetes has not been fully elucidated, hyperglycemia induced by diabetes is though to contribute to its development and maintaining good glycemic control could restrict the onset and progression of diabetic neuropathy.

2.2 Vascular complication

Hyperglycemia has a direct, harmful effect on the cardiovascular system requires, at the very least, a link between acute hyperglycemia and one or more risk factors for cardiovascular disease (CVD). Associated with obesity there is hyperinsulinemia, high circulating triglyceride and low HDL, and accelerated development of atherosclerosis. In diabetes, the plasma cholesterol level is usually elevated and this plays a role in the accelerated development of the atherosclerotic vascular disease that is a major long-term complication of diabetes in humans.

As usual diabetes is characterized by a high incidence of CVD, and poor control of hyperglycemia appears to play a significant role in the development of CVD in diabetes. Recently, there has been increasing evidence that the postprandial state is an important contributing factor to the development of atherosclerosis. In diabetes the postprandial phase is characterized by a rapid and large increase in blood glucose levels, and the possibility that these postprandial hyperglycemic spikes may be relevant to the pathophysiology of the late diabetes complications.

Insulin resistance (IR) has profound, negative effects on the function of arteries and arterioles throughout the body. In addition to the obvious link between IR and the development of type 2 diabetes, IR-associated dysfunction of resistance vessels is associated with arterial hypertension and vascular occlusive diseases. IR affects arteries and arterioles at both the endothelium and smooth muscle levels. For example, IR causes reduced responsiveness of vascular smooth muscle to dilator agents; predominantly due to impaired potassium channel function.

Vascular disease is one of the complicating features of diabetes mellitus. Several prospective studies have indicated that hypertension in diabetic patient's takes place at a rate more than twice compared to the normal population. The hypertension is also considered an independent risk factor for cardiovascular mortality in patients with diabetes. It has been suggested that alterations in the reactivity of blood vessels to neurotransmitters and circulating hormones are responsible for the cardiovascular complications of diabetes. Some studies showed that Ca/Mg ratio is a marker of vascular tone; its increase represents increased vascular reactivity and atherogenic risk. Atherogenic lesion is poorly correlated with serum cholesterol level and is highly dependent on plasma magnesium level and Ca/Mg ratio. Pervious studies showed that Ca/Mg ratio increase in diabetic case. Endothelial function is altered early in diabetes. It has been demonstrated that in diabetic subjects, the vasodilating response to stimuli is diminished and that this anomaly is related to glycemic control. In vivo studies have demonstrated that hyperglycemic spikes induce, in both diabetic and normal subjects, an endothelial dysfunction. This effect of hyperglycemia is probably linked with a reduced production/bioavailability of nitric oxide (NO), since hyperglycemia-induced endothelial dysfunction is counterbalanced by arginine. Furthermore, it is very interesting that a rapid decrease of flow-mediated vasodilation has been shown in the postprandial phase in type II diabetes patients and that the decrease correlated inversely with the magnitude of postprandial hyperglycemia.

3. Prevention of diabetes complications

Type I diabetes usually develops before the age 40, patients with this disease are not obese and they have a high incidence of ketosis and acidosis. Various anti-B cell antibodies are present in plasma, but the current thinking is that type I diabetes is primarily a T lymphocyte-mediated disease. But type II diabetes is the most common type of diabetes and is usually associated with obesity. It usually develops after age 40 and is not associated with total loss of the ability to secrete insulin. It has an insidious onset, is rarely associated with ketosis, and is usually associated with normal beta-cells morphology and insulin content if the beta-cells have not become exhausted. So it seems we should look for different methods for prevention of type I and II diabetes.

3.1 Diabetes diet

Several lifestyle factors affect the incidence of type 2 diabetes. Obesity and weight gain dramatically increase the risk, and physical inactivity further elevates the risk, independently of obesity. Cigarette smoking is associated with a small increase and moderate alcohol consumption with a decrease in the risk of diabetes. In addition, a low-fiber diet with a high glycemic index has been associated with an increased risk of diabetes, and specific dietary fatty acids may differentially affect insulin resistance and the risk of diabetes.

Excess body fat is the single most important determinant of type II diabetes. Weight control would be the most effective way to reduce the risk of type II diabetes, but current strategies have not been very successful on a population basis, and the prevalence of obesity continues to increase. The public generally does not recognize the connection between overweight or obesity and diabetes. Thus, greater efforts at education are needed.

Low-fat vegetarian and vegan diets are associated with reduced body weight, increased insulin sensitivity, and reductions in cardiovascular risk factors. The potential cardiovascular benefits of vegetarian and vegan diets may be especially important for individuals with diabetes, for whom cardiovascular disease is a main cause of premature mortality; the effects of such diets on cardiovascular risk factors appear to be similar in individuals with and without diabetes.

Prior studies have shown that near-vegetarian diets reduce the need for insulin and oral medications in individuals with type 2 diabetes. We previously reported that in individuals with type 2 diabetes, a low-fat, vegan diet was associated with improved glycemic control, weight loss, and improved plasma lipid control during a 22-wk study period. What is particularly critical in diabetes management is long-term improvement in clinical measures, particularly glycemia and cardiovascular risk factors. Well-planned low-fat vegan diets are nutritionally adequate and, in research studies, have shown acceptability comparable with that of other therapeutic diets, suggesting they are suitable for long-term use.

3.2 Immunosupression drug
If type one diabetic patient give immunosupression drugs like cyclosporine ameliorate early in the disease, before all beta cells are lost can be useful for prevention of disease. But chose the low fat and low carbohydrate diets could be useful for prevention of type 2 diabetes.

4. Magnesium

Some studies indicated that magnesium is a novel factor implicated in the pathogenesis of the complication of diabetes. Magnesium plays a fundamental role as a cofactor in various enzymatic reactions of energy metabolism. Magnesium is a cofactor in cell membrane glucose-transporting mechanisms, as well as in various enzymes in carbohydrate oxidation. It is also involved, at multiple levels, in insulin secretion, binding and activity. Magnesium deficit has been described in patients with type I diabetes. Hypomagnesemia can also be the cause or a result of diabetes complications. If it is followed by diabetes, osmotic diuresis may play a role in the mechanisms responsible for magnesium deficiency. Magnesium loss may be linked to the development of diabetes complications via a reduction in the rate of inositol transport and its subsequent intracellular depletion that might enhance the development of complications. Studies showed that the administration of magnesium corrected hyperglycemia and has brought blood glucose back to normal levels within 24 h of its administration. Moreover, magnesium appears to have some reparative effect on the pancrease of diabetic case. Accordingly, during long-term treatment, pancreatic repair may have an effective role in the control of plasma glucose levels. Magnesium also is a necessary cofactor for many enzymes which is involved in lipid metabolism. Mg-deficiency enhances catecholamine secretion which result in an increase in lipolysis and blood plasma magnesium has been shown to decrease when lipolysis is increased. Enhancement in lipolysis and subsequent elevation of plasma free fatty acids levels may lead to an increase in hepatic VLDL and triglycerides synthesis and secretion and elevated plasma triglyceride concentration. The hepato-biliary pathway is the main rout for removal of cholesterol from the body. Bile flow is significantly lower in Mg-deficient subject than in controls and the cholesterol concentration in bile is decreased. Magnesium administration could decrease triglycerides, cholesterol and LDL cholesterol and also increased HDL cholesterol. The decrease in serum triglycerides was associated with the change in serum total Mg concentration. Other supporting evidence is accumulating for the role of magnesium in the modulation of serum lipids and lipids uptake in macrophages. Studies showed that increase in plasma endothelin I due to magnesium deficiency and a direct effect of magnesium deficiency on vascular smooth muscle are involved in the elevation of vascular tone in diabetic pateint. Elevated vascular tone can contribute to increased blood pressure. Some studies have observed that systolic and diastolic blood pressure and mean arterial blood pressure in Mg-treated chronic diabetic subject are lower than in chronic diabetic. The administration of magnesium can decrease vascular bed sensitivity to phenylephrine and decrease Ca/Mg ratio. Studies also showed that magnesium decreases collagen thickness, intima/media thickness and the lumen/ media ratio in aorta. This suggests that the administration of magnesium can decrease blood pressure and prevent vascular morphological changes and decrease in vascular sensitivity to neurotransmitter. Hemoglobin deficiency is observed in diabetic subjects. This can probably be explained by the inhibition of ð-aminolevulinate dehydratase (ð-ALA-D) in diabetes. Studies have found that this enzyme is inhibited by glycation of the active site lysine residue involved in Schiff's base formation with the first ð-ALA-D molecule. Magnesium administration reduces this glycation via blood glucose reduction and, thus, prevents hemoglobin deficiency. So it seems that magnesium administration may play in the management of diabetes and the prevention of its vascular complications in diabetic patients.

5. Glucagone-like peptide-1 (GLP-1)

Type I diabetes is a complex disease that results from an autoimmune T-lymphocyte-dependent islet infiltration and destruction of islet beta- cells, with consequent insulin deficiency and dependence on exogenous insulin treatment. A strikingly decreased functional beta- cell mass owing to apoptosis constitutes the histopathological hallmark of the disease at diagnosis. Recently, strategies employing beta-cell growth factors to enhance functional beta-cell mass and restore insulin secretion have been proposed for the treatment and prevention of diabetes. One such promising beta-cell growth factor identified is glucagone-like peptide-1 (GLP-1). GLP-1 is an insulinotropic hormone that is secreted from intestinal L-cell in response to nutrient ingestion and promotes nutrient absorption via regulation of islet hormone secretion. GLP-1 receptor is expressed mainly by pancreatic beta-cells, and to some extent in other tissues like lung, kidney and brain. GLP-1 enhances pancreatic islet beta-cell proliferation and inhibits beta-cell apoptosis in a glucose-dependent fashion. Other actions of GLP-1 are to decrease glucagons secretion and gastric emptying. Together, all these actions tend to lower the plasma glucose concentration and to limit plasma glucose rises with meals. GLP-1 is another gastrointestinal hormone that is also expressed in the hypothalamus and brainstem. Their CNS actions are to decrease food intake, decrease water intake, and increase diuresis. However, native GLP-1 has a short circulating half-life (less than 2 min) that results mainly from rapid enzymatic inactivation by dipeptidyl-peptidase IV (DPP- IV), and/ or renal clearance. Therefore, continuous subcutaneous infusion by pump is necessary to maintain GLP-1 action. DPP- IV-resistant GLP-1 analogues and other formulations appear to be promising therapeutic drug candidates for the treatment and prevention of diabetes, but these peptides require once or twice-daily injections and/or combination therapies with oral diabetic medications. Scientifics recently developed a novel GLP-1 fusion peptide consisting of the active human GLP-1 molecule and the murine IgG1 constant heavy-chain (IgG-Fc). Plasmid-based, electroporation-enhanced intramuscular gene therapy with GLP-1/IgG-Fc improved insulin production and normalized glucose tolerance in type one or two diabetes.

6. Gama amino butyric acid (GABA)

Gama amino butyric acid (GABA) is an important neurotransmitter which was initially identified in the central nervous system and is also found in islet beta-cells. GABA has an important role in pathogenesis of diabetes. Excessive secretion of glucagon is a major contributor to the development of diabetic hyperglycemia. Secretion of glucagon is regulated by various nutrients, with glucose being a primary determinant of the rate of alpha-cell glucagon secretion. The intra-islet action of insulin is essential to exert of insulin, glucose is not able to suppress glucagons release in vivo. However, the precise mechanism by which insulin suppresses glucagon secretion from alpha-cells is unknown. Studies showed that insulin induces activation of GABAA Akt kinase-dependent pathway. This leads to membrane hyperpolarization in the alpha-cells and, ultimately, suppression of glucagon secretion. Researchers propose that defects in this pathway contribute to diabetic hyperglycemia. It is well known that the secretion of glucagon is abnormal in human type I diabetes patients. The patients do not secrete glucagon in response to hypoglycemia and they have an exaggerated response of glucagon to stimuli such as arginine infusion and a protein meal. In studies of patients with type I diabetes there are indications of an increase in alpha cell numbers. GABA decreases in diabetic patients. Some studies indicated that a reduction in cellular GABA level is more sensitive than insulin as a marker for the presence of dead beta-cells in isolated preparations. Pancreatic GABA content also rapidly decreased after diabetes induction and remained unaffected by 12 h of hyperglycemia. It seems that GABA therapy can has some beneficial effect to prevention or treatment type I diabetes.

7. Antioxidants

Increasing evidence in both experimental and clinical studies suggests that oxidative stress play a major role in the pathogenesis of both types of diabetes mellitus. Diabetes is usually accompanied by increased production of free radicals or impaired antioxidant defenses. Mechanisms by which increased oxidative stress is involved in the diabetic complication are partly known, including activation of transcription factors, advanced glycated end products (AGEs), and protein kinase C.

Excessively high levels of tree radicals cause damage to cellular proteins, membrane lipids and nucleic acids, and eventually cell death. Various mechanisms have been suggested to contribute to the formation of these reactive oxygen-free radicals. Glucose oxidation is believed to be the main source of free radicals. In its enediol form, glucose is oxidized in a transition-metal-dependent reaction to an enddiol radical anion that is converted into reactive ketoaldehydes and to superoxide anion radicals. The superoxide anion radicals undergo dismutation to hydrogen peroxide, which if not degraded by catalase or glutathione peroxidase, and in the presence of transition metals, can lead to production of extremely reactive hydroxyl radicals. Superoxide anion radicals can also react with nitric oxide to form reactive peroxynitrite radicals. Hyperglycemia is also found to promote lipid peroxidation of LDL by a superoxide- dependent pathway resulting in the generation of free radicals. Another important source of free radicals in diabetes is the interaction of glucose with proteins leading to the formation of Amadori product and then advanced glycation endproducts (AGEs). These AGEs, via their receptors (RAGEs), inactivate enzymes and alter their structures and functions, promote free radical formation, and quench and block antiproliferative effects of nitric oxide. By increasing intracellular oxidative stress, AGEs activate the transcription factor NF-kB, thus promoting up-regulation of various NF-kB controlled target genes. NF-kB enhances production of nitric oxide, which is believed to be a mediator of islet beta cell damage.

Considerable evidence also implicates activation of the sorbitol pathway by glucose as a component in the pathogenesis of diabetic complications, for example, in lens cataract formation or peripheral neuropathy. Efforts to understand cataract formation have provoked various hypotheses. In the aldose reductase osmotic hypothesis, accumulation of polyols initiates lenticular osmotic changes. In addition, oxidative stress is linked to decreased glutathione levels and depletion of NADPH levels. Alternatively, increased sorbitol dehydrogenase activity is associated with altered NAD^+ levels, which results in protein modification by nonenzymatic glycosylation of lens proteins.

Mechanisms linking the changes in diabetic neuropathy and induced sorbitol pathway are not well delineated. One possible mechanism, metabolic imbalances in the neural tissues, has been implicated in impaired neurotrophism, neurotrsnsmission changes, Schwann cell injury, and axonopathy.

While on the one hand hyperglycemia engenders free radicals, on the other hand it also impairs the endogenous antioxidant defense system in many ways during diabetes. Antioxidant defense mechanism involves both enzymatic and nonenzymatic strategies. Common antioxidants include the vitamins A, C and E, antioxidant minerals (copper, zinc, manganese, and selenium), and the cofactors (folic acid, vitamins B1, B2, B6, B12). They work in synergy with each other and against different types of free radicals. Vitamin E suppresses the propagation of lipid peroxidation; vitamin C with vitamin E inhibits hydroperoxide formation; metal complexing agents, such as penicillamine, bind transition metal involved in some reactions in lipid peroxidation and inhibit Fenton and Haber-weiss-type reactions; vitamins A and E scavenge free radicals.

8. Herbal medicine

Recently, the search for appropriate hypoglycemic agents has been focused on plants. Many herbal medicines have been recommended for the treatment of diabetes. Plant drugs are frequently considered to be less toxic and free from side effect than synthetic ones. The leaf of Psidium guava, Teucrium polium, Cinnamon and Garlic are used traditionally in many countries to manage, control and treat of diabetes. Some recent studies have shown that administration of Psidium guava or Teucrium polium leaves decrease blood glucose via enhance insulin secretion.

Psidium guajva Linn., commonly known as guava, is a native plant in tropical American and has long been naturalized in south east Asia and in south of Iran. Different parts of the plant are used in traditional medicine for the treatment of various human aliments such as wound, ulcers, bronchitis, cyesores and diarrhea. In folklore guava has been used for a long time as a medicinal herb to cure diabetes mellitus. Many people in some countries including Japan, Taiwan and Iran boil guava leaves in water and drink the exact as a folk medicine for diabetes and hypertension. Psidium guajava leaves have a beneficial effects on diabetes metabolic syndrome and vascular complications.

Photochemical analysis of Psidium guajava leaves have revealed the presence of flavonoids, which include quercetin and its derivatives (guajaverin, isoquercitrin, hyperin, quercitrin, avicularin), morin and its derivatives (morin-3-O-α-L-lixopyranoside and morin-3-O-α-Larabopyranoside), rutin, myricetin, luteolin and kaempferol. The leaves of the plant have also been shown to contain essential oil, fixed oil, volatile oil, saponin, resin, tannin, triterpenoids, asiatic acid and ellagic acid.

The relaxant effect of Psidium guajva Linn., on endothelium-intact aortic rings were only partially inhibited by N-nitro-L-arginine methyl ester (L-NAME), a nitric oxide synthase inhibitor, suggesting that the vasorelaxant effect of Psidium guajva Linn., on aortic rings is probably mediated via both endothelium-derived relaxing factor (EDRF)-dependent and EDRF-independent mechanisms but it seems this mechanism is not follow in diabetic rat vessel.

Teucrium polium L. is one of 300 species of the genus Teucrium and found mainly in the Mediterranean and Western Irano-Turanian sphere. It is widely distributed in Iran, Jordan and Palestine. The leaves 1-3 cm long, are sessile, oblong or linear, the stems are ending in a shortly paniculate or corymbose infoflorescences, corolla is white or pale cream colored. Several researchers have evaluated Teucrium polium grown in different geographic origin and it has flavonoids and iridoids. Hypoglycemic activity has been reported - in addition to the flavonoids- also for the volatile oils. Traditionally, especially in the Mediterranean countries and in Iran, Teucrium polium, is used for its antispasmodic and hypoglycemic activities by the native inhabitants and recommended by the herbalists. Anti-inflammatory, anti-hypertensive, antinociceptive, anti-ulcer and anorexic effects are other activities reported. Some investigators have reported reduction in blood glucose concentrations of animal diabetic model after treatment with a single i.v., i.p. and oral dose of Teucrium polium aqueous decoction. Some Iranian researchers have observed significant decrease in blood glucose in animal diabetic model after six weeks of consecutive oral treatment with ethanol/ water extract.

Spices such as Cinnamon display insulin-enhancing activity in vitro. Cinnamon can improve glucose metabolism and the overall condition of individuals with diabetes not only by hypoglycemic effects but also by improving lipid metabolism, antioxidant status, and capillary function. Aqueous extracts from Cinnamon have also been shown to increase in vitro glucose uptake and glycogen synthesis and to increase phosphorylation of the insulin receptor; in addition, these Cinnamon extracts are likely to aid in triggering the insulin cascade system. Because insulin also plays a key role in lipid metabolism, consumption of Cinnamon would lead to improved glucose and blood lipids in vitro. The mechanism of the effect of Cinnamon on glucose and blood lipids is not completely understood but the researchers believe that extracts of Cinnamon activated glycogen synthase, increased glucose uptake, and inhibited glycogen synthase kinase-3β. Extracts of Cinnamon also activated insulin receptor kinse and inhibited dephosphorylation of the insulin receptor, leading to maximal phosphorylation of the insulin receptor. All of these effects would lead to increased insulin sensitivity. The extract of Cinnamon also has function as potent antioxidants, which would lead to additional health benefits of this substance.

Garlic was known to be effective in decreasing, cholesterol and can inhibit LDL-Oxidation. Many clinical trials have been conducted to determine the lipid-lowering effects of fresh garlic and garlic supplements. Garlic consumption also can decrease blood glucose in diabetic patients and has beneficial effect on diabetic vessel. It seems that daily Garlic consumption can be useful to prevent of diabetes.

9. References

Abe A, Kawasoe C, Kondo Y, Sato K. 2003. Enhancement of norepinephrine-induced transient contraction in aortic smooth muscle of diabetic mice. Acta. Med. Okayama 57(1): 45-8

Adeghate E, Ponery AS. 2002. GABA in the endocrine pancreas: cellular localization and function in normal and diabetic rats. Tissue Cell. 34(1):1-6.

Afifi FU, Al-Khalidi B, Khalil E. 2005. Studies on the in vivo hypoglycemic activities of two medicinal plants used in the treatment of diabetes in Jordanian traditional medicine following intranasal administration. J. Ethnopharmacol. 100: 314-318

Ajay M, Achike FI, Mustafa AM, Mustafa MR. 2006. Effect of quercetin on altered vascular reactivity in aorta isolated from sterptozotocin-induced diabetic rats. Diabetes Res. Clin. Pract. 73: 1-7

Altura BM, Altura BT. 1995. Magnesium and cardiovascular biology an important link between cardiovascular risk factors and atherogenesis. Cellular and Molecular Bio. Research. 41(5): 245-271

Altura BM, Altura BT. 1991. Cardiovascular risk factors and magnesium: relationships to atherosclerosis, ischemic heart disease and hypertension. Magnes.Trace. Elem. 10: 182-192.

Anetor, JI, Senjobi A, Ajose OA, Agbedana, E.O. 2002. Decreased serum magnesium and zinc levels: atherogenic implications in type-2 diabetes mellitus in Nigerians. Nutr.Health 16: 291-300.

Anwar N, Mason DF. 1982. Two actions of gamma-aminobutyric acid on the responses of the isolated basilar artery from the rabbit. Br J Pharmacol. 75(1): 177-81.

Ashraf R, Aamir K, Shaikh AR, Ahmed T. 2005. Effect of Garlic on dyslipidemia in patients with type 2 diabetes mellitus. J Ayub Med Coll Abbottabad. 17(3): 1-5

Baluchnejadmojarad T, Roghani M, Homayounfar H, Hosseini M. 2003. Benefical effect of aqueous garlic extract on the vascular reactivity of streptozotocin-diabetic rats. J of Ethnopharmacol. 85: 139-144

Begum S, Hassan SI, Ali SN, Siddiqui BS. 2004. Chemical constituents from the leaves of psidium guajava. Nat Prod Res. 18: 135-140

Borboni P, Porzio O, Fusco A, Sesti G, Lauro R, Marlier LN. 1994. Molecular and cellular characterization of the GABAA receptor in the rat pancreas. Mol Cell Endocrinol. 103(1-2):157-63

Busija DW, Miller AW, Katakam P, Simandle S, Erdös B. 2004. Mechanisms of vascular dysfunctionin insulin resistance. Curr Opin Investig Drugs. 5(9): 929-35

Ceriello A. 2005. Postprandial hyperglycemia and diabetes complications. Is it time to treat? Diabetes. 54:1-7

Chiwororo DH, Ojewole J. 2008. Biphasic effect of psidium guajava Linn. (Myrtaceae) leaf aqueous extract on rat isolated vascular smooth muscle. Smooth Muscle Res. 44(6): 217-229

Corica F, Allegra A, Di BA, Giacobbe MS, Romano G, Cucinotta D, Buemi M, Ceruso D. 1994. Effects of oral magnesium supplementation on plasma lipid concentrations in patients with non-insulin-dependent diabetes mellitus. Magnes. Res. 7: 43-47 de Valk HW, Verkaaik R, van Rijn HJ, Geerdink RA, Struyvenberg A. 1998. Oral magnesium supplementation in insulin-requiring Type 2 diabetic patients. Diabet.Med. 15: 503-507

Diederich D, Skopec J, Diederich A, Dai FX. 1994. Endothelial dysfunction in mesenteric resistance arteries of diabetic rat: role of free radical. Am J. Physiol. 266: H1153-H1161

Djurhuus MS, Henriksen JE, Klitgaard NA, Blaabjerg O, Thye-Ronn P, Altura BM, Altura BT, Beck-Nielsen H. 1999. Effect of moderate improvement in metabolic control on magnesium and lipid concentrations in patients with type 1 diabetes. Diabetes Care. 22: 546-554.

Djurhuus MS, Klitgaard NAH, Pedersen KK, Blaabjerg O, Altura BM, Altura BT, Henriksen JE. 2001. Magnesium reduces insulin-stimulated glucose uptake and serum lipid concentrations in type 1 diabetes. Met.Clin. Exp 50: 1409-1417.

Dong H, Kumar M, Zhang Y, Gyulkhandanyan A, Xiang YY, Ye B. 2006. Gamma-aminobutyric acid up- and downregulates insulin secretion from beta cells in concert with changes in glucose concentration. Diabetologia. 49(4):697-705

Duarte J, Perez-Vizcaino F, Jimenez J, Tamargo J, Zarzuelo A. 1993. Vasodilatory effects of flavonoids in rat aortic smooth muscle. Structure-activity relationships. Gen. Pharmacol. 24: 857-862

Eidi A, Eidi M, Esmaeili E. 2006. Antidiabetic effect of garlic (Allium Sativum L.) in normal and sterptozotocin-induced diabetes rats. Phytomedicine. 13: 624-629

Ferriola PC, Cody V, Middleton EJR. 1989. Protein kinase C inhibition by flavonoids. Kinetic mechanism and structure-activity relationships. Biochem. Pharmacol. 38: 1617-1624

Franklin IK, Wollheim CB. 2004. GABA in the endocrine pancreas: its putative role as an islet cell paracrine-signalling molecule. J Gen Physiol. 123(3):185-90.

Giugliano D, Cericllo A, Paolisso G. 1996. Oxidative stress and diabetic vascular complication. Diabetes Care. 19: 257-267

Giugliano D, Marfella R, Coppola I, Verrazzo G, Acampora R, Giunta R, Nappo F, Lucarelli CD, Onofrio F. 1997. Vascular effects of acute hyperglycemia in humans are reversed by L-arginine evidence for reduced availability of nitric oxide during hyperglycemia. Circulation. 95:1783-1790

Gladkevich A, Korf J, Hakobyan Vp, Melkonyan KV. 2006. The peripheral GABAergic system as a target in endocrine disorders. Auton Neurosci. 124(1-2):1-8.

Gutierrez RMP, Mitchell S, Solie RV. 2008. Psidium guajava: a review of its traditional uses, phytochemistry and pharmacology. J. Ethnopharmacol. 117: 1-27

Hasanein P, Parviz M, Keshavarz M, Javanmardi K, Mansoori M, Soltani N. 2006. Oral magnesium administration prevents thermal hyperalgesia induced by diabetes in rats. Diabetes Res Clin Pract. 73(1): 17-22

Jarrett RJ. 1989. Cardiovascular disease and hypertension in diabetes mellitus. Diabetes/Metabolism Research and Reviews. 5: 547-558

Jenkins AJ, Klein RL, Chassereau CN, Hermayer KL, Lopes-Virella MF. 1996. LDL from patient with well-controlled IDDM is not more susceptible to in vitro oxidation. Diabetes. 45: 762-767

Jenkins AJ, Lyons T, Zheng DY, Otvos JD, Lackland DT, Mcgee D, Garvey WT, Klein RL. 2003. Serum lipoproteins in the diabetes control and complications trial/epidemiology of diabetes intervention and complications cohort - Associations with gender and glycemia. Diabetes Care 26: 810-818

Jensen KD, Jensen B, Lervang HH, Hejlesen OK. 2002. Diabetes patients' ability to estimate dietary carbohydrate content for use in a decision support system. Stud.Health Technol. Inform. 90: 649-654

Jorgensen RG, Russo I, Marttioli I, Moore WV. 1988. Early detection of vascular dysfunction in type I diabetes. Diabetes. 37:292-296

Kaneto H, Kajimoto Y, Miyagawa JI, Matsuoka TA, Fujitani Y, Umayahara Y, Hanafusa T, Matsuzawa Y, Yamasaki Y, Hori M. 1999. Beneficial effects of antioxidants in diabetes possible protection of pancreatic β-cells against glucose toxicity. Diabetes. 48: 2398-2406

Khan A, Khattak KN, Safdar M, Anderson R, Au Khan M. 2003. Cinnamon improves glucose and lipids of people with type 2 diabetes. Diabetes Care. 26(12): 3215-3218

Laight DW, Carrier MJ, Anggard EE. 2000. Antioxidant, diabetes and endothelial dysfunction. Cardiovasc. Res. 47: 457-464

Laires MJ, Moreira H, Monteiro CP, Sardinha L, Limao F, Veiga L, Goncalves A, Ferreira A, Bicho M. 2004. Magnesium, insulin resistance and body composition in healthy postmenopausal women. J. Am. College of Nutri 23: 510S-513S

Lal J, Vasudev K, Kela AK, Jain SK. 2003. Effect of oral magnesium supplementation on the lipid profile and blood glucose of patients with type 2 diabetes mellitus. J. Assoc. Physic. India. 51: 37-42

Laurant P, Touyz RM. 2000. Physiological and pathophysiological role of magnesium in the cardiovascular system: implications in hypertension. J. Hypertens. 18(9): 1177-91

Ligon B, Yang J, Morin SB, Ruberti MF, Steer ML. 2007. Regulation of pancreatic islet cell survival and replication by gamma-aminobutyric acid. Diabetologia. 50(4):764-73

Liu KH, Chan YL, Chan JC, Chan WB. 2005. Association of carotid intima-media thickness with mesenteric, preperitoneal and subcutaneous fat thickness. Atherosclerosis.179(2): 299-304

Liu KH, Chan Y.L, Chan WB, Chan JC, Chu CW. 2006. Mesenteric fat thickness is an independent dererminant of metabolic syndrome and identifies subjects with increased carotid intima-media thickness. Diabetes Care. 29(2): 379-84

Liu KH, Chan YL, Chan WB, Kong WL, Kong, MO, Chan JC. 2003. Sonographic measurement of mesenteric fat thickness is a good correlate with cardiovascular risk factors: comparison with subcutaneous and preperitoneal fat thickness, magnetic resonance imaging and anthropometric indexes. Int.J. Obes. Relat. Metab. Disord. 27: 1267-1273.

Maritim AC, Sanders RA, Watkins JB. 2003. Diabetes, oxidative stress and antioxidants: A review. J Biochem Molecular Toxicology. 17(1):24-38

Mirghazanfari SM, Keshavarz M, Nabavizadeh F, Soltani N, Kamalinejad M. 2010. The effect of Teucrium polium L. Extracts on insulin release from in situ isolated perfused rat pancrease in newly modified isolation method: the role of Ca and K channels. Iranian Biomedical Journal. 14(4):178-185

Narendhirakannan RT, Subtanman S, Kandaswamy M. 2006. Some commonly used Indian plants on sterptozotocine induced diabetes in experimental rats. Clin Exp Pharmacol Physol. 33: 1150-1157

Obatomi DK, Bikomo EO, Temple VJ. 1994. Anti- diabetic properties of African mistletoe in sterptozotocin-induced diabetic rats. J Ethnopharmacol. 43(1): 13-70

Ojewole JA. 2005. Hypoglycemic and hypotensive effects of Psidium guajava Linn. (myrtaceae) leaf aqueous extract. Methods Find Exp clin pharmacol. 27(10): 689-950

Okada Y, Taniguchi H, Schimada C. 1976. High concentration of GABA and high glutamate decarboxylase activity in rat pancreatic islets and human insulinoma. Science. 194(4265):620-2

Olatunji-Bello I, Odusanya AJ, Raji I, Ladipo CO. 2007. Contractile effect of aqueous extract of Psidium guajava leaves on aortic rings in rat. Fitoterapia 78: 241-243

Ozcelikay AT, Tay A, Guner S, Tasyaran V, Yildizoglu-Ar, N, Dincer UD, Altan VM. 2000. Reversal effects of L-arginine treatment on blood pressure and vascular responsiveness of streptozotocin-diabetic rats. Pharmacol. Res. 41(2): 201-9

Ozdem SS, Sadan G. 1999. Impairment of GABA-mediated contractions of rat isolated ileum by experimental diabetes. Pharmacology. 59: 165-170

Pari L, Umamaheswari J. 2000. Antihyperglycaemic activity of Musa Sapientum flowers: effect on lipid peroxidation in alloxan diabetic rats. Phytother. Res. 14: 1-3

Prudhomme GJ, Chang Y. 1999. Prevention of autoimmune diabetes by intramuscular gene therapy with a nonviral vector encoding an interferon-gamma receptor/ IgG1 fusion protein. Gene Therapy. 6: 771-777

Rasmussen H, Takuwa Y, Park S. 1987. Protein kinase C in the regulation of smooth muscle contraction. FSSEB J. 1: 177-185

Rayssiguier, Y, Gueux E, Durlach V, Durlach J, Nassir F, Mazur A. 1992. Magnesium and the cardiovascular system: I. New experimental data on magnesium and lipoproteins. In: Halpern,M.j. (Ed.), Molecular biology of atherosclerosis, Proceedings of the 57th European Atherosclerosis Society Meeting. John Libbey & Company Ltd, Eastleigh, pp. 507-512

Reetz A, Solimena M, Matteoli M, Folli F, Takei K, De Camilli P. 1991. GABA and pancreatic beta-cells: colocalization of glutamic acid decarboxylase (GAD) and GABA with synaptic-like microvesicles suggests their role in GABA storage and secretion. EMBO J. 10(5):1275-84.

Saad MF, Greco S, Osei K, Lewin AJ, Edwards C, Nunez M, Reinhardt RR. 2004. Ragaglitazar improves glycemic control and lipid profile in type 2 diabetic subjects: a 12-week, double-blind, placebo-controlled dose-ranging study with an open pioglitazone arm. Diabetes Care. 27(6): 1324-9

Shen SC, Cheng FC, Wu NJ. 2008. Effect of Guava (Psidium guajava Linn.) leaf soluble solids on glucose metabolism in type 2 diabetic rats. Phytother. Res. 22: 1458-1464

Shi Y, Kanaani J, Menard-Rose V, Ma YH, Chang PY, Hanahan D, et al. 2000. Increased expression of GAD65 and GABA in pancreatic beta-cells impairs first-phase insulin secretion. Am J Physiol Endocrinol Metab. 279 (3): E684-94

Singh RB, Rastogi SS, Mani UV, Seth J, Devi L. 1991. Does dietary magnesium modulate blood lipids? Biol. Trace. Elem. Res 30: 59-64.

Singh RB, Rastogi SS, Sharma VK, Saharia RB, Kulshretha SK. 1990. Can dietary magnesium modulate lipoprotein metabolism? Magnes.Trace. Elem. 9: 255-264

Soltani N, Keshavarz M, Dehpour AR. 2007. Effect of oral magnesium sulfate administration on blood pressure and lipid profile in streptozocin diabetic rat. Eur J Pharmacol. 560(2-3):201-5

Soltani N, Keshavarz M, Sohanaki H, Dehpour AR, Asl SZ. 2005. Oral magnesium administration prevents vascular complications in STZ-diabetic rats. Life Sci. 11 76(13): 1455-64

Soltani N, Kumar M, Glinka Y, Prud'homme GJ, Wang Q. 2007. Gene therapy of diabetes using a novel GLP-1/IgG1-Fc fusion construct normalizes glucose levels in db/db mice. Gene Ther. 14(2):162-72

Soltani N, Keshavarz M, Minaii B, Mirershadi F, Zahed Asl S, Dehpour AR. 2005. Effect of administration of oral magnesium on plasma glucose and pathological changes in the aorta and pancrease of diabetic rats. Clin Exp Pharmacol Physiol. 32(8): 604-10

Soltani N, Keshavarz M, Sohanaki H, Zahed Asl S, Dehpour AR. 2005. Relaxatory effect of magnesium on mesenteric vascular beds differs from normal and streptozotocin induced diabetic rats. Eur. J. Pharmacol 31 508(1-3): 177-81

Stamler J, Vaccaro O, Neaton JD, Wentworth D. 1993. The multiple risk factor intervention trial research group, diabetes, other risk factors and 12-yr cardiovascular mortality for men screened in the multiple risk factor intervention trial. Diabetes Care. 16:434-444

Sunagawa M, Shimada S, Zhang Z, Oonishi A, Nakamura M, Kosugi T. 2004. Plasma insulin concentration was increased by long-term ingestion of guava juice in spontaneous non-insulin-dependent diabetes mellitus (NIDDM) rats. Journal of health Sci. 50(6): 674-678

Suraez A. 1993. Decreased insulin sensitivity in skeletal muscle of hypomagnesium rats. Diabetologia. 36 (1): A82

Taniguchi H, Okada Y, Seguchi H, Shimada C, Seki M, Tsutou A. 1979. High concentration of gamma-aminobutyric acid in pancreatic beta cells. Diabetes. 28(7): 629-33

Tsai EC, Hirsch IB, Brunzell JD, Chait A. 1994. Reduced plasma peroxyl radical trapping capacity and increased susceptibility of LDL to oxidation in poorly controlled IDDM. Diabetes. 43: 1010-1014

Xu E, Kumar M, Zhang Y, Ju W, Obata T, Zhang N. 2006. Intra-islet insulin suppresses glucagon release via GABA-GABAA receptor system. Cell Metab. 3(1):47-58

Yajnik CS. 2001. The insulin resistance epidemic in India: fetal origins, later lifestyle, or both? Nutr. Rev. 59: 1-9

Zizzo MG, Mulè F, Serio R. 2007. Functional evidence for GABA as modulator of the contractility of the longitudinal muscle in mouse duodenum: role of GABA(A) and GABA(C) receptors. Neuropharmacology. 52(8):1685-90.

4

Perspectives of Cell Therapy in Type 1 Diabetes

Maria M. Zanone, Vincenzo Cantaluppi, Enrica Favaro,
Elisa Camussi, Maria Chiara Deregibus and Giovanni Camussi
*Renal and Vascular Physiopathology Laboratory, Department of Internal Medicine,
Molecular Biotechnology Centre and Research Centre for Molecular Medicine,
University of Torino,
Italy*

1. Introduction

Type 1 diabetes is an autoimmune disease leading to the destruction of pancreatic β cells. The reduction of β cell mass results in insulin deficiency that leads to a failure of glucose homeostasis with increased levels of glucose in blood. Hyperglycemia which *per se* is detrimental for the organism and may be life-threatening, may in the long term associate with chronic complications involving blood vessels and nerves. The gold standard treatment for diabetes patients aimed to reach a tight control of glycemia, relies on intensive insulin therapy based on multiple daily injections or continuous subcutaneous infusion of insulin. A tight control of glycemia reached with such regimens was shown to significantly reduce the incidence of microvascular complications in respect to the conventional insulin therapy. Nevertheless, to reach an optimal control of blood levels may prove to be difficult when compared to the physiological condition where this is guaranteed by the pancreatic β cells (Suckale, 2008). Therefore, preservation of β cell mass could be an important therapeutic target to reduce microvascular complications and to improve the glycemia control (Gonez & Knight, 2010). It is generally accepted that the endocrine pancreas has some regenerative capabilities, although it is still debated which cells are involved in β cell turnover. In rodents the capability of adult pancreas to increase β cell mass has been documented in physiological conditions and after injury. The understanding of mechanisms involved in β cell turnover may therefore be relevant to design new therapeutic strategies aimed to maintain a β cell mass or to favour regeneration of β cells. These strategies however, should take to account the problem of recurrent autoimmunity that in type 1 diabetes not only impairs the original β cell mass, but may also limit the regenerative process. Indeed, autoimmune T lymphocytes may kill the β cells newly formed in response to injury (Fan & Rudert, 2009).

2. β cell regeneration: Contribution of stem/progenitor cells or replication of β cell?

The physiological turnover of the long-lasting endocrine cells of pancreas requires the generation of new cells even with a very slow kinetic.

The organ growth after birth requires a coordinated increase in the number of constitutive cells. Moreover, in the adult body most of the tissues and organs have the ability to replace the cells that die for physiological senescence or following limited injury. The source of newly formed cells may derive from resident stem/progenitor cells or from the ability of differentiated cells to re-entry into cell cycle and replicate themselves. The prevalence of these two mechanisms varies in different organs and tissues; however, they may result in the restoration of the original tissue conformation and function. We therefore should expect that also the endocrine pancreas retains the ability of regeneration in appropriate physiological conditions. The nature and the location of the cells involved in such processes, as well as the mechanisms involved in the activation of the regenerative processes, still remain largely unknown.

The concept of "stem cell" implies the ability of unlimited self renewal and of high multilineage differentiation potential into different types of mature cells. Therefore, stem cells play fundamental roles in organogenesis during embryonic development, and in the adult are responsible for the growth, homeostasis and repair of many tissues.

In the haematopoietic system, the intestine and the skin, tissues that require a high cell turnover, the stem cells are critical for maintaining their homeostasis. However, adult stem/progenitor cells are present in the majority of tissues and organs of mammalian organisms, including the central nervous system (Reynolds & Weiss, 1992), retina (Tropepe et al., 2000), skeletal muscle (Jackson et al., 1999), liver (Herrera et al., 2006) and kidney (Bussolati et al., 2005).

In tissues with a low rate of cell turnover, such as the kidney, the lung, the skeletal muscle and the liver, the resident stem cells may activate after injury and participate in tissue repair. Tissue resident stem cells preferentially generate differentiated cells of the tissue of origin, suggesting a relevant role in the postnatal growth of organs, in physiological turnover and in tissue repair. Tissue-resident adult stem cells are thought to co-localize with supporting cells within specific regions or specialized microenvironments in each tissue/organ, called stem cell niche (Jones & Wagers, 2008; L. Li et al., 2005; Moore & Lemischka, 2006). In bone marrow the haematopoietic stem cells (HSC) are located in the endosteal niche, associated with the osteoblasts of the inner surface of the cavities of trabecular bone that could provide factors able to regulate number and function of HSC (Mitsiadis et al., 2007) and in the perivascular area of sinusoids that could ensure homeostatic blood cell production and prompt responses to haematological stresses (Kiel et al., 2005). The other stem cells present in bone marrow are the mesenchymal stem cells (MSC), undifferentiated adult stem cells of mesodermal origin, which localize in perivascular areas in the bone marrow in close association with HSC (Shi & Gronthos, 2003) and that have the capacity to differentiate into cells of connective tissue lineages, including bone, fat, cartilage and muscle (Y. Jiang et al., 2002).

Other stem cell niches detected in mammals (da Silva Meirelles et al., 2008; L. Li & Xie, 2005) are the epithelial stem cell niche in skin that resides in the bulge area of the hair follicle beneath the sebaceous gland (Cotsarelis et al., 1990; Niemann & Watt, 2002; Sun et al., 1991), the intestinal stem cell niche located at the fourth or fifth position above the Paneth cells from the crypt bottom (Booth & Potten, 2000; He et al., 2004; Sancho et al., 2004) and the neural stem cell niche at the subventricular zone and the subgranular zone of the hippocampus where neural stem cells could reside and support neurogenesis in the adult brain (Doetsch et al., 1999; Temple, 2001).

A problem in the identification of tissue resident stem cells is that we do not know specific markers allowing tracing of pluripotent stem cells in various tissues. Therefore, resident stem cells are mainly defined by functional *in vitro* assays using cultured cells, and their *in vivo* exact localization and function remains elusive. Several studies suggest that the adult tissue resident stem cells belong to the MSC lineage (da Silva Meirelles et al., 2006). The minimal criteria to define human MSC established by *Mesenchymal and Tissue Stem Cell Committee of the International Society for Cellular Therapy* (da Silva Meirelles et al., 2008; Dominici et al., 2006), include cell positivity for CD105, CD73, and CD90 and negativity for CD45, CD34, CD14 or CD11b, CD79a or CD19, and HLA-DR as well as osteo-, chondro-, and adipogenic-differentiation capabilities.

A perivascular location for MSC has been suggested, correlating these cells with pericytes providing an explanation for the presence of MSC virtually in all vascularized tissues (da Silva Meirelles et al., 2006). The perivascular zone may act as a MSC niche *in vivo*, where microenvironment factors may modulate their phenotype with transition to progenitor and mature cells. For many years the concept of niche has been associated with a hierarchical nature of stem cells that undergoing asymmetric division insure self-renewal and generation of a progeny with progressive loss of proliferative potential and gain of differentiated characteristics (Till et al., 1964). More recently, a continuum model of stem cell biology has been proposed (Colvin et al., 2004; Quesenberry et al., 2005). It has been postulated that the phenotype of stem cells is labile, it varies with position in the cell cycle and that it is reversible (Colvin et al., 2007). This cell-cycle reversibility is at the basis of the continuum model of stem cell biology, in which the phenotype of stem cells is reversibly changing during the cell cycle transit awaiting for a terminal-differentiating stimulus at a cycle-susceptible time. In this model the status of the cell cycle and the exposure to environmental factors play critical roles in the acquirement of different phenotypes by the same cell in different functional states (Quesenberry et al., 2007). Recently, Quesenberry and Aliotta proposed that the so-called niche consists in areas of influence which are continually adjusting to individual circumstances (Quesenberry & Aliotta, 2008). Based on these considerations, the refined regenerative system in mammalians does not need to position in each organ different stem cell types but it would be sufficient to maintain few undifferentiated cells with self-renewal capability that depending on the circumstances may vary their phenotype to replace the loss of differentiated cells. On the other hand, differentiated cells may re-acquire an undifferentiated phenotype and re-entry in to cell cycle first to restore the cell mass and subsequently to re-differentiate and restore functional integrity. In this context, the exchange of genetic information among cells by microvesicles in a defined environment plays a critical role in modulating plasticity of stem cells as well as the response of differentiated cells to injury (Deregibus et al., 2010).

Studies on β cell proliferation in humans are limited, but there is evidence that this process occurs at relatively high levels in the first 2 years of life declining thereafter with the possibility, at least in animals, of re-induction under conditions of insulin-resistance, such as pregnancy or obesity. (Meier et al., 2008). This suggests that β cells may retain an intrinsic capacity to replicate.

In the adult, endocrine pancreas β cells are considered to have a very low turnover. However, albeit quite slowly, β cells undergo senescence and should be continuously replaced by newly formed cells. By combining abdominal CT scans and morphometric analysis of human pancreatic tissue, Meier et al reported that the β cell mass expands by several fold from birth to adulthood as result of an expansion in size of islets rather than an increase in number of islets (Meier et al., 2008). The increase in β cell number per islet mainly occurs in young children in coincidence with the growth of the organ size. Cnop et al provided evidence for a long lifespan and low turnover of human islet β cells estimated by mathematical modelling of lipofuscin accumulation (Cnop et al., 2010). Human β cells, unlike those of young rodents, are long-lived and in the adult human β cell population is mainly established in the first 20 years of life. Dor et al using a method for genetic lineage tracing to determine the contribution of stem cells to pancreatic β cell neogenesis showed that pre-existing β cells, rather than pluripotent stem cells, are the major source of new β cells during adult life and after pancreatectomy in mice (Dor et al., 2004). These results suggest that terminally differentiated β cells retain, at least in mice, a significant proliferative capacity *in vivo*. Nir et al used a transgenic mouse model to study the dynamics of β cell regeneration from a transiently induced diabetic state (Nir et al., 2007). Lineage tracing analysis in this model indicated that enhanced proliferation of surviving β cells played the major role in regeneration. These studies provided evidence that adult pancreatic β cells are formed by self duplication rather than stem cell differentiation (Dor et al., 2004; Nir et al., 2007). On the other hand there are studies suggesting that regenerated β cells derive from precursors located within pancreatic ducts in the proximity of islets (Juhl et al., 2010). The origin from these precursors has been demonstrated in rodent models of pancreatic damage (Bonner-Weir et al., 2004; Xu et al., 2008). Monitoring the expression of Neurogenin 3 (Ngn3), the earliest islet cell-specific transcription factor in embryonic development, Xu et al showed activation of β cell progenitors located in the ductal lining in injured adult mouse pancreas (Xu et al., 2008). They found that differentiation of the adult progenitors is Ngn3 dependent and generates all islet cell types, including glucose responsive β cells that proliferate, both *in situ* and when cultured in embryonic pancreas explants. This study suggests that multipotent progenitor cells present in the pancreas of adult mice can increase the functional β cell mass by differentiation and proliferation rather than by self-duplication of pre-existing β cells only. Li et al investigated whether after partial pancreatectomy in adult rats, pancreatic-duct cells serve as a source of regeneration by undergoing a dedifferentiation and redifferentiation (W.C. Li et al., 2010). The Authors detected after pancreatectomy an early loss by the mature ducts of the ductal differentiation marker Hnf6, followed by the transient formation of areas composed of proliferating ductules, called foci of regeneration. These ductules expressed markers of the embryonic pancreatic epithelium Pdx1, Tcf2 and Sox9 (W.C. Li et al., 2010). Since foci subsequently form new pancreatic lobes, it was suggested that these cells act as progenitors of the regenerating pancreas. Islets in foci initially resemble embryonic islets as they transiently expressed the endocrine-lineage-specific transcription factor Ngn3 and lacked of MafA expression and contained low percentage of β cells. The numbers of MafA(+) insulin(+) cells progressively increased with the maturation of foci (W.C. Li et al., 2010). Based on these observations, it was suggested that adult pancreatic duct cells may recapitulate aspects of embryonic pancreas in response to injury (W.C. Li et al., 2010). This mechanism of regeneration implicates the plasticity of the differentiated cells within the pancreas.

As schematized in figure 1, after injury β cells may be replaced by replication of β cells or from differentiation of stem cells (SC) localized within the islets or in exocrine pancreatic tissues (ductal and acinal cells). After extreme loss of β cell mass, glucagon producing α cells may transdifferentiate in β cells. A possible contribution to β cell neogenesis comes from bone marrow derived stem cells of both haemopoietic (BM-derived HSC) and mesenchymal (BM-derived MSC) origin. These cells act by a paracrine mechanism releasing factors that favour tissue repair. Moreover, transdifferentiation of ductal and acinal cells may generate insulin secreting cells.

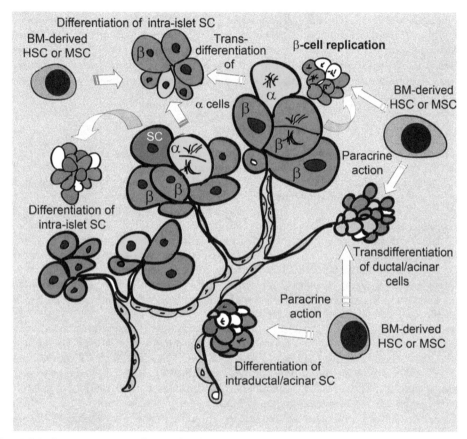

Fig. 1. Mechanisms potentially involved in β cell neogenesis.

The discrepancy in identification of cells that in the adult sustain β cell neogenesis, may result from the differential contribution in condition of physiological turnover and in condition of injury where the regenerative processes are accelerated and cells other than insulin producing β cells are involved to insure a reparative process. The study of Thorel et al showing the conversion of adult pancreatic α cells into β after extreme β cell loss stands in this line of interpretation (Thorel et al., 2010). In this study the Authors used *in vivo* genetic approaches to obtain near total β cell loss without autoimmunity combined with cell lineage tracing. For this purpose, they created a model of inducible, rapid β cell removal (>99%) by administration of diphtheria toxin (DT) in transgenic mice in which the DT receptor was expressed only in β cells (Thorel et al., 2010). In transgenic mice the systemic administration of DT permitted a specific cell ablation by apoptosis (Saito et al., 2001). In this model, β cell regeneration was monitored in combination with cell lineage tracing to investigate the origin of newly formed β cells. The results obtained showed that the adult pancreas can generate new β cells after their near total loss, mainly by the spontaneous reprogramming of glucagon-secreting α cells (Saito et al., 2001). Therefore, β cell replication may account for maintaining homeostasis, whereas transdifferentiation of other cell types could be required after injury to replace the lost cells.

Summarizing these studies, one can envisage a scenario in which β cells may replicate themselves to maintain homeostasis (Dor et al., 2004), tissue specific precursors localized within pancreatic ductal cells generate α and β cells after pancreatic injury and glucagon secreting α cells can transdifferentiate into β cells to repair an extremely severe selective β cell loss. Translation of these experimental studies in humans may be difficult without the help of lineage tracing or of specific cellular markers.

3. β cell mass in type 1 and type 2 diabetes

Despite the evidence of some turnover in adult humans and the apparent capacity of endocrine pancreatic β cells to regenerate throughout life, patients with type 1 as well as type 2 diabetes have substantial deficit in β cell mass, approximately 99% in long-standing type 1 diabetes and 65% in long-standing type 2 diabetes. This loss of β cells implies that restoration of endogenous insulin secretion might be accomplished through replacement or regeneration of islet cells.

The β cell deficit in type 1 diabetes is related to the established autoimmune destruction of the target cells. However, several lines of research indicate that some β cell regeneration may occur in recent onset type 1 diabetic patients (Willcox et al., 2010) and even in patients with long-standing type 1 diabetes (Meier et al., 2005). The failure of β cell regeneration in type 1 diabetes may be related to the increased vulnerability of the newly forming β cells to apoptosis induced by inflammatory cytokines (Meier et al., 2006).

Other mechanisms, involved in all forms of diabetes, include the hyperglycemic induction of the nitric oxide synthase (NOS)-dependent mechanisms in islet microendothelium, with production of the vasoactive mediator nitric oxide (NO) (Suschek et al., 1994), endothelial cell loss and vasculature disruption (Zanone et al., 2008). NO is in fact increased in hyperglycemic conditions, and has an established direct islet cytotoxicity and potentially impairs insulin release (Steiner et al, 1997; Suschek et al., 1994; Kröncke et al., 1993). Islet microendothelial cells are also source of the proinflammatory cytokine IL-1β under hypeglycemic conditions, independently of any viral or immune-mediated process. IL-1β impairs insulin release in human islet, induces Fas expression enabling Fas-mediated apoptosis and IL-1β is thus implicated as a mediator of glucotoxicity (Maedler et al., 2001; Loweth et al., 1998). The metabolic mechanisms by which hyperglycemia initiates apoptosis in vascular endothelium are incompletely understood. These mechanisms include oxidative stress, increased intracellular Ca++, mitocondrial dysfunction, changes in intracellular fatty-acid metabolism, and impaired phosphorylation of the protein kinase Akt (Favaro et al., 2008). Akt signaling pathway plays a pivotal role in preventing apoptosis in a variety of settings (Datta et al., 1999), and, in particular, Akt activation is crucial for the ability of factors such as insulin, IGF-I and VEGF to inhibit apoptosis in cultured endothelium (Jung et al., 2000). Recent data highlight the Akt role also in insulin-mediated glucose transport and pancreatic β cell mass and function (Bernal-Mizrachi et al., 2004; Elghazi et al., 2006). As for type 2 diabetes, the progressive increase in glucose levels that characterizes its natural history has been claimed to be due to gradual reduction of function and mass of β cells, and a significant reduction in β cell mass is clearly established in Type 2 diabetes (Donath & Halban, 2004; Weir & Bonner-Weir, 2004). The same mechanisms of glucotoxicity reported are involved, together with dyslipidaemia. In murine models of type 2 diabetes, short-term hyperglycemia has been shown to increase islet capillary blood pressure and perfusion, in a glucose dependent and reversible pathway, possibly mediated by a NOS–dependent mechanism (Bonner-Weir, 2004; Carlsson et al., 1998). However, with age, persistent hyperglycemia induces islet hypoperfusion. Inducible NOS (iNOS) increases the islet blood perfusion also in prediabetic low dose streptozotocin-treated mice, a model of type 1 diabetes (Carlsson et al., 2000). Increased islet capillary flow and pressure could, over time, contribute to the damage of the islet endothelium and thickening of the capillary wall, thus decreasing the islet perfusion. The hyperglycemia-induced NO production by the endothelium could also result cytotoxic to the islets and directly impair insulin release.

In Zucker diabetic fatty rats, a model of type 2 diabetes, it has been shown that changes in the islet vasculature play a key pathogenetic role in the development of diabetes (X. Li et al., 2006). In a biphasic pattern, an early vascular hyperplasia was followed by endothelial cell loss and vasculature disruption, in parallel to progressive islet failure.

4. Islet transplantation as strategy for β cell replacement

Allogenic pancreatic islet transplantation has become a suitable therapeutic option for the treatment of patients with unstable type I diabetes after the introduction of the Edmonton Protocol based on the optimization of islet isolation techniques and the development of a rapamycin-based glucocorticoid-free immunosuppressive regimen (Ricordi, 2003; Shapiro et al., 2000, 2003, 2006). However, after 5 years only 10% of the recipients were insulin independent (Ryan et al., 2005; Shapiro, 2006). In addition, although a sufficient islet mass can be obtained from good quality pancreata, to achieve insulin independence usually are needed islet preparations derived from multiple donors (Biancone & Ricordi, 2002). Therefore, this procedure is limited by the supply of cadaveric donors. Moreover, several factors may be responsible of the progressive dysfunction of transplanted islets. After an initial islet mass loss following the intraportal infusion, due to an inflammatory reaction, engraftment requires efficient islet revascularization by a chimeric vascular tree formed by host and recipient endothelial cells (Brissova et al., 2004). A poor vascular engraftment is one of the main causes of islet loss. Other factors that concur to islet loss include the exposure of islets to increased lipid levels, a side effect of immunosuppressive therapy based on mTOR inhibitors (Hafiz et al., 2005; Pileggi et al., 2006). Exposure to high-dose of calcineurin inhibitors (CNI) is recognized to induce direct β cell toxicity and functional impairment. The antiproliferative effects of mTOR inhibitors and CNI inhibit tissue remodelling and reduce β cell self-renewal (Nir et al., 2007). Moreover, the anti-angiogenic activity of rapamycin is a potential limitation of the current immunosuppressive protocols, that may be particularly detrimental in the early engraftment phase (Cantaluppi et al., 2006). Therefore, to overcome these problems it is necessary to improve the recovery and quality of islet cells from a single-donor pancreas and to develop strategies allowing the inhibition of inflammatory reactions, the improvement of islet vascularization and of islet engraftment using safer and less cytotoxic immunomodulatory approaches (Mineo et al., 2009; Pileggi et al., 2006; Ricordi, 2003). Recently, increased islet yields have been obtained by improving techniques of pancreas recovery and preservation and of islet isolation and purification (Pileggi et al., 2006;Ricordi, 2003). On the other hand, peritransplant interventions based on combination therapies have been proposed to inhibit allo- and auto-immune response minimizing the side effects and favoring development of T regulatory cells (Treg) to maintain long term tolerance and to favor β cell regeneration. Targeting the costimulatory molecules involved in T-cell activation and/or adhesion molecules by immunomodulatory agents now available for clinical applications could be an option to reduce the side effects of immunosuppression and the islet toxicity and to achieve specific immune tolerance (Ricordi & Strom, 2004). Several experimental studies suggest that a combined islet transplant and cell therapy with bone marrow–derived cells, mesenchymal cells, Treg, and tolerogenic dendritic cells may modulate recipient immune response and increase the engraftment and long term survival of islets (Mineo et al., 2008). This possibility is supported by recent clinical trials demonstrating stable mixed haematopoietic chimerism and/or improved tolerance in kidney allograft recipients using nonmyeloablative conditioning and donor haematopoietic stem cell infusion (Sykes, 2009).

Another factor limiting successful islet engraftment is the inflammatory reaction that takes place in the liver after portal vein infusion of islets. This observation led to experiments of co-transplantation of islets with bone marrow-derived mesenchymal stem cells to take advantage of the anti-inflammatory action of these cells (Ito et al., 2010).

To improve islet vascularization is also a must for a better engraftment of islets. It has been shown that bone marrow-derived endothelial progenitor cells (EPC) isolated from peripheral blood specifically localize within sites of endothelial injury inducing a regenerative program. EPC are able to chimerize with donor vessels in transplanted organs, suggesting a putative role of these cells in graft revascularization (Schuh et al., 2008, Koopmans et al., 2006). EPC are recruited to the pancreas in response to islet injury and EPC-mediated pancreas neovascularization may facilitate the recovery of injured β cells improving islet allograft function (Mathews et al., 2004). In a murine model of islet transplantation, the increase of EPC in the peripheral circulation obtained by mobilization with granulocyte-macrophage colony-stimulating factor has been associated with higher vascular density and engraftment (Contreras et al., 2003). Therefore, the identification of factors able to enhance neoangiogenesis may increase the success of islet transplantation.

Another goal of combination therapies is to preserve islet function after detection of graft dysfunction (Froud et al., 2008). For this purpose it has been suggested, for instance, the use of exenatide, glucagon-like peptide synthetic analog, anti-tumor necrosis factor α agents or immunomodulatory therapy (Faradji et al., 2008; Froud et al., 2008). However, the recently released results of two trials addressing strategies of combination therapies are disappointing. The phase three trial based on combination of anti-CD25 mAb (Daclizumab) that blocks IL-2 signalling pathway in activated T cells without interfering with Treg, in combination with mycophenolate mofetil that bloks the *de novo* purine synthesis in T and B lymphocytes, reported no improvement of β cell preservation (Gottlieb et al., 2010). The anti-CD25 mAb was tested in another trial in association with exenatide. Also in this trial the improvement of β cell function was not observed (Rother et al., 2009). Several other phase II-III National Institutes of Health (NIH)–sponsored randomized trials in islet transplantation alone and in islet-after-kidney transplantation are currently under evaluation by the Clinical Islet Transplantation Consortium (http://www.citisletstudy.org/). An alternative to allow long term survival of islets after transplantation is the development of efficient encapsulation techniques aimed to guarantee immune-isolation, an adequate exchange of nutrients to islet cells and release of insulin (Calafiore et al., 2006). This kind of approach may protect from cell-mediated rejection of implanted islets, although soluble mediators may still reach β cells and induce cell death. On the other hand, this strategy might allow full maturation of embryonic stem cells into glucose sensitive insulin secreting β cells. Indeed, human embryonic stem cells differentiated into pancreatic endoderm could be encapsulated in a protective device before transplantation (D'Amour et al., 2005; Kroon et al., 2008). Experiments in NOD mice demonstrated that encapsulated human β cell precursors may generate functional insulin producing cells after implantation improving diabetes (S.H. Lee et al., 2009). As an alternative, ongoing studies are evaluating the use of encapsulated porcine islets to correct type 1 diabetes (Elliott et al., 2007). Preliminary studies in humans showed long term survival of xenotransplantation of porcine neonatal islets and Sertoli cells using a technology to provide an immune protective environment (Valdes-Gonzales et al., 2005). A vascularized chamber model allowing tissue growth in threedimension under influence of hypoxia that triggers angiogenesis has been developped in mouse (Cronin et al., 2004) and rat (Mian et al., 2000; Tanaka et al., 2000). Vascularized chambers containing syngenic islets were used to improve glucose control in diabetic mice (Hussey et al., 2009). In this study islets were transplanted into prevascularized chambers implanted on the epigastric pedicle in the groin of diabetic mice resulting in a significant reduction in blood glucose levels and improvement of glycemic control. This study suggests that islet survival and function are enhanced by prevascularization of tissue engineering chambers before islet transplantation (Hussey et al., 2009). Opara et al. reported a new design of a bioartificial pancreas comprising islets co-encapsulated with angiogenic protein in permselective multilayer alginate-poly-L-ornithine-alginate microcapsules and transplanted in an omentum pouch in diabetic experimental animals (Opara et al., 2010). A great effort is invested to improve the encapsulation techniques to avoid clogging of the device that may reduce the influx of nutrients and glucose and impair the insulin efflux. Teramura & Iwata recently reviewed the obstacles and the new techniques to overcome these problems, such as conformal coating and islet enclosure with cells (Teramura & Iwata, 2010).

In consideration of the shortage of pancreata for islet transplantation and of the side effects of current immunosuppressive protocols, the research has been focused on the possible development of alternative sources of functional β cells. The ideal approach to overcome the current inadequate supply of human pancreatic islet cells for transplantation is the availability of an unlimited source of transplantable insulin-producing cells. The potential of adult and embryonic stem cells to generate islet cells as well as development of appropriate conditions for expansion and differentiation to β cells of pancreatic islet cell precursors or of cells that share common embryonic origin such as liver cells is under intense investigation (Mineo et al., 2009). Finally, xenogeneic islet transplantation remains a viable therapeutic option for the future (Ricordi, 2003).

5. In search for alternative sources of β cells

The consideration that stem cells play a crucial role to self-renewal in physiologic and pathologic conditions in the endocrine pancreas (Bouvens, 2006; Sarvetnick et al., 2007a, 2007b) prompted researchers to develop SC-based therapy to stimulate β cell regeneration.

In the last years, a variety of approaches have been employed to induce β cell neogenesis using pluripotent stem cells (embryonic stem cells or induced pluripotent stem cells), multipotent adult stem cells such as the hepatic oval cells or terminally differentiated cells such as the exocrine pancreatic cells (Yechoor & Chan, 2010). Brolén et al investigated the potential of human embryonic stem cells to differentiate into β cells (Brolen et al., 2005). They found that signals from the embryonic mouse pancreas induce differentiation of human embryonic stem cells into insulin-producing β cell-like cells. Human embryonic stem cells (hESC) under two-dimensional growth conditions spontaneously differentiated in Pdx1(+)/Foxa2(+) pancreatic progenitors and Pdx1(+)/Isl1(+) endocrine progenitors but not in insulin-producing cells. The differentiation of β cell-like cell clusters required co-transplantation with the dorsal pancreas from mouse embryos. hESC-derived insulin(+) cell clusters exhibited several features of normal β cells, such as synthesis (proinsulin) and processing (C-peptide) of insulin and nuclear localization of key β cell transcription factors, including Foxa2, Pdx1, and Isl1 (Brolén et al., 2005). Insulin-producing islet-like cells were also generated from human embryonic stem cells under feeder-free conditions (Jiang et al., 2007). Cell aggregates formed in the presence of epidermal growth factor, basic fibroblast growth factor, and noggin were finally matured in the presence of insulin-like growth factor II and nicotinamide. The temporal kinetic of pancreas-specific gene expression was considerably similar to that of *in vivo* pancreas development. The final population contained cells representative of the ductal, exocrine, and endocrine pancreas. Ricordi et al reported a diabetes reversal in mice by embryonic-derived stem cells (Ricordi & Edlund, 2008). They showed that endodermal-derived embryonic stem cells were able to differentiate into cells that expressed typical pancreatic endodermal markers and, once transplanted in diabetic mice, these cells showed a diffuse staining for insulin, other hormones and markers of fully differentiated β cells (Ricordi & Edlund, 2008). The therapy with embryonic stem cells represents an exciting approach towards β cell regeneration and function. So far, the most promising data are from a group of NovoCell who demonstrated the generation of glucose-responsive insulin-secreting cells *in vivo* by pancreatic endoderm derived from human embryonic stem cells into immune-deficient mice (Kroon et al., 2008). However, several problems remain to be solved, such as the reproducibility of the advance, the protection of the engrafted cells against tumor formation and immune-protection that could be achieved by encapsulation devices. Recently, Matveyenko et al tried to reproduce and extend the studies of NovoCell by the implantation of human embryonic stem cell-derived pancreatic endoderm into athimic nude rats, analysing the metabolic parameters of insulin sensitivity and glucose-stimulated insulin secretion to verify the development of viable glucose-responsive insulin secreting cells. The implantation was assessed into the epididymal fat pads of the athymic nude rats or subcutaneously into Theracyte encapsulation devices for 20 weeks (Matveyenko et al., 2010). The data resulting from this study not completely confirmed the development of islet-like structures from human embryonic stem cells differentiated to pancreatic endoderm, since the extent of endocrine cell formation and secretory function was insufficient to be clinically relevant given that human C-peptide and insulin were detectable at very low levels, no increase in human C-peptide/insulin levels after glucose challenge and no development of viable pancreatic tissue or efficient insulin secretion by implantation in the encapsulation devices were present (Matveyenko et al., 2010).

Nevertheless, because the use of embryonic stem cells is burdened with the limited access to embryonic tissues and with the complex ethical concerns involved with the use of embryonic cells, more attention has been focused on adult stem cells. We found that stem cells derived from normal adult human liver (HLSC) with multiple differentiating capabilities distinct from those of oval stem cells may generate islet-like structures. HLSC expressed several MSC markers such as CD73, CD90, CD29, CD44 and the stem cell marker nestin (Herrera et al., 2006). At variance of MSC, HLSC did not express α-SMA and expressed liver tissue-specific proteins such as AFP, a marker of hepatocyte precursors, and human albumin, suggesting a partial hepatocyte commitment. At variance with oval cells, the HLSC isolated from normal adult liver, did not express the CD34, c-kit and CK19 markers, and were pluripotent. Moreover, the HLSC were able to differentiate in appropriate conditions into pancreatic insulin producing cells (Herrera et al., 2006). When cultured in DMEM with high glucose content (23mM) for one month followed by 5-7 days of culture in the presence of 10 mM nicotinamide, HLSC formed small spheroid cell clusters positive for human insulin and Glut2 which is a glucose transporter that has been suggested to function as a glucose sensor in pancreatic β cells (L. Yang et al., 2002). Moreover, HLSC under this differentiating condition, were positively stained with the Zn-chelating agent dithizone, that is specific for the insulin containing granules (Shiroi et al., 2002). It has been recently shown that adult human pancreas contains rare multipotent stem cells that express insulin (Smukler et al., 2011).

Several studies demonstrate that the β cell phenotype can be induced both *in vitro* and *in vivo* by transfection of pancreatic transcription factors into the liver that develops from the same embryological origin of pancreas (Kojima et al., 2003; Lemaigre & Zaret, 2004; Nagaya et al., 2009).

The potential of bone marrow derived MSC has also been explored. Genetically modified MSC by recombinant PDX-1 adenovirus or by non-virus gene transfection, were able to express insulin sufficient to reduce blood glucose in the streptozotocin mouse model of diabetes (Y. Li et al., 2007). The differentiated PDX-1+ human MSC expressed multiple islet-cell genes such as neurogenin3 (Ngn3), insulin, GK, Glut2, and glucagon, produced and released insulin/C-peptide. After transplatation into STZ-induced diabetic mice the differentiated PDX-1+ human MSC induced within 2 weeks euglycemia and maintained it for at least 42 days. These findings suggest that appropriately modified MSC may allow enrichment of human β cells and represent a possible source for cell replacement therapy in diabetes (Y. Li et al., 2007).

Human umbilical cord blood contains several types of stem/precursor cells. Recent studies indicate the possibility to obtain multipotent stem cells from umbilical cord blood able to confer protection to β cells and to stimulate β cell neogenesis (Zhao & Mazzone, 2010). Islet-like cell clusters were obtained from MSC derived from humbilical cord vein. However, they secreted very low amounts of insulin in vitro (Chao, 2008). Denner et al showed that directed engineering of human cord blood stem cells may produce C-peptide and insulin (Denner et al., 2007).

A better understanding of the mechanisms of β cell regeneration may provide further insight for development of cell based therapeutic approaches. Besides the potential contribution of circulating and resident stem cells, the transdifferentiation of existing pancreatic cells such as pancreatic ductal/acinar cells into insulin secreting cells could be potentially exploited (Baeyens et al., 2005; Cantaluppi et al., 2008; Minami et al., 2005; Rosenberg, 1995).

The successful differentiation of stem cells into β cells may prove not to be easy. The secretion of insulin in physiological concentration in response to glucose concentration is the goal to be achieved. One of the more difficult tasks is to maintain an intact coupling of stimulus-secretion in order to obtain a regulated insulin secretion to keep physiological glucose concentration.

Another pre-requisite for β cell replacement therapy is to obtain a non limiting source of cells possibly derived from the patient himself to avoid the allo-immune response (Wagner et al., 2010). The possibility of reprogramming patient's own cells could be an approach to these requirements. This was rendered possible by the discovery that induced pluripotent stem cells (iPS) can be generated from adult human somatic cells such as fibroblasts by transfection with selected genes encoding for transcription factors able to confer the characteristics of pluripotency to cells (Takahashi & Yamanaka, 2006; Yamanaka et al., 2007). iPS share the same differentiation potential of embryonic stem cells and they can differentiate into cells of different lineages including insulin producing cells. Tateishi et al tried to generate human iPS cells by retroviral expression of human Oct4, Sox2, Klf4 and c-Myc in the human foreskin fibroblast cells and tested the differentiation potential of human iPS cells into insulin secreting islet-like clusters, demonstrating that iPS cells derived from human skin cells can be differentiated into pancreatic islet-like cluster cells. These cluster cells were shown to contain C-peptide-positive and glucagon-positive cells and, more importantly, to release the C-peptide upon glucose stimulation (Tateishi et al., 2008). iPS cells were also generated from patients with type 1 diabetes by reprogramming their adult fibroblasts with three transcription factors (*OCT4, SOX2, KLF4*). The iPS generated from patients were shown to differentiate into insulin-producing cells (Maehr et al., 2009). A proof of principle for potential clinical applications of reprogrammed somatic cells in the treatment of diabetes type 1 or 2 was provided by Alipio et al who were able to reverse hyperglycemia in diabetic mouse models using iPS-derived pancreatic β like cells (Alipio et al., 2010). iPS could overcome the ethical issues and the immunogenicity of embryonic stem cells. The possibility to use iPS individually tailored for each patient is certainly appealing. However, several problems of bio-safety must be solved before iPS enter in clinical use. These include an aberrant or incomplete differentiation and a tumorigenic potential. Reprogramming cells typically requires integration of genes such as *c-MYC, OCT4 AND KLF4* that are known to be oncogenic and may favour development of tumors (Miura et al., 2009). Although after reprogramming the transgenes undergo silencing, it is always possible a reactivation. Therefore, the research in this field is actively searching for alternative strategies to induce pluripotency.

6. Stem cell therapy to counteract the autoimmune destruction of β cells

Assuming that we could generate pluripotent stem cell lines for each individual patient and that after infusion they would be able to restore the β cell mass, we still have to face the problem of recurrent autoimmunity. The autoimmune destruction of islet β cells by reactive T lymphocytes not only plays a role in the establishment of type 1 diabetes but also impairs an efficient regenerative process. Newly forming β cells show increased vulnerability to apoptosis induced by inflammatory cytokines (Meier et al., 2006), explaining the failure of β cell regeneration in type 1 diabetes. Therefore, newly generated β cells are systematically killed as they acquire the mature phenotype, thus impairing the regenerative attempts in type 1 diabetic patients. Furthermore, therapeutic intervention studies in new onset type 1 diabetes involving broadly immunosuppressive agents, such as cyclosporin A, failed to produce lasting remission, demonstrating the inherent tendency of the autoimmune effector response in humans to recur. Therefore, it is critical that any immunemodulatory therapy induces tolerance to β cell antigens, while minimizing detrimental effects on host defence. This is strengthened by recurrence of type 1 diabetes in syngenic pancreas transplantation (Sutherland et al., 1984).

Cell-based therapeutic strategies for immunemodulation that answer to the requirement of safety and effectiveness are under development. The intravenous use of humanized antibodies against CD3 (part of the T-cell receptor complex) soon after the initial onset of diabetic clinical symptoms decreased the insulin requirement compared to controls without this monoclonal antibody therapy. However, this therapy is burdened by several adverse effects (Keymeulen et al., 2005; Herold et al., 2002; McDevitt & Unanue, 2008).

Other approaches of immunemodulation included subcutaneous administration of heat-shock protein (Raz et al., 2001) or intravenous injection of rabbit polyclonal anti T-cell globulin (Saudek et al., 2004). In many of these studies a short term effective preservation of β cell function was observed; however, only few patients no longer required insulin treatment. Using human recombinant glutamic acid decarboxylase (GAD65) as therapeutic vaccine it was observed a preservation of C-peptide levels and a decrease in insulin dose requirement only in patients with very recent-onset of diabetes (Ludvigsson et al., 2008; Uibo and Lernmark 2008). Compelling evidence indicates the relevant role of Treg in the inhibition of autoimmune response. A decreased number and function of Treg have been reported in patients with type 1 diabetes (Roncarolo & Battaglia, 2007). Therefore, intervention to restore Treg function in diabetic patients is an attractive therapeutic strategy. Nevertheless, only few studies have shown re-establishment of Treg function in diabetes. Zhao et al demonstrated the possibility to correct functional defects of CD4+ CD62L Treg using human cord blood stem cells. This strategy allowed reversal of autoimmune diabetes in NOD mice (Y. Zhao et al., 2009) providing proof of principle that cord blood stem cells can correct function of Treg.

Treg may act by producing IL-10 and in particular transforming growth factor-β1 (TGFβ1), cytokines that are known to contribute to the induction of immunetolerance. It has been suggested that protection of newly generated β cells achieved by treatment with Treg depends on the formation of TGFβ1 cell ring surrounding pancreatic islands and conferring protection against autoimmune T lymphocytes inducing their apoptosis (Y. Zhao et al., 2009). In a pilot study in Type 1 diabetic children based on administration of autologous umbilical cord blood shortly after disease onset a lower level of HbA1c and a reduced insulin requirement was reported. However, none of the patients achieved insulin-treatment independency (Haller et al., 2007).

Recent studies raised great interest on the immunemodulatory potential of mesenchymal stem cells (Le Blanc & Pittenger, 2005). MSC can modulate several T cell functions exerting an immunesuppressive effect. MSC that lack MHC class II molecules and do not express key costimulatory molecules B7-1, B7-2, CD40 and CD40L, were shown to reduce the expression of several lymphocyte activation markers (Aggarwal & Pittenger, 2005). The mechanism has been related to the induction of an anti-inflammatory phenotype in dendritic cells, naive and activated T cells and NK cells, and to an increase of the regulatory T cell population. This results not only in the inhibition of T cell proliferation to polyclonal stimuli, but also in inhibition of naive and memory antigen-specific T cells response to their cognate peptide (Krampera et al., 2003). The MSC-induced suppression has been ascribed to several soluble factors, including hepatocyte growth factor (HGF), TGF-β1 and prostaglandin E_2 (PGE$_2$) (Aggarwal & Pittenger, 2005). Moreover, MSC have been shown to induce mature dendritic cells type 2 (DC2) to increase IL-10 secretion thus promoting anti-infammatory DC2 signaling. Several studies suggest that MSC improve the outcome of allogenic transplantation and hamper graft-versus-host disease (Le Blanc et al., 2004; Ringden et al.,

2006). Studies on the immunemodulatory potential of MSC in human type 1 diabetes are still lacking but it has been reported their regenerative potential in diabetic NOD/SCID mice leading to an increased number of pancreatic islets and β cells (R.H. Lee et al., 2006). We recently demonstrated that human allogenic bone marrow derived MSC can abrogate *in vitro* a pro-inflammatory Th1 response to islet antigen GAD in new onset type 1 diabetes, by impairing the production of IFN-γ and by inducing anti-inflammatory IL-4 production (Zanone et al., 2010). These data stimulate further studies on MSC immunemodulation in diabetes and open a perspective for immune-intervention strategies. The mechanisms of MSC interaction with the immune system cells are still controversial (van Laar & Tyndall, 2006; Abdi et al., 2008), and include reduction of the expression of lymphocyte activation markers, change of the cytokine profile of dendritic cells, naive and activated T cells and NK cells to an anti-inflammatory phenotype, and increase of the regulatory T cell population (Aggarwal & Pittenger, 2005; Le Blanc et al., 2004). In the reported study in type 1 diabetes, MSC induced in peripheral blood mononuclear cells (PBMC) of responder patients IL-4 producing cells and IL-4 secretion, suggesting a possible switch to an anti-inflammatory Th2 signalling of T cells (Zanone et al., 2010). Increased IL-4 secretion has been shown in studies of MSC cocultured with subpopulations of PHA-stimulated immune cells (Aggarwal & Pittenger, 2005) but not in studies of T cells activated by encephalitogenic peptide (Zappia et al., 2005). Lymphocyte activation is extremely complex and it is likely that several mechanisms are involved in the MSC-mediated immunesuppression and that the specific factors may depend on the lymphocyte population tested, the stimulus used, the timing of analysis and the context of the immune disease.

Further, inhibition of PGE$_2$ production abrogated the MSC-mediated IFN-γ suppression, indicating that PGE$_2$ secretion plays a key role in MSC-mediated immune effects, and the contact between MSC and PBMC enhances the production of prostaglandin E2 (Zanone et al., 2010). This observation suggests the requirement of both soluble factors and cell-contact in line with the interpretation that the immunemodulatory effects of MSC might require an initial cell-contact phase (Krampera et al., 2003). Nevertheless, the requirement of cell contact for MSC to operate their inhibition is a controversial issue, and the results reported in the literature may depend on the species and the type of stimulus.

Other studies in murine diabetic models on the regenerative capabilities of MSC, showed that injection of MSC into immunodeficient diabetic NOD/SCID mice resulted in the selective homing of MSC to pancreatic islets and in an increased number of pancreatic islets and functioning β cells (R.H. Lee et al., 2006). Further, MSC can be influenced to differentiate into cells with properties of the β cell phenotype, becoming more efficient after transplantation in mice (M. Zhao et al., 2008). Indeed, genetically modified MSC by recombinant Pdx-1 adenovirus or by non-virus gene transfection, were able to express insulin sufficient to reduce blood glucose in the streptozocin mouse model of diabetes (Karnieli et al., 2007; M. Zhao et al., 2008). More recently, allogenic MSC obtained from diabetes-prone as well as -resistant mice and injected into NOD mice, have been shown to delay the onset of diabetes or to reverse hyperglycemia (Fiorina et al., 2009). This study indicates that the beneficial effects observed could also be ascribed to the immunemodulatory capacities of MSC, as for other studies focusing on MSC-induced repair of cell injury (Abdi et al., 2008; Morigi et al., 2004; Duffield et al., 2005).

Studies on *ex vivo* expanded MSC to improve the outcome of allogenic transplantation and of acute graft-versus-host disease paved the way for the clinical use of MSC also in autoimmune diseases. In experimental autoimmune encephalomyelitis, animal model of multiple sclerosis mediated by autoreactive T cells, injected MSC home to lymphoid organs where they cluster around T cells, and ameliorate the disease onset (Gerdoni et al., 2007). In this setting, MSC induce peripheral tolerance, impairing both the cellular and humoral arm of the encephalitogenic immune response, without evidence of transdifferentiation into neural cells (Zappia et al., 2005; Gerdoni et al., 2007). Furthermore, in a murine model of rheumatoid arthritis MSC have been demonstrated to exert an immunemodulatory effect by educating antigen-specific regulatory T cells (Augello et al., 2007). MSCs are also able to inhibit autoreactive T and B cells in experimental models of systemic lupus erythematosus (Deng et al., 2005). Overall, studies on murine models of type 1 diabetes (Fiorina et al., 2009; Madec et al., 2009) and multiple sclerosis (Zappia et al., 2005) as well as non-autoimmune diseases (Herrera et al., 2007) indicate that a key feature of MSC is their ability to selectively migrate into sites of injury, where they are likely to interact with activated T cells. Diabetogenic T cells are generated in pancreatic lymph nodes where they are introduced to antigens by dendritic cells. The preferential homing of MSC to pancreatic lympho nodes (Fiorina et al., 2009; Madec et al., 2009), supports the hypothesis that these cells could directly suppress autoreactive T cells *in vivo* within the pancreatic environment. Further, the desired therapeutic effects could be achieved by modulation of chemokines/receptors to promote the homing of MSC to specific anatomical sites (Sackstein et al., 2008). The first report on transplantation of human allogenic MSC, into a patient with autoimmune systemic sclerosis, indicates its safety and, notably, striking efficacy by selective immunesuppression and regeneration of impaired endothelial progenitors (Christopeit et al., 2008). Thus, results on the use of MSC infusion for treatment of severe graft-versus-host disease or autoimmune diseases (Lazarus et al., 2005; Fouillard et al., 2003; Le Blanc et al., 2004; Ringden et al., 2006; Christopeit et al., 2008) suggest a potential use in patients at risk of type 1 diabetes or at disease onset, to preserve or reduce loss of ß cells (Abdi et al., 2008; Staeva-Vieira et al., 2007).

7. MSC treatment of complications of diabetes mellitus

The ability of MSC to differentiate into tissue of mesodermal origin makes them attractive also as therapeutic agents for a number of complications of diabetes, including cardiomyopathy, nephropathy, polyneuropathy and diabetic wounds. MSC have been shown to differentiate into several cell types, including cardiomyocytes, endothelial cells, neurons, hepatocytes, epithelial cells and adipocytes, characteristics coupled with capacity of self renewal.

Chronic hyperglycemia is responsible for myocardial remodelling leading to ventricular dysfunction with hypertrophy and apoptosis of cardiomyocytes, microcirculatory defects, altered extracellular matrix and matrix metalloproteinasis (Jesmin et al., 2003). MSC can induce myogenesis and angiogenesis by different mitogenic, angiogenic and antiapoptotic factors, such as VEGF, IGF-1 and HGF (Zhang et al., 2008). In a diabetic rat model, intravenous MSC have been shown to improve cardiac function, potentially by differentiation into cardiomyocytes and improvement of myogenesis and angiogenesis. Metalloproteinase activity was also modulated, leading to increased arteriolar density and decreased collagen volume. Cardioprotection is probably more mediated by release of paracrine factors by MSC. These include VEGF, HGF, Bcl-2, Hsp20, activation of Akt

(Wang et al., 2009), which can affect remodelling, repair and neovascularization. Intravenous autologous MSC in post-infarction patients have indeed been shown to reduce episodes of ventricular tachycardia and to increase ventricular ejection fraction (R.H. Lee et al., 2010).

Diabetic limb ischemia could also be improved by MSC-derived pro-angiogenic factors (Comerota et al., 2010).

MSC have also been used for treatment of diabetic nephropathy in NOD/SCID and streptozocin C57B1/6 mice (R.H. Lee et al., 2006). The injected cells engraft in damaged kidneys, potentially differentiate into renal cells and endothelial cells and can regulate the immune response. This resulted in improved kidney function and regeneration of glomerular structure. MSC, however, were unable to proliferate; therefore, it is conceivable that MSC contribute to the repair by releasing paracrine factors that promote neovasculatization and limit cytotoxic injury.

As for diabetic polyneuropathy, in diabetic rats, intramuscular injection of MSC led to increased ratio of capillaries to muscle fibers, improvement of hyperalgesia and function of neural fibers. MSC settled in the gap between muscle fibers at the transplanted site, and produced VEGF and basic bFGF, without differentiating into neural cells (Shibata et al., 2008).

By releasing paracrine factors and by differentiation into photoreceptor and glial-like cells in the retina, transplanted MSC have also been shown to improve the integrity of the blood-retinal barrier, ameliorating diabetic retinopathy in streptozocin diabetic rats (Z. Yang et al., 2010).

Prolonged and uncompleted wound healing can complicate the diabetic condition. Injection of MSC in animal models of diabetes improved wound healing, with increase of collagen levels and of wound-breaking strength, together with increased levels of TFGβ, KGF, EGF, PDGF, VEGF, all involved in repair (Wu et al., 2007). Besides these paracrine effects MSC were shown to differentiate and regenerate damaged epithelium.

Limitation of the potential therapeutic use of MSC also for diabetic chronic complications are, at present, mainly the poor engraftment and the limited differentiation under *in vivo* conditions, together with the potential differentiation into unwanted mesenchymal lineages.

8. Conclusion

A number of issues should be addressed before a cell based therapy may come to a clinical setting. The first challenge is to define which kind of cells are more suitable for β cell substitution. This implies to develop efficient strategies of stem cell differentiation that lead to cells that produce and secrete insulin in physiological amounts under the control of glycemia. Moreover, safety of a cell based therapy remains a critical point, as any precursor or stem cell types might induce tumor formation. Whether the achievement of fully differentiated cells would reduce this risk remains to be proved. Another relevant point is to define the strategies that allow an immune modulation to avoid the recurrence of autoimmune destruction of newly formed β cells.

9. Acknowledgement

Funded by Regione Piemonte, Piattaforme Biotecnologiche, Pi-Stem project.

10. References

Abdi, R., Fiorina, P., Adra, C.N., Atkinson, M. & Sayegh, M.H. (2008). Immunomodulation by mesenchymal stem cells: a potential therapeutic strategy for type 1 diabetes. *Diabetes*, Vol. 57, No. 7, (July 2008), pp. 1759-1767, ISSN 0012-1797.

Aggarwal, S. & Pittenger, M.F. (2005). Human mesenchymal stem cells modulate allogeneic immune cell responses. *Blood*, Vol. 105, No. 4, (February 2005), pp. 1815-1822, ISSN 0006-4971

Alipio, Z., Liao, W., Roemer, E.J., Waner, M., Fink, L.M., Ward, D.C. & Ma, Y. (2010). Reversal of hyperglycemia in diabetic Augello mouse models using induced-pluripotent stem (iPS)-derived pancreatic beta-like cells. *Proc Natl Acad Sci U S A*, Vol. 107, No. 30, (July 2010), pp. 13426-13431, ISSN 0027-8424

Augello, A., Tasso.,R., Negrini, S.M., Cancedda, R. & Pennesi, G. (2007). Cell therapy using allogeneic bone marrow mesenchymal stem cells prevents tissue damage in collagen-induced arthritis. *Arthritis Rheum*, Vol. 56, No. 4, (April 2007), pp. 1175-1186, ISSN 00043591

Baeyens, L., De Breuck, S., Lardon, J., Mfopou, J.K., Rooman, I. & Bouwens, L. (2005). In vitro generation of insulin-producing beta cells from adult exocrine pancreatic cells. *Diabetologia*, Vol. 48, No. 1, (January 2005), pp. 49-57, ISSN 0012-186X

Bernal-Mizrachi, E., Fatrai, S., Johnson, J.D., Ohsugi, M., Otani, K., Han, Z., Polonsky, K.S. & Permutt, M.A. (2004). Defective insulin secretion and increased susceptibility to experimental diabetes are induced by reduced Akt activity in pancreatic islet beta cells. *J Clin Invest*, Vol. 114, No. 7, (October 2004), pp. 928-936, ISSN 0021-9738

Biancone, L. & Ricordi, C. (2002). Pancreatic islet transplantation: an update. *Cell Transplant*, Vol. 11, No. 4, pp. 309-311, ISSN 0963-6897

Bonner-Weir, S., Toschi, E., Inada, A., Reitz, P., Fonseca, S.Y., Aye, T. & Sharma, A. (2004). The pancreatic ductal epithelium serves as a potential pool of progenitor cells. *Pediatr Diabetes*, Vol. 5, Suppl 2, pp. 16-22, ISSN 1399-543X

Booth, C. & Potten, C.S. (2000). Gut instincts: thoughts on intestinal epithelial stem cells. *J Clin Invest*, Vol. 105, No. 11, (June 2000), pp. 1493-1499, ISSN 0021-9738

Bouvens, L. (2006). Beta cell regeneration. *Curr Diabetes Rev*, Vol. 2, pp. 3-9 ISSN 1573-3998

Brissova, M., Fowler, M., Wiebe, P., Shostak, A., Shiota, M., Radhika, A., Lin, P.C., Gannon, M. & Powers, A.C. (2004). Intraislet endothelial cells contribute to revascularization of transplanted pancreatic islets. *Diabetes*, Vol. 53, No. 5, (May 2004), pp. 1318-1325, ISSN 0012-1797

Brolén, G.K., Heins, N., Edsbagge, J. & Semb, H. (2005). Signals from the embryonic mouse pancreas induce differentiation of human embryonic stem cells into insulin-producing beta-cell-like cells. *Diabetes*, Vol. 54, No. 10, (October 2005), pp. 2867-2874, ISSN 0012-1797

Bussolati, B., Bruno, S., Grange, C., Buttiglieri, S., Deregibus, M.C., Cantino, D. & Camussi, G. (2005). Isolation of renal progenitor cells from adult human kidney. *Am J Pathol*, Vol. 166, No. 2, (February 2005), pp. 545-555, ISSN 0002-9440

Calafiore, R., Basta, G., Luca, G., Lemmi, A., Montanucci, M.P., Calabrese, G., Racanicchi, L., Mancuso, F. & Brunetti, P. (2006). Microencapsulated pancreatic islet allografts into nonimmunosuppressed patients with type 1 diabetes: first two cases. *Diabetes Care*, Vol. 29, No. 1, (January 2006), pp. 137-138, ISSN 0149-5992

Cantaluppi, V., Biancone, L., Romanazzi, G.M., Figliolini, F., Beltramo, S., Ninniri, M.S., Galimi, F., Romagnoli, R., Franchello, A., Salizzoni, M., Perin, P.C., Ricordi, C., Segoloni, G.P. & Camussi, G. (2006). Antiangiogenic and immunomodulatory effects of rapamycin on islet endothelium: relevance for islet transplantation. *Am J Transplant*, Vol. 6, No. 11, (November 2006), pp. 2601-2611, ISSN 1600-6135

Cantaluppi, V., Bruno, S. & Camussi, G. (2008). Pancreatic ductal transdifferentiation for β-cell neogenesis. *Expert Opin Ther Patents*, Vol. 18, No. 8, pp. 1-5, ISSN 1354-3776

Carlsson, P.O., Andersson, A. & Jansson, L. (1998). Influence of age, hyperglycemia, leptin, and NPY on islet blood flow in obese-hyperglycemic mice. *Am J Physiol*, Vol. 275, No. 4 Pt 1, (October 1998), pp. E594-601, ISSN 0002-9513

Carlsson, P.O., Flodström, M. & Sandler, S. (2000). Islet blood flow in multiple low dose streptozotocin-treated wild-type and inducible nitric oxide synthase-deficient mice. *Endocrinology*, Vol. 141, No. 8, (August 2000), pp. 2752-2757, ISSN 0013-7227

Chao, K.C., Chao, K.F., Fu, Y.S. & Liu, S.H. (2008). Islet-like clusters derived from mesenchymal stem cells in Wharton's Jelly of the human umbilical cord for transplantation to control type 1 diabetes. *PLoS One*, Vol. 3, No. 1, (January 2008), pp. e1451, ISSN 1932-6203

Christopeit, M., Schendel, M., Föll, J., Müller, L.P., Keysser, G. & Behre, G. (2008). Marked improvement of severe progressive systemic sclerosis after transplantation of mesenchymal stem cells from an allogeneic haploidentical-related donor mediated by ligation of CD137L. *Leukemia*, Vol. 22, No. 5, (May 2008), pp. 1062-1064, ISSN 0887-6924

Cnop, M., Hughes, S.J., Igoillo-Esteve, M., Hoppa, M.B., Sayyed, F., van de Laar, L., Gunter, J.H., de Koning, E.J., Walls, G.V., Gray, D.W., Johnson, P.R., Hansen, B.C., Morris, J.F., Pipeleers-Marichal, M., Cnop, I. & Clark, A. (2010). The long lifespan and low turnover of human islet beta cells estimated by mathematical modelling of lipofuscin accumulation. *Diabetologia*, Vol. 53, No. 2, (February 2010), pp. 321-330, ISSN 0012-186X

Colvin, G.A., Lambert, J.F., Moore, B.E., Carlson, J.E., Dooner, M.S., Abedi, M., Cerny, J. & Quesenberry, P.J. (2004). Intrinsic hematopoietic stem cell/progenitor plasticity: Inversions. *J Cell Physiol*, Vol. 199, No. 1, (April 2004), pp. 20-31, ISSN 0021-9541

Colvin, G.A., Dooner, M.S., Dooner, G.J., Sanchez-Guijo, F.M., Demers, D.A., Abedi, M., Ramanathan, M., Chung, S., Pascual, S. & Quesenberry, P.J. (2007). Stem cell continuum: directed differentiation hotspots. *Exp Hematol*, Vol. 35, No. 1, (January 2007), pp. 96-107, ISSN 0301-472X

Comerota, A.J., Link, A., Douville, J. & Burchardt, E.R. (2010). Upper extremity ischemia treated with tissue repair cells from adult bone marrow. *J Vasc Surg*, Vol. 52, No. 3, (September 2010), pp. 723-729, ISSN 0741-5214

Contreras, J.L., Smyth, C.A., Eckstein, C., Bilbao, G., Thompson, J.A., Young, C.J. & Eckhoff, D.E. (2003). Peripheral mobilization of recipient bone marrow-derived endothelial progenitor cells enhances pancreatic islet revascularization and engraftment after intraportal transplantation. *Surgery*, Vol. 134, No. 2, (August 2003), pp. 390-398, ISSN 0039-6060

Cotsarelis, G., Sun, T.T. & Lavker, R.M. (1990). Label-retaining cells reside in the bulge area of pilosebaceous unit: implications for follicular stem cells, hair cycle, and skin carcinogenesis. *Cell*, Vol. 61, No. 7, (June 1990), pp. 1329-1337, ISSN 0092-8674

Cronin, K.J., Messina, A., Knight, K.R., Cooper-White, J.J., Stevens, G.W., Penington, A.J. & Morrison, W.A. (2004). New murine model of spontaneous autologous tissue engineering, combining an arteriovenous pedicle with matrix materials. *Plast Reconstr Surg*, Vol. 113, No. 1, (January 2004), pp. 260-269, ISSN 0032-1052

D'Amour, K.A., Agulnick, A.D., Eliazer, S., Kelly, O.G., Kroon, E. & Baetge, E.E. (2005). Efficient differentiation of human embryonic stem cells to definitive endoderm. *Nat Biotechnol*, Vol. 23, No. 12, (December 2005), pp. 1534-1541, ISSN 1087-0156

da Silva Meirelles, L., Chagastelles, P.C. & Nardi, N.B. (2006). Mesenchymal stem cells reside in virtually all post-natal organs and tissues. *J Cell Sci*, Vol. 119, No. 11, (June 2006), pp. 2204-2213, ISSN 0021-9533

da Silva Meirelles, L., Caplan, A.I. & Nardi, N.B. (2008). In search of the in vivo identity of mesenchymal stem cells. *Stem Cells*, Vol. 26, No. 9, (September 2008), pp. 2287-2299, ISSN 1066-5099

Datta, S.R., Brunet, A. & Greenberg, M.E. (1999). Cellular survival: a play in three Akts. *Genes Dev*, Vol. 13, No. 22, (November 1999), pp. 2905-2927, ISSN 0890-9369

Deng, W., Han, Q., Liao, L., You, S., Deng, H. & Zhao, R.C. (2005). Effects of allogeneic bone marrow-derived mesenchymal stem cells on T and B lymphocytes from BXSB mice. *DNA Cell Biol*, Vol. 24, No. 7, (July 2005), pp. 458-463, ISSN 1044-5498

Denner, L., Bodenburg, Y., Zhao, J.G., Howe, M., Cappo, J., Tilton, R.G., Copland, J.A., Forraz, N., McGuckin, C. & Urban, R. (2007). Directed engineering of umbilical cord blood stem cells to produce C-peptide and insulin. *Cell Prolif*, Vol. 40, No. 3, (June 2007), pp. 367-380, ISSN 0960-7722

Deregibus, M.C., Tetta, C. & Camussi, G. (2010). The dynamic stem cell microenvironment is orchestrated by microvesicle-mediated transfer of genetic information. *Histol Histopathol*, Vol. 25, No. 3, (March 2010), pp. 397-404, ISSN 0213-3911

Doetsch, F., Caillé, I., Lim, D.A., García-Verdugo, J.M. & Alvarez-Buylla, A. (1999). Subventricular zone astrocytes are neural stem cells in the adult mammalian brain. *Cell*, Vol. 97, No. 6, (June 1999), pp. 703-716, ISSN 0092-8674

Dominici, M., Le Blanc, K., Mueller, I., Slaper-Cortenbach, I., Marini, F., Krause, D., Deans, R., Keating, A., Prockop, D.J. & Horwitz, E. (2006). Minimal criteria for defining multipotent mesenchymal stromal cells. The International Society for Cellular Therapy position statement. *Cytotherapy*, Vol. 8, No. 4, pp. 315-317, ISSN 1465-3249

Donath, M.Y. & Halban, P.A. (2004). Decreased beta-cell mass in diabetes: significance, mechanisms and therapeutic implications. *Diabetologia*, Vol. 47, No. 3, (March 2004), pp. 581-589, ISSN 0012-186X

Dor, Y., Brown, J., Martinez, O.I. & Melton, D.A. (2004). Adult pancreatic beta-cells are formed by self-duplication rather than stem-cell differentiation. *Nature*, Vol. 429, No. 6987, (May 2004), pp. 41-46, ISSN 0028-0836

Duffield, J.S., Park, K.M., Hsiao, L.L., Kelley, V.R., Scadden, D.T., Ichimura, T. & Bonventre, J.V. (2005). Restoration of tubular epithelial cells during repair of the postischemic kidney occurs independently of bone marrow-derived stem cells. *J Clin Invest*, Vol. 115, No. 7, (July 2005), pp. 1743-1755, ISSN 0021-9738

Elghazi, L., Balcazar, N. & Bernal-Mizrachi, E. (2006). Emerging role of protein kinase B/Akt signaling in pancreatic beta-cell mass and function. *Int J Biochem Cell Biol*, Vol. 38, No. 2, (February 2006), pp. 157-163, ISSN 1357-2725

Elliott, R.B., Terán, L. & White, D.J. (2005). Xenotransplantation of porcine neonatal islets of Langerhans and Sertoli cells: a 4-year study. *Eur J Endocrinol*, Vol. 153, No. 3, (September 2005), pp. 419-427, ISSN 0804-4643

Elliott, R.B., Escobar, L., Tan, P.L., Muzina, M., Zwain, S. & Buchanan, C. (2007). Live encapsulated porcine islets from a type 1 diabetic patient 9.5 yr after xenotransplantation. *Xenotransplantation*, Vol. 14, No. 2, (March 2007), pp. 157-161, ISSN 0908-665X

Fan, Y., Rudert, W.A., Grupillo, M., He, J., Sisino, G. & Trucco, M. (2009). Thymus-specific deletion of insulin induces autoimmune diabetes. *EMBO J*, Vol. 28, No. 18, (September 2009), pp. 2812-24, ISSN 0261-4189

Faradji, R.N., Tharavanij, T., Messinger, S., Froud, T., Pileggi, A., Monroy, K., Mineo, D., Baidal, D.A., Cure, P., Ponte, G., Mendez, A.J., Selvaggi, G., Ricordi, C. & Alejandro, R. (2008). Long-term insulin independence and improvement in insulin secretion after supplemental islet infusion under exenatide and etanercept. *Transplantation*, Vol. 86, No. 12, (December 2008), pp. 1658-65, ISSN 0041-1337

Favaro, E., Miceli, I., Bussolanti, B., Schmitt-Ney, M., Cavallo Perin, P., Camusi, G. & Zanone, M.M. (2008). Hyperglycemia induces apoptosis of human pancreatic islet endothelial cells: effects of pravastatin on the Akt survival pathway. *Am J Pathol*, Vol. 173, No. 2, (August 2008), pp. 442-450, ISSN 0002-9440

Fiorina, P., Jurewicz, M., Augello, A., Vergani, A., Dada, S., La Rosa, S., Selig, M., Godwin, J., Law, K., Placidi, C., Smith, R.N., Capella, C., Rodig, S., Adra, C.N., Atkinson, M., Sayegh, M.H. & Abdi, R. (2009). Immunomodulatory function of bone marrow-derived mesenchymal stem cells in experimental autoimmune type 1 diabetes. *J Immunol*, Vol. 183, No. 2, (July 2009), pp. 993-1004, ISSN 0022-1767

Fouillard, L., Bensidhoum, M., Bories, D., Bonte, H., Lopez, M., Moseley, A.M., Smith, A., Lesage, S., Beaujean, F., Thierry, D., Gourmelon, P., Najman, A. & Gorin, N.C. (2003). Engraftment of allogeneic mesenchymal stem cells in the bone marrow of a patient with severe idiopathic aplastic anemia improves stroma. *Leukemia*, Vol. 17, No. 2, (February 2003), pp. 474-476, ISSN 0887-6924

Froud, T., Faradji, R.N., Pileggi, A., Messinger, S., Baidal, D.A., Ponte, G.M., Cure, P.E., Monroy, K., Mendez, A., Selvaggi, G., Ricordi, C. & Alejandro, R. (2008). The use of exenatide in islet transplant recipients with chronic allograft dysfunction: safety, efficacy, and metabolic effects. *Transplantation*, Vol. 86, No. 1, (July 2008), pp. 36-45, ISSN 0041-1337

Gerdoni, E., Gallo, B., Casazza, S., Musio, S., Bonanni, I., Pedemonte, E., Mantegazza, R., Frassoni, F., Mancardi, G., Pedotti, R. & Uccelli, A. (2007). Mesenchymal stem cells effectively modulate pathogenic immune response in experimental autoimmune encephalomyelitis. *Ann Neurol*, Vol. 61, No. 3, (March 2007), pp. 219-227, ISSN 0364-5134

Gonez, L.J. & Knight, K.R. (2010). Cell therapy for diabetes: stem cells, progenitors or beta-cell replication? *Mol Cell Endocrinol*, Vol. 323, No. 1, (July 2010), pp. 55-61, ISSN 0303-7207

Gottlieb, P.A., Quinlan, S., Krause-Steinrauf, H., Greenbaum, C.J., Wilson, D.M., Rodriguez, H., Schatz, D.A., Moran, A.M., Lachin, J.M. & Skyler, J.S. (2010). Type 1 Diabetes TrialNet MMF/DZB Study Group. Failure to preserve beta-cell function with mycophenolate mofetil and daclizumab combined therapy in patients with new-onset type 1 diabetes. *Diabetes Care*, Vol. 33, No. 4, (April 2010), pp. 826-832, ISSN 0149-5992

Hafiz, M.M., Faradji, R.N., Froud, T., Pileggi, A., Baidal, D.A., Cure, P., Ponte, G., Poggioli, R., Cornejo, A., Messinger, S., Ricordi, C. & Alejandro, R. (2005). Immunosuppression and procedure-related complications in 26 patients with type 1 diabetes mellitus receiving allogeneic islet cell transplantation. *Transplantation*, Vol. 80, No. 12, (December 2005), pp. 1718-1728, ISSN 0041-1337

Haller, M.J., Viener, H.L., Brusko, T., Wasserfall, C., McGrail, K., Staba, S. & Cogle, C., Atkinson, M. & Schatz, D.A. (2007). Insulin requirements, HbA1c, and stimulated C-peptide following autologous umbilical cord blood transfusion in children with T1D. *Diabetes*, Vol. 56, No. A82 Suppl. 1 (June 2007), ISSN 0012-1797

He, X.C., Zhang, J., Tong, W.G., Tawfik, O., Ross, J., Scoville, D.H., Tian, Q., Zeng, X., He, X., Wiedemann, L.M., Mishina, Y. & Li, L. (2004). BMP signaling inhibits intestinal stem cell self-renewal through suppression of Wnt-beta-catenin signaling. *Nat Genet*, Vol. 36, No. 10, (October 2004), pp. 1117-1121, ISSN 1061-4036

Herold, K.C., Hagopian, W., Auger, J.A., Poumian-Ruiz, E., Taylor, L., Donaldson, D., Gitelman, S.E., Harlan, D.M., Xu, D., Zivin, R.A. & Bluestone J.A. (2002). Anti-CD3 monoclonal antibody in new-onset type 1 diabetes mellitus. *N Engl J Med*, Vol. 346, No. 22, (May 2002), pp. 1692-1698, ISSN 0028-4793

Herrera, M.B., Bruno, S., Buttiglieri, S., Tetta, C., Gatti, S., Deregibus, M.C., Bussolati, B. & Camussi, G. (2006). Isolation and characterization of a stem cell population from adult human liver. *Stem Cells*, Vol. 24, No. 12, (December 2006), pp. 2840-2850, ISSN 1066-5099

Herrera, M.B., Bussolati, B., Bruno, S., Morando, L., Mauriello-Romanazzi, G., Sanavio, F., Stamenkovic, I., Biancone, L. & Camussi, G. (2007). Exogenous mesenchymal stem cells localize to the kidney by means of CD44 following acute tubular injury. *Kidney Int*, Vol. 72, No. 4, (August 2007), pp. 430-441, ISSN 0085-2538

Hussey, A.J., Winardi, M., Han, X.L., Thomas, G.P., Penington, A.J., Morrison, W.A., Knight, K.R. & Feeney, S.J. (2009). Seeding of pancreatic islets into prevascularized tissue engineering chambers. *Tissue Eng Part A*, Vol. 15, No. 12, (December 2009), pp. 3823-3833, ISSN 2152-4947

Ito, T., Itakura, S., Todorov, I., Rawson, J., Asari, S., Shintaku, J., Nair, I., Ferreri, K., Kandeel, F. & Mullen, Y. (2010). Mesenchymal stem cell and islet co-transplantation promotes graft revascularization and function. *Transplantation*, Vol. 89, No. 12, (June 2010), pp. 1438-1445, ISSN 0041-1337

Jackson, K.A., Mi, T. & Goodell, M.A. (1999).Hematopoietic potential of stem cells isolated from murine skeletal muscle. *Proc Natl Acad Sci U S A*, Vol. 96, No. 25, (December 1999), pp. 14482-14486, ISSN 0027-8424

Jesmin, S., Sakuma, I., Hattori, Y. & Kitabatake, A. (2003). Role of angiotensin II in altered expression of molecules responsible for coronary matrix remodeling in insulin-resistant diabetic rats. *Arterioscler Thromb Vasc Biol*, Vol. 23, No. 11, (November 2003), pp. 2021-2026, ISSN 1079-5642

Jiang, J., Au, M., Lu, K., Eshpeter, A., Korbutt, G., Fisk, G. & Majumdar, A.S. (2007). Generation of insulin-producing islet-like clusters from human embryonic stem cells. *Stem Cells*, Vol. 25, No. 8, (August 2007), pp. 1940-1953, ISSN 1066-5099

Jiang, Y., Jahagirdar, B.N., Reinhardt, R.L., Schwartz, R.E., Keene, C.D., Ortiz-Gonzalez, X.R., Reyes, M., Lenvik, T., Lund, T., Blackstad, M., Du, J., Aldrich, S., Lisberg, A., Low, W.C., Largaespada, D.A. & Verfaillie, C.M. (2002). Pluripotency of mesenchymal stem cells derived from adult marrow. *Nature*, Vol. 418, No. 6893, (July 2002), pp. 41-49, ISSN 0028-0836

Jones, D.L. & Wagers, A.J. (2008). No place like home: anatomy and function of the stem cell niche. *Nat Rev Mol Cell Biol*, Vol. 9, No. 1, (January 2008), pp. 11-21, ISSN 1083-8791

Juhl, K., Bonner-Weir, S. & Sharma, A. (2010). Regenerating pancreatic beta-cells: plasticity of adult pancreatic cells and the feasibility of in-vivo neogenesis. *Curr Opin Organ Transplant*, Vol. 15, No. 1,(February 2010), pp. 79-85, ISSN 1531-7013

Jung, F., Haendeler, J., Goebel, C., Zeiher, A.M. & Dimmeler, S. (2000). Growth factor-induced phosphoinositide 3-OH kinase/Akt phosphorylation in smooth muscle cells: induction of cell proliferation and inhibition of cell death. *Cardiovasc Res*, Vol. 48, No. 1, (October 2000), pp. 148-57, ISSN 0008-6363

Karnieli, O., Izhar-Prato, Y., Bulvik, S. & Efrat, S. (2007). Generation of insulin-producing cells from human bone marrow mesenchymal stem cells by genetic manipulation. *Stem Cells*, Vol. 25, No. 11, (November 2007), pp. 2837-2844, ISSN 1066-5099

Keymeulen, B., Vandemeulebroucke, E., Ziegler, A.G., Mathieu, C., Kaufman, L., Hale, G., Gorus, F., Goldman, M., Walter, M., Candon, S., Schandene, L., Crenier, L., De Block, C., Seigneurin, J.M., De Pauw, P., Pierard, D., Weets, I., Rebello, P., Bird, P., Berrie, E., Frewin, M., Waldmann, H., Bach, J.F., Pipeleers, D. & Chatenoud, L. (2005). Insulin needs after CD3-antibody therapy in new-onset type 1 diabetes. *N Engl J Med*, Vol. 352, No. 25, (June 2005), pp. 2598-2608, ISSN 0028-4793

Kiel, M.J., Yilmaz, O.H., Iwashita, T., Yilmaz, O.H., Terhorst, C. & Morrison, S.J. (2005). SLAM family receptors distinguish hematopoietic stem and progenitor cells and reveal endothelial niches for stem cells. *Cell*, Vol. 121, No. 7, (July 2005), pp. 1109-1121, ISSN 0092-8674

Kojima, H., Fujimiya, M., Matsumura, K., Younan, P., Imaeda, H., Maeda, M. & Chan, L. (2003). NeuroD-betacellulin gene therapy induces islet neogenesis in the liver and reverses diabetes in mice. *Nat Med*, Vol. 9, No. 5, (May 2003), pp. 596-603, ISSN 1078-8956

Koopmans, M., Kremer Hovinga, I.C., Baelde, H.J., de Heer, E., Bruijn, J.A. & Bajema, I.M. Endothelial chimerism in transplantation: Looking for needles in a haystack. *Transplantation*, Vol. 82 Suppl. 1, pp. S25-S29, ISSN 0041-1337

Krampera, M., Glennie, S., Dyson, J., Scott, D., Laylor R, Simpson, E. & Dazzi, F. (2003). Bone marrow mesenchymal stem cells inhibit the response of naive and memory antigen-specific T cells to their cognate peptide. *Blood*, Vol. 101, No. 9, (May 2003), pp. 3722-3729, ISSN 0006-4971

Kröncke, K.D., Rodriguez, M.L., Kolb, H. & Kolb-Bachofen, V. (1993). Cytotoxicity of activated rat macrophages against syngeneic islet cells is arginine-dependent, correlates with citrulline and nitrite concentrations and is identical to lysis by the nitric oxide donor nitroprusside. *Diabetologia*, Vol. 36, No. 1, (January 1993), pp. 17-24, ISSN 0012-186X

Kroon, E., Martinson, L.A., Kadoya, K., Bang, A.G., Kelly, O.G., Eliazer, S., Young, H., Richardson, M., Smart, N.G., Cunningham, J., Agulnick, A.D., D'Amour, K.A., Carpenter, M.K. & Baetge, E.E. (2008). Pancreatic endoderm derived from human embryonic stem cells generates glucose-responsive insulin-secreting cells in vivo. *Nat Biotechnol*, Vol. 26, No. 4, (April 2008), pp. 443-452, ISSN 1087-0156

Lazarus, H.M., Koc, O.N., Devine, S.M., Curtin, P., Maziarz, R.T., Holland, H.K., Shpall, E.J., McCarthy, P., Atkinson, K., Cooper, B.W., Gerson, S.L., Laughlin, M.J., Loberiza, F.R. Jr, Moseley, A.B. & Bacigalupo, A. (2005). Cotransplantation of HLA-identical sibling culture-expanded mesenchymal stem cells and hematopoietic stem cells in hematologic malignancy patients. *Biol Blood Marrow Transplant*, Vol. 11, No. 5, (May 2005), pp. 389-398, ISSN 1083-8791

Le Blanc, K., Rasmusson, I., Sundberg, B., Götherström, C., Hassan, M., Uzunel, M. & Ringdén, O. (2004). Treatment of severe acute graft-versus-host disease with third party haploidentical mesenchymal stem cells. *Lancet*, Vol. 363, No. 9419, (May 2004), pp. 1439-1441, ISSN 0140-6736

Le Blanc, K., Rasmusson, I., Götherström, C., Seidel, C., Sundberg, B., Sundin, M., Rosendahl, K., Tammik, C. & Ringdén, O. (2004). Mesenchymal stem cells inhibit the expression of CD25 (interleukin-2 receptor) and CD38 on phytohaemagglutinin-activated lymphocytes. *Scand J Immunol*, Vol. 60, No. 3, (September 2004), pp. 307-315, ISSN 0300-9475

Le Blanc, K. & Pittenger M. (2005). Mesenchymal stem cells: progress toward promise. *Cytotherapy*, Vol. 7, No. 1, pp. 36-45, ISSN 1465-3249

Lee, J.S., Hong, J.M., Moon, G.J., Lee, P.H., Ahn, Y.H. & Bang, O.Y.; STARTING collaborators. (2010). A long-term follow-up study of intravenous autologous mesenchymal stem cell transplantation in patients with ischemic stroke. *Stem Cells*, Vol. 28, No. 6, (June 2010), pp. 1099-1106, ISSN 1066-5099

Lee, R.H., Seo, M.J., Reger, R.L., Spees, J.L., Pulin, A.A., Olson, S.D. & Prockop, D.J. (2006). Multipotent stromal cells from human marrow home to and promote repair of pancreatic islets and renal glomeruli in diabetic NOD/scid mice. *Proc Natl Acad Sci U S A*, Vol. 103, No. 46, (November 2006), pp. 17438-17443, ISSN 0027-8424

Lee, S.H., Hao, E., Savinov, A.Y., Geron, I., Strongin, A.Y. & Itkin-Ansari, P. (2009). Human beta-cell precursors mature into functional insulin-producing cells in an immunoisolation device: implications for diabetes cell therapies. *Transplantation*, Vol. 87, No. 7, (April 2009), pp. 983-991, ISSN 0041-1337

Lemaigre, F. & Zaret, K.S. (2004). Liver development update: new embryo models, cell lineage control, and morphogenesis. *Curr Opin Genet Dev*, Vol. 14, No. 5, (October 2004), pp. 582-590, ISSN 0959-437X

Li, L. & Xie, T. (2002). Stem cell niche: structure and function. *Annu Rev Cell Dev Biol*, Vol. 21, pp. 605-631, ISSN 1081-0706

Niemann, C. & Watt, F.M. (2002). Designer skin: lineage commitment in postnatal epidermis. *Trends Cell Biol*, Vol. 12, No. 4, (April 2002), pp. 185-192, ISSN 0962-8924

Li, L. & Xie T. (2005). Stem cell niche: structure and function. *Annu Rev Cell Dev Biol*, Vol. 21, pp. 605-631, ISSN 1081-0706

Li, W.C., Rukstalis, J.M., Nishimura, W., Tchipashvili, V., Habener, J.F., Sharma, A. & Bonner-Weir, S. (2010). Activation of pancreatic-duct-derived progenitor cells during pancreas regeneration in adult rats. *J Cell Sci*, Vol. 123, Pt16, (August 2010), pp. 2792-2802, ISSN 0021-9533

Li, X., Zhang, L., Meshinchi, S., Dias-Leme, C., Raffin, D., Johnson, J.D., Treutelaar, M.K. & Burant, C.F. (2006). Islet microvasculature in islet hyperplasia and failure in a model of type 2 diabetes. *Diabetes*, Vol. 55, No. 11, (November 2006), pp. 2965-2973, ISSN 0012-1797

Li, Y., Zhang, R., Qiao, H., Zhang, H., Wang, Y., Yuan, H., Liu, Q., Liu, D., Chen, L. & Pei, X. (2007). Generation of insulin-producing cells from PDX-1 gene-modified human mesenchymal stem cells. *J Cell Physiol*, Vol. 211, No. 1, (April 2007), pp. 36-44, ISSN 0021-9541

Loweth, A.C., Williams, G.T., James, R.F., Scarpello, J.H. & Morgan, N.G. (1998). Human islets of Langerhans express Fas ligand and undergo apoptosis in response to interleukin-1beta and Fas ligation. *Diabetes*, Vol. 47, No. 5, (May 1998), pp. 727-732, ISSN 0012-1797

Ludvigsson, J., Faresjö, M., Hjorth, M., Axelsson, S., Chéramy, M., Pihl, M., Vaarala, O., Forsander, G., Ivarsson, S., Johansson, C., Lindh, A., Nilsson, N.O., Aman, J., Ortqvist, E., Zerhouni, P. & Casas, R. (2008). GAD treatment and insulin secretion in recent-onset type 1 diabetes. *N Engl J Med*, Vol. 359, No. 18, (October 2008), pp. 1909-1920, ISSN 0028-4793

Madec, A.M., Mallone, R., Afonso, G., Abou Mrad, E., Mesnier, A., Eljaafari, A. & Thivolet, C. (2009). Mesenchymal stem cells protect NOD mice from diabetes by inducing regulatory T cells. *Diabetologia*, Vol. 52, No. 7, (July 2009), pp. 1391-1399, ISSN 0012-186X

Maedler, K., Spinas, G.A., Lehmann, R., Sergeev, P., Weber, M., Fontana, A., Kaiser, N. & Donath, M.Y. (2001). Glucose induces beta-cell apoptosis via upregulation of the Fas receptor in human islets. *Diabetes*, Vol. 50, No. 8, (August 2001), pp. 1683-1690, ISSN 0012-1797

Maehr, R., Chen, S., Snitow, M., Ludwig, T., Yagasaki, L., Goland, R., Leibel, R.L. & Melton, D.A. (2009). Generation of pluripotent stem cells from patients with type 1 diabetes. *Proc Natl Acad Sci U S A*, Vol. 106, No. 37, (September 2009), pp. 15768-15773, ISSN 0027-8424

Mathews, V., Hanson, P.T., Ford, E., Fujita, J., Polonsky, K.S. & Graubert, T.A. (2004). Recruitment of bone marrow-derived endothelial cells to sites of pancreatic beta-cell injury. *Diabetes*, Vol. 53, No. 1, pp. 91-98, ISSN 0012-1797

Matveyenko, A.V., Georgia, S., Bhushan, A. & Butler, P.C. (2010). Inconsistent formation and nonfunction of insulin-positive cells from pancreatic endoderm derived from human embryonic stem cells in athymic nude rats. *Am J Physiol Endocrinol Metab*, Vol. 299, No. 5, (November 2010), pp. E713-E720, ISSN 0193-1849

McDevitt, H.O. & Unanue, E.R. (2008). Autoimmune diabetes mellitus--much progress, but challenges. *Adv Immunol*, Vol. 100, pp. 1-12, ISSN 0065-2776

Meier, J.J., Bhushan, A., Butler, A.E., Rizza, R.A. & Butler, P.C. (2005). Sustained beta cell apoptosis in patients with long-standing type 1 diabetes: indirect evidence for islet regeneration? *Diabetologia*, Vol. 48, No. 11, (November 2005), pp. 2221-2228, ISSN 0012-186X

Meier, J.J., Ritzel, R.A., Maedler, K., Gurlo, T. & Butler, P.C. (2006). Increased vulnerability of newly forming beta cells to cytokine-induced cell death. *Diabetologia*, Vol. 49, No. 1, (January 2006), pp. 83-89, ISSN 0012-186X

Meier, J.J., Butler, A.E., Saisho, Y., Monchamp, T., Galasso, R., Bhushan, A., Rizza, R.A. & Butler, P.C. (2008). Beta-cell replication is the primary mechanism subserving the postnatal expansion of beta-cell mass in humans. *Diabetes*, Vol. 57, No. 6, (June 2008), pp. 1584-1594, ISSN 0012-1797

Mian, R., Morrison, W.A., Hurley, J.V., Penington, A.J., Romeo, R., Tanaka, Y. & Knight, K.R. (2000). Formation of new tissue from an arteriovenous loop in the absence of added extracellular matrix. *Tissue Eng*, Vol. 6, No. 6, (December 2000), pp. 595-603, ISSN 1076-3279

Minami, K., Okuno, M., Miyawaki, K., Okumachi, A., Ishizaki, K., Oyama, K., Kawaguchi, M., Ishizuka, N., Iwanaga, T. & Seino, S. (2005). Lineage tracing and characterization of insulin-secreting cells generated from adult pancreatic acinar cells. *Proc Natl Acad Sci U S A*, Vol. 102, No. 42, (October 2005), pp. 15116-15121, ISSN 0027-8424

Mineo, D., Ricordi, C., Xu, X., Pileggi, A., Garcia-Morales, R., Khan, A., Baidal, D.A., Han, D., Monroy, K., Miller, J., Pugliese, A., Froud, T., Inverardi, L., Kenyon, N.S. & Alejandro, R. (2008). Combined islet and hematopoietic stem cell allotransplantation: a clinical pilot trial to induce chimerism and graft tolerance. *Am J Transplant*, Vol. 8, No. 6, (June 2008), pp. 1262-1274, ISSN 1600-6135

Mineo, D., Pileggi, A., Alejandro, R. & Ricordi, C. (2009). Point: steady progress and current challenges in clinical islet transplantation. *Diabetes Care*, Vol. 32, No. 8, (August 2009), pp. 1563-1569, ISSN 0149-5992

Mitsiadis, T.A., Barrandon, O., Rochat, A., Barrandon, Y. & De Bari, C. (2007). Stem cell niches in mammals. *Exp Cell Res*, Vol. 313, No. 16, (October 2007), pp. 3377-3385, ISSN 0014-4827

Miura, K., Okada, Y., Aoi, T., Okada, A., Takahashi, K., Okita, K., Nakagawa, M., Koyanagi, M., Tanabe, K., Ohnuki, M., Ogawa, D., Ikeda, E., Okano, H. & Yamanaka, S. (2009). Variation in the safety of induced luripotent stem cell lines. *Nat Biotechnol*, Vol. 27, No. 8, (August 2009), pp. 743-745, ISSN 1087-0156

Moore, K.A. & Lemischka, I.R. (2006). Stem cells and their niches. *Science*, Vol. 311, No. 5769, (March 2006), pp. 1880-1885, ISSN 0036-8075

Morigi, M., Imberti, B., Zoja, C., Corna, D., Tomasoni, S., Abbate, M., Rottoli, D., Angioletti, S., Benigni, A., Perico, N., Alison, M. & Remuzzi, G. (2004). Mesenchymal stem cells are renotropic, helping to repair the kidney and improve function in acute renal failure. *J Am Soc Nephrol*, Vol. 15, No. 7, (July 2004), pp. 1794-1804, ISSN 1046-6673

Nagaya, M., Katsuta, H., Kaneto, H., Bonner-Weir, S. & Weir, G.C. (2009). Adult mouse intrahepatic biliary epithelial cells induced in vitro to become insulin-producing cells. *J Endocrinol*, Vol. 201, No. 1, (April 2009), pp. 37-47, ISSN 0022-0795

Nir, T., Melton, D.A. & Dor, Y. (2007). Recovery from diabetes in mice by beta cell regeneration. *J Clin Invest*, Vol. 117, No. 9, (September 2007), pp. 2553-2561, ISSN 0021-9738

Opara, E.C., Mirmalek-Sani, S.H., Khanna, O., Moya, M.L. & Brey, E.M. (2010). Design of a bioartificial pancreas(+). *J Investig Med*, Vol. 58, No. 7, (October 2010), pp. 831-837, ISSN 1081-5589

Pileggi, A., Cobianchi, L., Inverardi, L. & Ricordi, C. (2006). Overcoming the challenges now limiting islet transplantation: a sequential, integrated approach. *Ann N Y Acad Sci*, Vol. 1079, (October 2006), pp. 383-398, ISSN 0077-8923

Quesenberry, P., Abedi, M., Dooner, M., Colvin, G., Sanchez-Guijo, F.M., Aliotta, J., Pimentel, J., Dooner, G., Greer, D., Demers, D., Keaney, P., Peterson, A., Luo, L. &

Foster, B. (2005). The marrow cell continuum: stochastic determinism. *Folia Histochem Cytobiol*, Vol. 43, No. 4, pp. 187-190, ISSN 1897-5631

Quesenberry, P.J., Colvin, G., Dooner, G., Dooner, M., Aliotta, J.M. & Johnson, K. (2007). The stem cell continuum: cell cycle, injury, and phenotype lability. *Ann N Y Acad Sci*, Vol. 1106, (June 2007), pp. 20-29, ISSN 0077-8923

Quesenberry, P.J. & Aliotta, J.M. (2008). The paradoxical dynamism of marrow stem cells: considerations of stem cells, niches, and microvesicles. *Stem Cell Rev*, Vol. 4, No. 3 (September 2008), pp. 137-147, ISSN 1550-8943

Raz, I., Elias, D., Avron, A., Tamir, M., Metzger, M. & Cohen, I.R. (2001). Beta-cell function in new-onset type 1 diabetes and immunomodulation with a heat-shock protein peptide (DiaPep277): a randomised, double-blind, phase II trial. *Lancet*, Vol. 358, No. 9295, (November 2001), pp. 1749-1753, ISSN 1550-8943

Reynolds, B.A. & Weiss, S. (1992). Generation of neurons and astrocytes from isolated cells of the adult mammalian central nervous system. *Science*, Vol. 255, No. 5052, (March 1992), pp. 1707-1710, ISSN 0036-8075

Ricordi, C. (2003). Islet transplantation: a brave new world. *Diabetes*, Vol. 52, pp. 1595-1603, ISSN 0012-1797

Ricordi, C. & Strom, T.B. (2004). Clinical islet transplantation: advances and immunological challenges. *Nat Rev Immunol*, Vol. 4, No. 4, (April 2004), pp. 259-268, ISSN 1474-1733

Ricordi, C. & Edlund, H. (2008). Toward a renewable source of pancreatic beta-cells. *Nat Biotechnol*, Vol. 26, No. 4, (April 2008), pp. 397-398, ISSN 1087-0156

Ringdén, O., Uzunel, M., Rasmusson, I., Remberger, M., Sundberg, B., Lönnies, H., Marschall, H.U., Dlugosz, A., Szakos, A., Hassan, Z., Omazic, B., Aschan, J., Barkholt, L. & Le Blanc, K. Mesenchymal stem cells for treatment of therapy-resistant graft-versus-host disease. (2006). *Transplantation*, Vol. 81, No. 10, (May 2006), pp. 1390-1397, ISSN 0041-1337

Roncarolo, M.G. & Battaglia, M. (2007). Regulatory T-cell immunotherapy for tolerance to self antigens and alloantigens in humans. *Nat Rev Immunol*, Vol. 7, No. 8, (August 2007), pp. 585-598, ISSN 1474-1733

Rosenberg, L. (1995). In vivo cell transformation: neogenesis of beta cells from pancreatic ductal cells. *Cell Transplant*, Vol. 4, No. 4, (July-August 1995), pp. 371-383, ISSN 0963-6897

Rother, K.I., Spain, L.M., Wesley, R.A., Digon, B.J. 3rd, Baron, A., Chen, K., Nelson, P., Dosch, H.M., Palmer, J.P., Brooks-Worrell, B., Ring, M. & Harlan, D.M. (2009). Effects of exenatide alone and in combination with daclizumab on beta-cell function in long-standing type 1 diabetes. *Diabetes Care*, Vol. 32, No. 12, (December 2009), pp. 2251-2257, ISSN 0149-5992

Ryan, E.A., Paty, B.W., Senior, P.A., Bigam, D., Alfadhli, E., Kneteman, N.M., Lakey, J.R. & Shapiro, A.M. (2005). Five-year follow-up after clinical islet transplantation. *Diabetes*, Vol. 54, No. 7, (July 2005), pp. 2060-2069, ISSN 0012-1797

Sackstein, R., Merzaban, J.S., Cain, D.W., Dagia, N.M., Spencer, J.A., Lin, C.P. & Wohlgemuth, R. (2008). Ex vivo glycan engineering of CD44 programs human multipotent mesenchymal stromal cell trafficking to bone. *Nat Med*, Vol. 14, No. 2, (February 2008), pp. 181-187, ISSN 1078-8956

Saito, M., Iwawaki, T., Taya, C., Yonekawa, H., Noda, M., Inui, Y., Mekada, E., Kimata, Y., Tsuru, A. & Kohno, K. (2001). Diphtheria toxin receptor-mediated conditional and targeted cell ablation in transgenic mice. *Nat Biotechnol*, Vol. 19, No. 8, (August 2001), pp. 746-750, ISSN 1087-0156

Sancho, E., Batlle, E. & Clevers, H. (2004). Signaling pathways in intestinal development and cancer. *Annu Rev Cell Dev Biol*, Vol. 20, pp. 695-723, ISSN 1081-0706

Sarvetnick, N., Krakowki, M.L. & Kritzik, M.R. (2007). An animal model for identifying a common stem/progenitor to liver cells and pancreatic cells. Patent: EP1857546; 2007a.

Sarvetnick, N., Krakowki, M.L. & Kritzik, M.R. Pancreatic progenitor cells and methods for isolating the same. Patent: US2007148706; 2007b.

Saudek, F., Havrdova, T., Boucek, P., Karasova, L,, Novota, P. & Skibova, J. (2004). Polyclonal anti-T-cell therapy for type 1 diabetes mellitus of recent onset. *Rev Diabet Stud*, Vol. 1, No. 2, (Summer 2004), pp. 80-88, ISSN 1614-0575

Schuh, A., Liehn, E.A., Sasse, A., Hristov, M., Sobota, R., Kelm, M., Merx, M.W. & Weber, C. (2008). Transplantation of endothelial progenitor cells improves neovascularization and left ventricular function after myocardial infarction in a rat model. *Basic Res Cardiol*, Vol. 103, No. 1, (January 2008), pp. 69-77, ISSN 0300-8428

Shapiro, A.M., Lakey, J.R., Ryan, E.A., Korbutt, G.S., Toth, E., Warnock, G.L., Kneteman, N.M. & Rajotte, R.V. (2000). Islet transplantation in seven patients with type 1 diabetes mellitus using a glucocorticoid-free immunosuppressive regimen. *N Engl J Med*, Vol. 343, No. 4, (July 2000), pp. 230-238, ISSN 0028-4793

Shapiro, A.M., Ricordi, C. & Hering, B. (2003). Edmonton's islet success has indeed been replicated elsewhere. *Lancet*, Vol. 362, No. 9391, (October 2003), pp. 1242, ISSN 0140-6736

Shapiro, A.M., Ricordi, C., Hering, B.J., Auchincloss, H., Lindblad, R., Robertson, R.P., Secchi, A., Brendel, M.D., Berney, T., Brennan, D.C., Cagliero, E., Alejandro, R., Ryan, E.A., DiMercurio, B., Morel, P., Polonsky, K.S., Reems, J.A., Bretzel, R.G., Bertuzzi, F., Froud, T., Kandaswamy, R., Sutherland, D.E., Eisenbarth, G., Segal, M., Preiksaitis, J., Korbutt, G.S., Barton, F.B., Viviano, L., Seyfert-Margolis, V., Bluestone, J. & Lakey, J.R. (2006). International trial of the Edmonton protocol for islet transplantation. *N Engl J Med*, Vol. 355, No. 13, (September 2006), pp. 1318-1330, ISSN 0028-4793

Shi, S. & Gronthos, S. (2003). Perivascular niche of postnatal mesenchymal stem cells in human bone marrow and dental pulp. *J Bone Miner Res*, Vol. 18, No. 4, (April 2003), pp. 696-704, ISSN 0884-0431

Shibata, T., Naruse, K., Kamiya, H., Kozakae, M., Kondo, M., Yasuda, Y., Nakamura, N., Ota, K., Tosaki, T., Matsuki, T., Nakashima, E., Hamada, Y., Oiso, Y. & Nakamura, J. (2008). Transplantation of bone marrow-derived mesenchymal stem cells improves diabetic polyneuropathy in rats. *Diabetes*, Vol. 57, No. 11, (November 2008), pp. 3099-3107, ISSN 0012-1797

Shiroi, A., Yoshikawa, M., Yokota, H., Fukui, H., Ishizaka, S., Tatsumi, K. & Takahashi, Y. (2002). Identification of insulin-producing cells derived from embryonic stem cells by zinc-chelating dithizone. *Stem Cells*, Vol. 20, No. 4, pp. 284-292, ISSN 1066-5099

Smukler, S.R., Arntfield, M.E., Razavi, R., Bikopoulos, G., Karpowicz, P., Seaberg, R., Dai, F,, Lee, S., Ahrens, R., Fraser, P.E., Wheeler, M.B. & van der Kooy, D. (2011). The adult mouse and human pancreas contain rare multipotent stem cells that express insulin. Cell Stem Cell, Vol. 8, No. 3, (March 2011), pp. 281-93, ISSN 1934-5909

Staeva-Vieira, T., Peakman, M. & von Herrath, M. (2007). Translational mini-review series on type 1 diabetes: Immune-based therapeutic approaches for type 1 diabetes. *Clin Exp Immunol*, Vol. 148, No. 1, (April 2007), pp. 17-31, ISSN 0009-9104

Steiner L, Kröncke K, Fehsel K, & Kolb-Bachofen V. (1997). Endothelial cells as cytotoxic effector cells: cytokine-activated rat islet endothelial cells lyse syngeneic islet cells via nitric oxide. *Diabetologia*, Vol. 40, No. 2, (February 1997), pp. 150-155, ISSN 0012-186X

Suckale, J. & Solimena, M. (2008). Pancreas islets in metabolic signalling focus on the beta-cell. *Front Biosci*, Vol. 13, (May 2008), pp. 7156-7171, ISSN 1093-9946

Sun, T.T., Cotsarelis, G. & Lavker, R.M. (1991). Hair follicular stem cells: the bulge-activation hypothesis. *J Invest Dermatol*, Vol. 96, No. 5, (May 1991), pp. 77S-78S, ISSN 0022-202X

Suschek, C., Fehsel, K., Kröncke, K.D., Sommer, A. & Kolb-Bachofen, V. (1994). Primary cultures of rat islet capillary endothelial cells. Constitutive and cytokine-inducible macrophagelike nitric oxide synthases are expressed and activities regulated by glucose concentration. *Am J Pathol*, Vol. 145, No. 3, (September 1994), pp. 685-695, ISSN 0002-9440

Sutherland, D.E., Sibley, R., Xu, X.Z., Michael, A., Srikanta, A.M., Taub, F., Najarian, J. & Goetz, F.C. (1984). Twin-to-twin pancreas transplantation: reversal and reenactment of the pathogenesis of type I diabetes. *Trans Assoc Am Physicians*, Vol.97, pp. 80-87, ISSN 0066-9458

Sykes, M. (2009). Hematopoietic cell transplantation for tolerance induction: animal models to clinical trials. *Transplantation*, Vol. 87, No. 3, (February 2009), pp. 309-316, ISSN 0041-1337

Takahashi, K. & Yamanaka, S. (2006). Induction of pluripotent stem cells from mouse embryonic and adult fibroblast cultures by defined factors. *Cell*, Vol. 126, No. 4, (August 2006), pp. 663-676, ISSN 0092-8674

Takahashi, K., Tanabe, K., Ohnuki, M., Narita, M., Ichisaka, T., Tomoda, K. & Yamanaka, S. (2007). Induction of pluripotent stem cells from adult human fibroblasts by defined factors. *Cell*, Vol. 131, No. 5, (November 2007), pp. 861-872, ISSN 0092-8674

Tanaka, Y., Tsutsumi, A., Crowe, D.M., Tajima, S. & Morrison, W.A. (2000). Generation of an autologous tissue (matrix) flap by combining an arteriovenous shunt loop with artificial skin in rats: preliminary report. *Br J Plast Surg*, Vol. 53, No. 1, (January 2000), pp. 51-57, ISSN 0007-1226

Tateishi, K., He, J., Taranova, O., Liang, G., D'Alessio, A.C. & Zhang, Y. (2008). Generation of insulin-secreting islet-like clusters from human skin fibroblasts. *J Biol Chem*, Vol. 283, No. 46, (November 2008), pp. 31601-31607, ISSN 0021-9258

Temple S. (2001). The development of neural stem cells. *Nature*, Vol. 414, No. 6859, (November 2001), pp. 112-117, ISSN

Teramura, Y. & Iwata, H. (2010). Bioartificial pancreas microencapsulation and conformal coating of islet of Langerhans. *Adv Drug Deliv Rev*, Vol. 62, No. 7-8, (June 2010), pp. 827-840, ISSN 0021-9258

Till, J.E., McCulloch, E.A. & Siminovitch, L. (1964). A stochastic model of stem cell proliferation, based on the growth of spleen colony-forming cells. *Proc Natl Acad Sci U S A*, Vol. 51, (January 1964), pp. 29-36, ISSN 0027-8424

Smukler, S.R., Arntfield, M.E., Razavi, R., Bikopoulos, G., Karpowicz, P., Seaberg, R., Dai, F., Lee, S., Ahrens, R., Fraser, P.E., Wheeler, M.B. & van der Kooy, D. (2011). The adult mouse and human pancreas contain rare multipotent stem cells that express insulin. Cell Stem Cell vol. 8, No., 3 (Mar 2011), pp. 281-293, ISSN 1934-5909

Thorel, F., Népote, V., Avril, I., Kohno, K., Desgraz, R., Chera, S. & Herrera, P.L. (2010). Conversion of adult pancreatic alpha-cells to beta-cells after extreme beta-cell loss. *Nature*, Vol. 464, No. 7292, (April 2010), pp. 1149-1154, ISSN 0028-0836

Tropepe, V., Coles, B.L., Chiasson, B.J., Horsford, D.J., Elia, A.J., McInnes, R.R. & van der Kooy, D. (2000). Retinal stem cells in the adult mammalian eye. *Science*, Vol. 287, No. 5460, (March 2000), pp. 2032-2036, ISSN 0036-8075

Uibo, R. & Lernmark, A. (2008). GAD65 autoimmunity-clinical studies. *Adv Immunol*, Vol. 100, pp. 39-78, ISSN 0065-2776

Valdés-González, R.A., Dorantes, L.M., Garibay, G.N., Bracho-Blanchet, E., Mendez, A.J., Dávila-Pérez, R., Yechoor, V. & Chan, L. (2010). Minireview: beta-cell replacement therapy for diabetes in the 21st century: manipulation of cell fate by directed differentiation. *Mol Endocrinol*, Vol. 24, No. 8, (August 2010), pp. 1501, ISSN 0888-8809

van Laar, J.M. & Tyndall A. (2006). Adult stem cells in the treatment of autoimmune diseases. *Rheumatology (Oxford)*, Vol. 45, No. 10, (October 2006), pp. 1187-1193, ISSN 1462-0324

Wagner, R.T., Lewis, J., Cooney, A. & Chan, L. (2010). Stem cell approaches for the treatment of type 1 diabetes mellitus. *Transl Res*, Vol. 156, No. 3, (September 2010), pp. 169-179, ISSN 1931-5244

Wang, X., Zhao, T., Huang, W., Wang, T., Qian, J., Xu, M., Kranias, E.G., Wang, Y. & Fan, G.C. (2009). Hsp20-engineered mesenchymal stem cells are resistant to oxidative stress via enhanced activation of Akt and increased secretion of growth factors. *Stem Cells*, Vol. 27, No. 12, (December 2009), pp. 3021-3031, ISSN1066-5099

Weir, G.C. & Bonner-Weir, S. (2004). Five stages of evolving beta-cell dysfunction during progression to diabetes. *Diabetes*, Vol. 53 Suppl 3, (December 2004), S16-21, ISSN 0012-1797

Willcox, A., Richardson, S.J., Bone, A.J., Foulis, A.K. & Morgan, N.G. (2010). Evidence of increased islet cell proliferation in patients with recent-onset type 1 diabetes. *Diabetologia*, Vol. 53, No. 9, (September 2010), pp. 2020-2028, ISSN 0012-186X

Wu, Y., Chen, L., Scott, P.G. & Tredget, E.E. (2007). Mesenchymal stem cells enhance wound healing through differentiation and angiogenesis. *Stem Cells*, Vol. 25, No. 10, (October 2007), pp. 2648-2659, ISSN 1066-5099

Xu, X., D'Hoker, J., Stangé, G., Bonné, S., De Leu, N., Xiao, X., Van de Casteele, M., Mellitzer, G., Ling, Z., Pipeleers, D., Bouwens, L., Scharfmann, R., Gradwohl, G. & Heimberg, H. (2008). Beta cells can be generated from endogenous progenitors in injured adult mouse pancreas. *Cell*, Vol. 132, No. 2, (January 2008), pp.197-207, ISSN 0092-8674

Yang, L., Li, S., Hatch, H., Ahrens, K., Cornelius, J.G., Petersen, B.E., Peck, A.B. (2002). In vitro trans-differentiation of adult hepatic stem cells into pancreatic endocrine hormone-producing cells. *Proc Natl Acad Sci U S A*, Vol. 99, No. 12, (June 2002), pp. 8078-8083, ISSN 0027-8424

Yang, Z., Li, K., Yan, X., Dong, F. & Zhao, C. (2010). Amelioration of diabetic retinopathy by engrafted human adipose-derived mesenchymal stem cells in streptozotocin diabetic rats. *Graefes Arch Clin Exp Ophthalmol*, Vol. 248, No. 10, (October 2010), pp. 1415-1422, ISSN 0721-832X

Zappia, E., Casazza, S., Pedemonte, E., Benvenuto, F., Bonanni, I., Gerdoni, E., Giunti, D., Ceravolo, A., Cazzanti, F., Frassoni, F., Mancardi, G. & Uccelli, A. (2005). Mesenchymal stem cells ameliorate experimental autoimmune encephalomyelitis inducing T-cell anergy. *Blood*, Vol. 106, No. 5, (September 2005), pp. 1755-1761, ISSN 0006-4971

Zhang, N., Li, J., Luo, R., Jiang, J. & Wang, J.A. (2008). Bone marrow mesenchymal stem cells induce angiogenesis and attenuate the remodeling of diabetic cardiomyopathy. *Exp Clin Endocrinol Diabetes*, Vol. 116, No. 2, (February 2008), pp. 104-111, ISSN 0947-7349

Zhao, M., Amiel, S.A., Ajami, S., Jiang, J., Rela, M., Heaton, N. & Huang, G.C. (2008). Amelioration of streptozotocin-induced diabetes in mice with cells derived from human marrow stromal cells. *PLoS One*, Vol. 3, No. 7, (July 2008), pp. e2666, ISSN 1932-6203

Zhao, Y., Lin, B., Darflinger, R., Zhang, Y., Holterman, M.J. & Skidgel, R.A. (2009). Human cord blood stem cell-modulated regulatory T lymphocytes reverse the autoimmune-caused type 1 diabetes in nonobese diabetic (NOD) mice. *PLoS One*, Vol. 4, No. 1, (January 2009), pp. e4226, ISSN 1932-6203

Zhao, Y. & Mazzone, T. (2010). Human cord blood stem cells and the journey to a cure for type 1 diabetes. *Autoimmun Rev*, Vol. 10, No. 2, (December 2010), pp. 103-107, ISSN 1568-9972

Zanone, M.M., Favaro, E. & Camussi, G. (2008). From endothelial to beta cells: insights into pancreatic islet microendothelium. *Curr Diabetes Rev*, Vol. 4, No. 1, (February 2008), pp. 1-9, ISSN 1573-3998

Zanone, M.M., Favaro, E., Miceli, I., Grassi, G., Camussi, E., Caorsi, C., Amoroso, A., Giovarelli, M., Perin, P.C. & Camussi, G. (2010). Human mesenchymal stem cells modulate cellular immune response to islet antigen glutamic acid decarboxylase in type 1 diabetes. *J Clin Endocrinol Metab*, Vol. 95, No. 8, (August 2010), pp. 3788-97, ISSN 0021-972X

5

The Enigma of β-Cell Regeneration in the Adult Pancreas: Self-Renewal Versus Neogenesis

A. Criscimanna[1,2,3], S. Bertera[1], F. Esni[3], M. Trucco[1] and R. Bottino[1]

[1]*Division of Immunogenetics, Department of Pediatrics, Children's Hospital of Pittsburgh,*
University of Pittsburgh
[2]*Division of Endocrinology, DOSAC, Universita' degli Studi di Palermo*
[3]*Department of Surgery, Children's Hospital of Pittsburgh*
University of Pittsburgh
[1,3]*USA*
[2]*Italy*

1. Introduction

The pancreas is constituted by two distinctly different tissues: the exocrine component, i.e., pancreatic acinar cells that secrete digestive enzymes; and the endocrine component, the islets of Langerhans, constituted by hormone secreting cells. In the islet, the α-cells produce glucagon; the β-cells, insulin; the δ-cells, somatostatin; γ-cells, pancreatic polypeptide (Figure 1). Diabetes is caused either by an absolute (type 1) or relative (type 2) defect of insulin-producing β-cells in the pancreas. Therefore, regardless of the different pathogenesis, diabetes is the perfect candidate for cell replacement therapy. Currently the two available alternatives for β-cell replacement therapy are whole pancreas or isolated islet transplantation (Shapiro et al., 2000). However, these approaches are severely limited by a shortage of human organ donors and the need of lifelong immunosuppressive therapy. In the absence of other clearly suitable and renewable sources of surrogate β-cells, an alternative strategy to exogenous cell replacement therapy might be fostering endogenous β-cell regeneration. Therefore, knowledge of the mechanisms regulating β-cell plasticity in both embryonic and adult life, as well as in pathological conditions, is of particular interest.

During pancreatic development, β-cells derive from a population of endocrine precursors arising from the pancreatic epithelium (Gittes, 2009). Activation of cell-specific transcription factors guides the initially multipotent progenitors and determines their differentiation into mature β-cells. The final size of the endocrine pancreas is limited by the size of the progenitor cell pool in the developing pancreatic bud (Stanger et al., 2007). After birth, most β-cells are considered quiescent, however, it has been shown that the β-cell mass can adaptively expand under some physiologic or pathologic circumstances, such as pregnancy and obesity, both in mammals and rodents (Bernard-Kargar & Ktorza, 2001).

In mouse models there is also evidence that the pancreas preserves the ability to regenerate its β-cell mass in response to several non-physiological injuries, such as selective chemical destruction or surgical excision (Trucco, 2005; Thorel, 2010). Furthermore, in non-obese diabetic mice (NOD) it has been shown that recovery of sufficient endogenous insulin production is possible via combination of strategies involving reversal of the autoimmune attack (Zorina et al., 2003; Kodama et al., 2003; Suri et al., 2006; Chong et al., 2006; Nishio et al., 2006).

In humans it is still debated whether this recovery is possible and, if so, to what extent it is feasible. Spontaneous recovery of β-cell function has been reported in patients with recent onset type 1 diabetes, suggesting that β-cells can regenerate despite underlying autoimmunity (Karges et al., 2004, 2006; Meier et al., 2006a; Butler et al., 2007). Additionally, the observation that people with long-standing type 1 diabetes still possess β-cells despite their destruction by the enduring autoimmunity and glucotoxicity, suggests that new β-cell formation might occur throughout life [Meier et al., 2005]. However, it remains largely unclear through which molecular and cellular mechanisms it occurs.

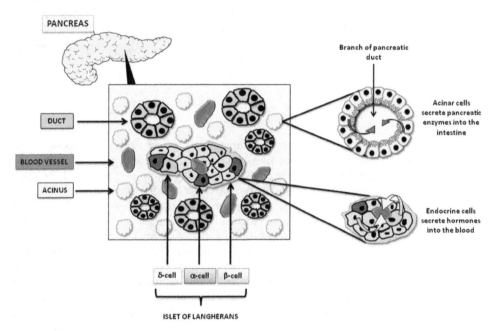

Fig. 1. Cells of the pancreas

The pancreas houses two different tissues. Its bulk is comprised of exocrine tissue, which is made up of acinar cells. These cells secrete pancreatic enzymes delivered to the intestine to facilitate the digestion of food. Scattered throughout the exocrine tissue are many thousands of clusters of endocrine cells known as islets of Langerhans. Within the islet, α-cells produce glucagon; β-cells, insulin; δ-cells, somatostatin; and γ-cells, pancreatic polypeptide — all of which are delivered into the blood stream.

2. Can the endocrine pancreas regenerate? Models of artificially induced diabetes

To address the question whether the pancreas possesses the ability to regenerate, several models have been used to artificially reduce the β-cell mass in order to stimulate a pancreatic response. Most of these models allow exploring the plasticity of the pancreas in the absence of concurrent autoimmunity, which might prevent or block any attempt of β-cell restoration.

2.1 Partial pancreatectomy

Partial pancreatectomy (>90% removal) was shown to induce limited re-growth of the remnant organ in rats (Pearson et al., 1977). In comparison to liver regeneration second to partial hepatectomy, subtotal pancreatectomy is followed only by a limited regenerative growth that is proportional to the size of the excision. In addition, regeneration is mostly related to the exocrine tissue, while the endocrine part was shown to rescue, at its best, only approximately 30% of its initial mass (De Leon et al., 2003). The extent of the surgical intervention seems to be important, and could explain discrepancies in some reports describing absent (Dor et al., 2004) or vigorous pancreatic regeneration [Bonner-Weir et al., 1993] after 70% and 90% organ resection, respectively. In addition, hyperglycemia, which is present only in the latter case, could act as co-stimulator.

2.2 Pancreatic duct ligation

Pancreatic duct ligation (PDL) was also used to determine obstruction and consequently local inflammation and stimulation of pancreatic regeneration. During the first week post-ligation an increase in the β-cell number and the presence of intermediate ductal/endocrine (Wang et al., 1995) or acinar/endocrine phenotypes (Bertelli & Bendayan, 1997; Inada et al., 2008) has been observed. Additional stimulation of the expansion of the β-cell mass following PDL can be achieved by gastrin infusion (Rooman et al., 2002).

2.3 Wrapping of the pancreas with cellophane

Wrapping the pancreas with cellophane has also been used to induce islet neogenesis from ducts, and it has been reported to reverse streptozotocin-induced diabetes in hamsters (Rosenberg et al., 1996).

2.4 Selective β-cell destruction

Selective β-cell destruction can be obtained by chemical ablation with streptozotocin or alloxan, alone and in combination with pancreatectomy (Finegood et al., 1999; Wang et al., 1996; Rood et al., 2006). Streptozotocin (STZ) is a drug that leads to cell death by DNA alkylation, while alloxan is a generator of oxygen free radicals causing extensive DNA damage. Adult mice rendered diabetic with a high dose of STZ or alloxan are unable to recover endogenous β-cell function (Szkudelski, 2001). Interestingly, β-cell neogenesis can be stimulated in STZ-diabetic newborn rats by administration of the hormone glucagon-like peptide-1 (GLP-1), resulting in improved glucose homeostasis persisting at adult age (Tourrel et al., 2001). In another murine experimental model of alloxan-induced beta-cell destruction, treatment with gastrin and epidermal growth factor (EGF) was found to restore glycemic control and 30–40% of the normal beta-cell mass within 7 days (Rooman & Bouwens, 2004). Combination of the same growth factors proved to be effective also in facilitating islet β-cell neogeneisis in NOD mice with autoimmune diabetes (Suarez-Pinzon et al., 2005). In addition, rescue of endogenous islet function was shown in STZ-diabetic mice after removal of the kidney bearing syngeneic islets, which temporarily maintained mice normoglicemic (Yin et al., 2006), thus indicating that glucose control might be relevant to facilitate the regenerative process. On the other hand, the possibility that recovery of the endogenous β-cell function may occur independently of glucose control exists, i.e., by the mediation of cytokines, which may activate residual β-cell proliferation or progenitor cell differentiation. To note, in the study by Yin et al., a facilitating role was exerted by the presence of the spleen, which probably plays an indirect role as modulator of the inflammatory process in the pancreas, thereby stimulating recovery of the STZ-damaged islets. STZ seems to trigger a pancreatic regenerative response also in non-human primate models, although it does not lead to a substantial endogenous β-cell recovery in absence of additional stimuli, like the failure of exogenous islet transplantation in the liver (Bottino et al., 2009).

Method	Target Cells	Potential Mechanism for Regeneration
Pancreatectomy	Endocrine	Replication of pre-existing β-cells
	Exocrine	Reactivation of embryonic program
Pancreatic duct ligation	Endocrine	Regeneration through Ngn3+ precursors
	Exocrine	Regeneration through Ca-II and Sox-9+ progenitors
Streptozotocin	β-cell	β-cell neogenesis from ductal cells
Alloxan	β-cell	β-cell neogenesis from ductal cells

CA-II: carbonic anhydrase II

Table 1. Summary of the models used to investigate pancreatic regeneration.

3. Lineage tracing techniques

Lineage tracing techniques have been widely used to investigate both the ontogeny of pancreatic cell fates during mouse embryogenesis as well as the identification of progenitor cells *in vivo* during regeneration (see Figure 2 and 3 for further explanations).

In lineage analysis, specific cells are labeled or marked so that their progeny can be identified later during development. In the pancreas, lineage analysis has been used to recognize not only the progenitor cells giving rise to mature endocrine and exocrine cells, but also the stage at which each set of progenitors is restricted to a particular cell fate. Lineage tracing is also useful to label and isolate marked cells in order to study their gene expression profile and *in vitro* differentiation.

In pancreatic lineage analysis, cells can be labeled using distinct approaches. A physical label - such as dye or a replication-incompetent retrovirus - can be directly injected into embryos to label cells within a tissue. The tissue is allowed to mature *in vivo* or in culture, and the cell types that become labeled reveal the lineage of the starting cells. However, since this method marks cells indiscriminately, in most tissues it cannot be used to label specific sub-populations. A more reliable approach is to genetically mark progenitor cells using endogenous gene expression patterns. This method selectively labels cells that express a particular gene, thus revealing the fate of their progeny. In most cases, a tissue specific promoter (for example Pdx-1) driving Cre recombinase is used to irreversibly tag cells. Other options include the use of a transgene driven by a specific promoter within different cell types, and lineage ablation, either using gene-inactivation mutants (knockout) or transgenic expression of cellular toxins. All these approaches have been used to follow pancreatic cell lineages (reviewed in Gu et al. 2003).

3.1 Cre/LoxP system

Cells can be irreversibly marked using the Cre/LoxP system, thus permitting detection of progeny cells that no longer express the gene of interest. This system uses two transgenic mouse lines, the "reporter" and the "deletor" (Figure 2).

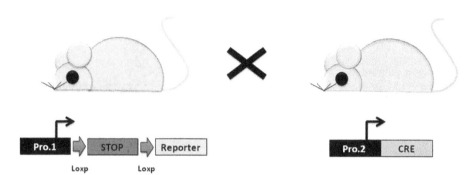

The reporter line uses promoter 1 (Pro.1, black rectangle) to drive reporter gene expression (green rectangle). Upstream of the reporter gene coding region is a STOP cassette made of three repeats of a polyadenilation signal (red rectangle). Flanking the blocking signal are two LoxP sites (blue arrows). Promoter 1 can be tissue specific or ubiquitous. In the deletor line, another tissue specific promoter (Pro. 2, black rectangle) is used to drive the expression of *Cre* recombinase (yellow rectangle). When the two mouse lines are crossed, CRE is expressed in the cells in which promoter 2 is active, thus deleting the blocking signal. This results in the expression of the reporter gene in cells that also express promoter 1.

Fig. 2. Design plan for direct cell lineage analysis.

The first transgenic mouse uses a promoter (promoter 1), which can be tissue specific or ubiquitous, to drive the expression of a reporter gene, such as LacZ or green fluorescent protein (GFP). The second mouse carries a transgene that uses a different tissue specific promoter (promoter 2) to drive the expression of Cre recombinase. In the absence of the Cre deletor transgene, the expression of the reporter protein is prevented by a STOP cassette (multiple repeats of a poly-adenylation signal) upstream of the reporter coding sequence. However, in the presence of Cre recombinase, two LoxP sites flanking the blocking sequence permit this block to be removed. Thus, in double transgenic animals, the reporter gene will be expressed in cells following the excision event, thereby labeling all progeny derived from those precursors that express the deletor transgene.

A fine-tuning of the Cre/LoxP system can be achieved with the CRE-ER™ recombinase, which is a fusion between the catalytic domain of the CRE recombinase and the ligand-binding domain of a modified estrogen receptor. The CRE-ER™ protein requires an artificial ligand, tamoxifen, to catalyze LoxP mediated recombination. Because tamoxifen is active within mouse embryos for less than 48 h, cells expressing Cre-ER™ at a specific developmental stage can be selectively labeled by administration of tamoxifen during that stage. After tamoxifen treatment, the conventional CRE recombinase activates the reporter transgene expression as soon as CRE protein is generated, and labeled cells accumulate in any lineage where Cre has been expressed. This type of recombinase can be used to follow selectively the progeny of cells born at defined developmental stages, including postnatal growth and during regeneration.

3.2 Lineage analysis based on simple transgenes

A simpler transgenic approach drives expression of a reporter gene, such as LacZ or green fluorescent protein (GFP), under the promoter of interest. The drawback of this approach is that any progeny of these cells, which cease expression of the chosen protein cannot be followed. In addition, since this method marks cells from the first time the promoter is activated, and as these cells accumulate during development, it becomes impossible to distinguish new members of the population. Thus, one cannot distinguish the progeny of cells born during embryogenesis from those born in adults.

3.3 Lineage analysis based on cell ablation

Another method to investigate lineage relationship is cell ablation. This can be accomplished by specific gene inactivation mutations (knockout), such as in the *Pdx1* knockout mouse, which has no mature pancreatic cells. Alternatively, a tissue specific promoter can be used to drive the expression of a cellular toxin, such as the Diphtheria Toxin A (DTA) subunit. In these transgenic animals, the DTA subunit will kill those cells whose progenitors express that specific transgene. A similar approach is represented by the Diphtheria Toxin Receptor (DTR)-mediated conditional cell ablation model. DTR is a membrane-anchored form of the heparin-binding EGF-like growth factor (HB-EGF precursor). The human and simian HB-EGF precursors bind DT and function as toxin receptors, whereas HB-EGF from mice and rats do not bind the toxin and therefore remain insensitive to DT. Thus, transgenic expression of the simian or human DTR in mice can render cells DT-sensitive. Recently, a mouse strain was generated (iDTR), in which the gene encoding DTR has been introduced into the *ROSA26* locus (R26^{DTR}), but its expression is dependent on the Cre-mediated removal of a transcriptional STOP cassette. Therefore, only Cre-expressing cells and their progeny will undergo Cre-recombinase activity and subsequently will transcribe DTR. Although viable and normally functioning, these cells are rapidly killed upon DT administration (Figure 3) (Buch et al. 2003).

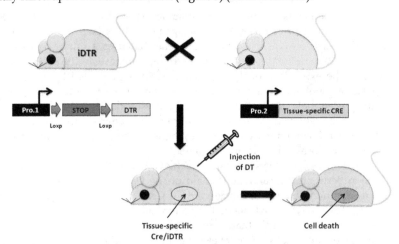

The STOP cassette, which prohibits DTR expression, is removed by crossing the iDTR strain to a tissue-specific Cre-expressing mouse strain. Consecutive expression of the DTR renders the respective tissues sensitive to cell death induced by injection of diphtheria toxin. Filled rectangles, *loxP* sites; arrows, transcriptional activity; open ovals, promoter.

Fig. 3. Design plan of the inducible DTR mouse strain (iDTR).

4. Evidence of pancreatic endocrine progenitors/stem cells in the pancreas

Several cells in the pancreas have been described as potential sources of β-cell renewal.

4.1 Pancreatic ductal progenitor cells

During pancreatic organogenesis, stem cells within the duct pancreatic epithelium give rise to both the endocrine and acinar cells (Gittes, 2009). Therefore it seems reasonable to think that the regeneration process could start within the ductal compartment, recapitulating embryonic and fetal development. In addition, there are similarities between islet regeneration and embryonic pancreas development at the gene expression level. Evidence of adult duct cells harboring stem cells capable of differentiating into β-cells was reported both *in vivo* and *in vitro* (Dudek et al., 1991; Ramiya et al., 2000; Bonner-Weir et al., 2000, 2008; Gao et al., 2003). In 2000 Ramiya et al. claimed that long-term cultivation of pancreatic ductal epithelial cells isolated from pre-diabetic, adult, non-obese diabetic mice contained nestin-positive stem cells able to differentiate into islets of Langerhans (Ramiya et al., 2000). These "surrogate" islets responded *in vitro* to glucose challenge, and reversed insulin-dependent diabetes after being implanted into diabetic NOD mice. Similar observations were reported using more defined culture conditions in which isolated human pancreatic duct preparations led to formation and propagation of human islet-like structures (Bonner-Weir et al., 2000, 2008; Gao et al., 2003). Ogata et al. also derived a similar subset of islet-like insulin secreting cells from pancreatic ducts of neonatal rats (Ogata et al., 2004). After incubation with activin A and betacellulin, cells showed tolbutamide- and glucose-responsive insulin secretion. Transplantation of these pseudo-islets in STZ-diabetic NOD mice improved blood glucose levels. Hao et al. confirmed the existence of endocrine stem or progenitor cells within the epithelial compartment of the adult human pancreas, by isolating stem cells from the non-endocrine fraction after islet separation of adult human pancreas digests (Hao et al., 2006). Following elimination of the contaminating mesenchymal cells, the highly purified population of non-endocrine pancreatic epithelial cells (NEPECs) was transplanted under the kidney capsule of immunodeficient (SCID) mice. Although NEPECs produced only low amounts of insulin, when co-transplanted with fetal pancreatic cells, they were capable of endocrine differentiation. No evidence of β-cell replication or cell fusion was observed. To directly test whether ductal cells serve as pancreatic progenitors after birth and give rise to new islets, a transgenic mouse expressing human carbonic anhydrase II (CAII) promoter was generated. This study showed that CAII-expressing cells within the pancreas act as progenitors that give rise to both new islets and acini normally after birth and after injury (PDL) (Inada et al., 2008).

Additional evidence of the existence of endocrine precursor cells within the ductal compartment come from the detection of the nuclear transcription factor Neurogenin-3 (Ngn3) in the ducts during regeneration after STZ. Ngn3 is a basic helix–loop–helix transcription factor, which is able to commit pancreatic cells to an endocrine cell fate (Schwitzgebel et al., 2000). Lack of Ngn3 leads to an absence of islets (Gradwhol et al., 2000); its ectopic expression determines premature over-commission towards the endocrine lineage (Apelqvist et al., 1999). Presence of Ngn3 is very convincing evidence that pancreatic regeneration starts from pancreatic progenitors and mimics the same pathway followed during normal development (Figure 4). By using an inducible Cre-ERTM-LoxP system to

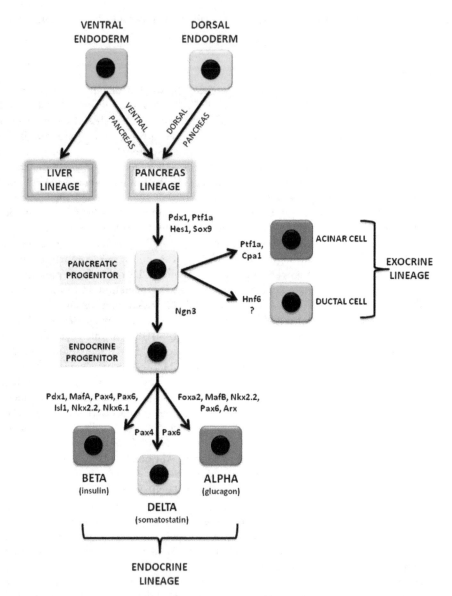

Fig. 4. Regulatory nuclear transcription factors controlling cell type lineages during embryonic pancreas development.

mark the progeny of cells expressing either Ngn3 or Pdx1 at different stages of development, Gu et al. showed that endocrine/exocrine and ductal lineages are separated before E12.5 (Gu et al., 2002). Authors demonstrate that, while cells expressing Pdx1 give rise to all three types of pancreatic tissue (exocrine, endocrine and duct), only the subset Pdx 1/Ngn3+ cells are islet progenitors. The duct cells that do not contain progeny of

Ngn3[+] cells presumably give rise to the adult duct system and account for the heterogeneity in developmental potential among 'duct-like structures'. Kodama et al. also suggested that in STZ-treated mice, regeneration occurs mainly from intra-islet Ngn3[+] progenitor cells rather than from ductal precursors (Kodama et al., 2005). Recently, Xu et al. showed that PDL in the pancreatic tail resulted in some β-cell proliferation and, more strikingly, in a large upregulation of Ngn3 gene expression (Xu et al., 2008). Ngn3 positive cells were found to be closely associated with ducts, and possibly cells of the ductal lineage themselves. After isolation, these cells could give rise to all islet cell types, including glucose responsive β-cells, both *in situ* and when cultured in Ngn3[-/-] embryonic pancreas explants. In addition, White et al. utilized a system based on Ngn3–enhanced green fluorescent protein knock-in mouse model to isolate endocrine progenitor cells from embryonic pancreata to generate an ample gene expression profile of these progenitors and their immediate descendants (White et al., 2008). On the other hand, a recent publication reported low level expression of Ngn3 in adult endocrine cells, raising concerns about using Ngn3 expression as a marker of endocrine progenitors and neogenesis in the adult pancreas (Wang et al., 2009). Furthermore, another study indicates that although PDL leads to Ngn3 expression in a sub-population of cells within the ducts, it does not induce appropriate cues to allow for completion of the entire β-cell neogenesis program (Kopp et al., 2011).

The potential for the pancreatic organ to recover the endocrine function after injury has been also investigated in non-human primates, where a ductal involvement was observed in STZ-diabetic monkeys that recovered endogenous β-cell function following pig islet transplantation in the liver (Bottino et al., 2009).

Further evidence that hormone-positive cells arise from the ducts comes from the comparison of 16 donor pancreas specimens and pancreas biopsies from 8 simultaneous pancreas/kidney transplantations (Martin-Pagoda et al., 2008). While in the donor pancreas the frequency of insulin[+] duct cells was low (0.45%), in five pancreatic transplants with recurrent autoimmunity, 57.5% of the duct cells expressed insulin protein. If new islets were generated from pre-existing ductal tissue, transient co-expression of hormones and residual duct markers could be expected. Indeed, this has been demonstrated in grafts of purified human duct cells (Yatoh et al., 2007).

4.2 Pancreatic non-ductal progenitor cells

Besides ductal progenitors, other groups proposed that pancreatic stem cells may also reside within the islets or in the acinar compartment.

4.2.1 Acinar cells

Acinar cells, which represent the main portion of pancreatic tissue, have been shown to transdifferentiate into islet cells *in vivo* and *in vitro*, through the generation of duct cells as an intermediate step (Lardon et al., 2004; Baeyens et al., 2005; Rooman et al., 2000; Lipsett et al., 2007). Lineage tracing has been used *in vitro* to further strengthen the conclusion that endocrine cells can be generated from exocrine cells via transdifferentiation [Minami et al., 2005]. Earlier *in vivo* lineage tracing experiments in mice showed that acinar cells scarcely contribute to generate new β-cells and duct cells (Desai et al., 2007). However, more recent studies by Collombat et al. demonstrated that upon expression of Pax4, adult α-cells can transdifferentiate to β-cells (Collombat et al., 2009). The ectopic expression of Pax4 forces endocrine precursor cells as well as mature α-cells, to adopt a β-cell fate. In addition, since α-cells were constantly recruited and converted to β-cells, the resulting glucagon deficiency provoked a compensatory and continuous glucagon⁺ cell neogenesis through Ngn3⁺ precursors. On the other hand, Arx misexpression in β-cells, using either an Ins^Cre or in adult β-cells using an inducible Pdx1^CreERT system reduced insulin-expressing cells and increased alpha and PP-positive cells (Collombat et al., 2007).

Alpha-to-Beta-cell transdifferentiation was also recently described in a transgenic model of diphtheria-toxin-induced acute selective near-total β-cell ablation (Thorel et al., 2010). Lineage-tracing to label the glucagon-producing α-cells before β-cell ablation, tracked large fractions of regenerated β-cells as deriving from α-cells, revealing a previously unknown flexibility in the functioning of the pancreas in relation to hormone secretion, with the potential for exploiting it to cure diabetes.

Generation of β-cells from α-cells has also been shown with a unique model that combines PDL with alloxan-mediated β-cells destruction (Chung et al., 2010). In this model, large numbers of β-cells were generated primarily from α-cells by two mechanisms: the first involved extensive α-cell proliferation, which provided a large pool of precursors that, in turn, would become β-cells via asymmetric division; the second demonstrated that β-cells could form directly from α-cells via transdifferentiation. This latter mechanism was put forward by the finding of intermediate cells co-expressing α- and β-cell-specific markers. Double-positive cells were detectable in the first week after injury, but their number gradually declined and by the second week some converted into mature β-cells, as shown by loss of glucagon and new expression of MafA, a β-cell-specific transcriptional activator.

4.2.2 Nestin-positive cells

Nestin-positive cells have been identified within adult rat islets as being capable of differentiating into insulin-positive cells *in vitro* (Zulewski et al., 2001). Nestin is an intermediate filament protein expressed by the neural lineage, which, according to some groups can be found in the pancreas (Edlund, 2002), in contrast to others that could not find its expression during development of the human pancreatic epithelium (Piper et al., 2002). More recent lineage-tracing experiments showed that nestin-positive cells contribute to the vasculature as well as acinar lineages but not to the endocrine lineage (Treutelaar et al., 2003; Esni et al., 2004; Delacour et al., 2004).

4.2.3 Proliferative human islet precursor cells (hIPCs)

Proliferative human islet precursor cells (hIPCs) were obtained *in vitro* from preparations of adult human islets after extensive *in vitro* proliferation (Gershengorn et al., 2004). Authors believed that these cells, showing a mesenchymal phenotype, derived from insulin-expressing cells undergoing epithelial-to-mesenchymal transition (EMT). hIPCs could be re-differentiated into insulin-expressing islet-like cell aggregates (ICAs) and secreted insulin when transplanted under the kidney capsule of immunodeficient mice. However, many criticisms were advanced from other groups, claiming that, at least in mouse pancreatic cultures, islet-derived fibroblast-like cells are not generated via EMT from pancreatic β-cells (Chase et al., 2007; Atouf et al., 2007). Later, Gershengorn et al. further confirmed the basic differences between human and mouse cultures, and claimed that hIPCs are a special kind of pancreatic mesenchymal stromal cells (Morton et al., 2007). More recently, using a lineage-tracing *in vitro* technique, Russ et al. found evidence for massive proliferation of cells derived from human β-cells. Nevertheless, it appears that induction of significant replication *in vitro* results in dedifferentiation. (Russ et al, 2008).

5. Evidence of pancreatic progenitors/stem cells outside the pancreas

In addition to pancreatic progenitors, cells from other organs, such as liver, spleen, bone marrow, adipose tissue and limbus have been identified as either new sources of islets or stimulators of islet regeneration.

5.1 Liver stem cells

Pancreas and liver share the same origin from the embryonic endoderm (Zaret, 2000). It has been reported that transdifferentiation of pancreas into liver occurs both *in vitro* and *in vivo* in animal models after a number of experimental treatments (Rao et al., 1986, 1995; Dabeva et al., 1997; Kralowski et al., 1999; Shen et al., 2000). The opposite conversion of liver into pancreas is also possible (Horb et al., 2003). Zalzman et al. were able to immortalize a population of human fetal liver epithelial progenitor cells that, once transfected with the Pdx1 gene, generated a stable population of insulin-producing cells (Zalzman et al., 2003). Intraperitoneal transplantation of these cells into immunodeficient mice led to reversal of diabetes for 80 days. However, Yang et al. showed that expression of Pdx1 in hepatocytes does not result in the formation of functional endocrine pancreas in Pdx1 deficient mice, thus suggesting that Pdx1 is necessary but not sufficient to induce differentiation of the pancreatic tissue (Yang et al., 2002).

5.2 Splenic stem cells

The hypothesis that the spleen may harbor stem cells capable of differentiating into β-cells has also been investigated. Faustman and colleagues initially showed that splenocytes contributed to the reversal of autoimmunity in the NOD mouse model when injected with Freund's complete adjuvant (Ryu et al., 2001). Later they also suggested that splenocytes may directly contribute to islet regeneration by differentiation into β-cells (Kodama et al., 2003). However, these findings proved to be controversial. Indeed several other groups, confirming a partial recovery from the autoimmune attack following splenocyte injections, actually failed to display evidence of a direct contribution of donor cells to β-cell regeneration (Suri et al., 2006; Chong et al., 2006; Nishio et al., 2006). Nonetheless, Yin and colleagues supported a facilitating role of the spleen in the regeneration of endogenous β-cell mass (Yin et al., 2006).

5.3 Mesenchymal stem cells

There are numerous reports suggesting that the bone marrow not only harbors haemopoietic stem cells, which are committed to differentiate into blood cells, but also mesenchymal stem cells (MSCs), capable of differentiation into β-cells (Oh et al., 2004; Moriscot et al., 2005). MSCs were reported to differentiate *in vivo* into glucose-competent pancreatic endocrine cells when transplanted in NOD mice (Ianus et al., 2003). However, following studies resulted in controversial outcomes, suggesting that MSCs do not become *per se* insulin producing cells, rather they take part in islet vascularization, eventually promoting β-cell regeneration (Hess et al., 2003 Chamson-Reig et al., 2010). Transplantation of human MSCs was also shown to induce repair of pancreatic islets and renal glomeruli in immunodeficient mice (NOD/SCID) suffering from STZ-induced diabetes (Lee et al., 2006). The role exerted by bone marrow cells by quenching autoimmunity allowing therefore functional recovery of residual β-cell mass in the pancreas, has been proven by Zorina et al. (Zorina et al., 2003). In the NOD autoimmune diabetes mouse model" in place of, restoration of endogenous β-cell function to physiologically sufficient levels was achievable after allogeneic bone marrow transplantation. Abrogation of autoimmunity and consequent β-cell mass recovery interestingly occurred even when allogeneic bone marrow cell tranplantation was performed after the clinical onset of diabetes. A recent study has suggested that bone marrow cells might have a role in permitting survival of endogenous β-cells also in humans (Voltarelli et al., 2007). Authors reported insulin independence for up to a year in more than half the cases of a small number of patients with recent-onset type 1 diabetes. Patients were administered high-dose immunosuppressive therapy to kill autoreactive T cell clones followed by autologous non-myeloablative stem cell transplantation. Nonetheless, because autologous bone marrow cell transplantation could not change indefinitely the genetic susceptibility to develop autoimmune diabetes, autoimmunity recurred soon after full immunocompetence was re-established. Therefore, different approaches should be used to obtain durable abrogation of β-cell specific autoimmunity, and allow recovery of insulin production (Giannoukakis et al., 2008).

Collectively these series of reports suggest that bone marrow cells do not give rise directly to new insulin producing cells - however they can indirectly facilitate regeneration of the endocrine pancreas, perhaps by secreting appropriate regenerative factors that still need to be characterized.

Other mesenchymal stem cells have been taken into consideration as a potential source of β-cells. Human and rat multipotent adipose tissue-derived stem cells (ADSCs) have been reported to generate insulin-producing cells after transduction with Pdx1 gene. The surrogate β-cells improved glucose sensitivity when transplanted under the renal capsule of STZ-induced diabetic rats [Lin et al., 2009]. In addition, intraportal infusion of human ADSCs together with bone marrow stem cells could increase endogenous insulin levels reducing exogenous insulin requirements in patients affected by type 1 diabetes (Trivedi et al., 2008).

The human limbus has also been indicated as a source of stem cells. The limbus is a highly specialized region of the eye hosting a well-recognized population of epithelial stem cells, which continuously renew the corneal surface. Additionally, the limbal niche also hosts stromal fibroblast-like stem cells (f-LSCs), with multilineage transdifferentiation potential. f-LSCs were able to generate functional pancreatic hormone-expressing cells *in vitro* recapitulating pancreatic organogenesis (Criscimanna et al., 2011).

6. Evidence of β-cell regeneration via proliferation of pre-existing β-cells

During the fetal stage, differentiation from precursor cells is the major mechanism by which β-cells are formed, while β-cells replication is enhanced during the perinatal and neonatal period. Lineage-tracing experiments in rodents provided convincing proof to the theory that adult β-cells predominantly arise from other β-cells without significant contributions from underlying stem or progenitor cell populations (Cano et al., 2008). Several studies conducted by the group of Melton and colleagues showed that, after pancreatic resection (Dor et al., 2004), or in a diabetic status induced by transgenic expression of diphtheria toxin (Nir et al., 2007), mouse β-cells possess significant capacity for spontaneous regeneration, sufficient to recover from overt diabetes. Authors claim that failure of β-cell regeneration in both autoimmune and pharmacological models of diabetes is due to confounding factors disguising the innate regenerative response, such as the persistence of circulating autoreactive T cells. To further sustain this hypothesis, it has been demonstrated how therapeutic protocols intended at blocking autoimmunity in NOD mice (Chatenoud et al., 1994) and in humans with type 1 diabetes (Herold et al., 2002, 2005, Bresson et al., 2006) resulted in partial remission from the disease. Whether this is due to a true regeneration process or just recovery of dysfunctional β-cells is still debated.

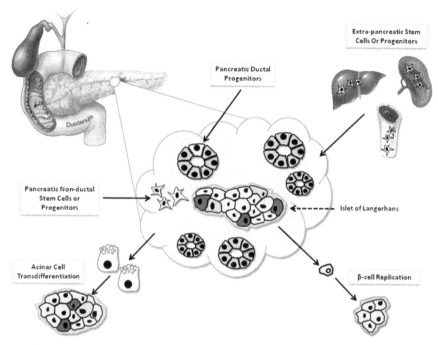

Fig. 5. Schematic illustration of potential cell sources for postnatal ß cell regeneration

Recently, Brennand et al. also demonstrated that in adult mice all β-cells, not just a subpopulation, equally contribute to islet growth and maintenance (Brennand et al., 2007). Two approaches were performed to address this issue. First, evaluation of the replicative potential of the entire β-cell mass was performed by monitoring the disappearance of a fluorescent marker accompanying cell division. Second, clonal analysis of dividing β-cells was completed. Because a uniform loss of label (cell division) across the entire cell population was observed, and all clones were of comparable size, authors conclude that the β-cell pool homogeneously possesses replication ability.

In humans, increased β-cell replication has been documented adjacent to intrapancreatic gastrinomas, suggesting that adult human β-cells can be driven, under specific circumstances, into the cell cycle (Meier et al., 2006b). Support to this remark was also given by another study, which demonstrated that β-cell replication is the primary mechanism responsible for the postnatal expansion of the β-cell mass in a population of young non-diabetic individuals [Meier et al., 2008]. In particular, it was shown that β-cell mass is able to (1) expand by several folds from birth to adulthood, (2) this is accomplished by an increase in number of β-cells per islet with a concomitant expansion in islet size (3) the relative rate of β-cell growth is higher in infancy and gradually declines thereafter to adulthood with no secondary accelerated growth phase during adolescence, (4) β-cell mass (and presumably growth) is highly variable between individuals, (5) a high rate of β-cell replication is coincident with the major postnatal expansion of β-cell mass. A summary of the theories on β-cell origin is presented in Figure 5.

7. The chronic pancreatitis model

Regenerative responses from the pancreatic tissue can be the result of a surgical or inflammatory injury. It has been described that pancreatic stellate cells, the star shaped cells representing approximately 4% of the resident pancreatic cell pool, are involved in fibrogenesis and pancreas regeneration. In chronic pancreatitis, these cells undergo transformation from quiescent to activated myofibroblast-like cells. Upon activation, which can be triggered by reactive oxygen intermediates, ethanol, Transforming Growth Factor (TGF) α and - β1, they can disclose special features, including the capability to increase the synthesis of collagen, fibronectins, in addition to cytokines. Interestingly TGF-β_1 is expressed by ductal cells in chronic pancreatitis, with a role in development of fibrosis and glandular atrophy (Demois et al. 2002). Recently it has been shown in the adult human pancreas of patients with chronic pancreatitis increased numbers of insulin as well as glucagon -containing cells in the ducts, in addition to other cells containing endocrine and exocrine markers. Such findings were also associated to higher numbers of proliferating cells (Ki67 positive) and Pdx1[+] cells, suggestive of a "metaplastic" status (Philips et al.,2007).

In our own experience as a reference center for the isolation of human islet cells, we observed peculiar morphological features in the pancreatic sections in patients with chronic pancreatitis. Not only did we find a higher density of islets, probably due to the destruction of the surrounding exocrine tissue (Figure 6), but, interestingly, we found that the intra-islet β-cell area relative to the α-cell area was significantly higher in chronic pancreatitis patients. Co-expression of the epithelial marker CK19, typical of ductal cells, with Ngn3, a transcription factor expressed in endocrine-committed cells during pancreatic development (Figure 7) was also identified.

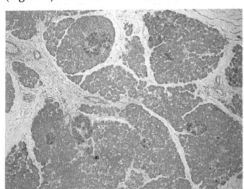 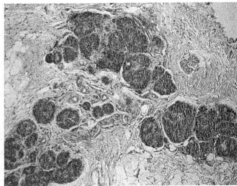

Fig. 6. Histological pancreatic features in chronic pancreatitis.

Islets of Langerhans (immunostained for insulin in brown/red) of a healthy individual (left) in comparison with those of a patient affected by chronic pancreatitis (right).

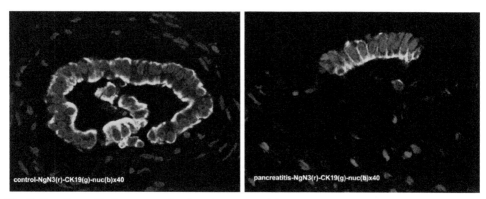

control-NgN3(r)-CK19(g)-nuc(b)x40   pancreatitis-NgN3(r)-CK19(g)-nuc(b)x40

Fig. 7. Peculiar cell phenotypes in chronic pancreatitis.

Co-expression of the epithelial marker CK19 (green) and Ngn3 (red), a transcription factor typically expressed in progenitor cells committed to the endocrine lineage in the pancreas of a patient with chronic pancreatitis (right panel). Control healthy pancreas (left panel).

A number of questions can be asked regarding the process by which damage, and pancreatitis specifically, mobilize these cells. For example, what is the potential role of the immune response to a damage signal in the pancreas in the differentiation of ductal and exocrine cells towards the endocrine lineage? Do immune cells produce soluble factors that facilitate the process of differentiation? What are the characteristics of differentiating non-endocrine and endocrine cells in response to pancreatitis? Can endocrine progenitor cells be better characterized using pancreatitis as an inductive event? Would isolation of such progenitor cells offer a framework for *in vitro* genetic manipulation to further differentiate such cells into defined and fully functional endocrine cells? Would *in vivo* genetic manipulation of the microenvironment exhibiting differentiation processes in response to pancreatitis offer a framework to direct such cells into endocrine lineages? These questions are important in the context of identifying progenitor cells that can serve as the source of endocrine cells, especially insulin-producing β-cells.

8. Conclusions

In conclusion, caution is required in interpreting studies unraveling the mechanisms involved in the maintenance of the β-cell mass. The extrapolation of information from animal studies can be misleading and not necessarily indicative for regenerative therapy in diabetic patients because mechanisms of regeneration/maintenance of the β-cell mass might be different across species (Hanley et al., 2008). For example, in obese rodents, an increment in β-cell mass is achieved by a massive increase of islet size and β-cell number per islet, consistent with a predominant mechanism of β-cell replication. On the contrary, in obese humans, islets are only modestly increased in size, consistent with minor involvement of β-cell replication (Butler et al., 2003). Also, a 90% pancreatectomy performed in young rodents leads to transient diabetes and regeneration of β-cell mass of ~50% within 2 weeks (Bonner-Weir et al., 1983, 1994), while only a 50% pancreatectomy is sufficient to determine diabetic status in adult humans who afterward became obese too. Certainly, one potential explanation for the reported differences between rodents and humans could be that rodents are more frequently studied at 1–3 months of age, when there is a high capacity for β-cell replication, whereas human pancreatic tissue is primarily studied in adults. It is therefore of great value to investigate the potential of pancreatic tissue to recover endogenous endocrine function after injury in animal models more similar to humans, such as non-human primates. However, even if the mechanisms regulating the maintenance of the β-cell mass in physiologic conditions are the same in humans, monkeys and rodents, we cannot exclude that during pathological conditions different pathways, species-specific and injury-specific (for type and magnitude), might be activated. For example, although the potential of acinar, duct (epithelial) and mesenchymal cells to differentiate into other cell types has been demonstrated *in vitro*, the mechanisms *in vivo* may be totally different. These discrepancies would not be surprising as cells taken into a foreign environment commonly behave differently than when residing in their natural niche. Another consideration is that, if regeneration occurs by recapitulation of fetal development, adult precursors should respond to fetal inductive signals. Conversely, if regeneration occurs by a different pathway, it is less likely that the process would be influenced by the same signals. The study of the factor(s) secreted by bone marrow precursors may shed some light on these aspects of the regenerative process as well.

In conclusion, the debate between the supporters of neogenesis and self-renewal for maintenance and replacement of β-cells is still open. It is perhaps acceptable to conclude that there is some truth in both proposed hypothesis, and that one does not exclude the other. Understanding the potential contribution of each mechanism will be crucial to find better curative approaches for diabetes.

9. References

Apelqvist A, Li H, Sommer L, Beatus P, Anderson DJ, Honjo T, Hrabe de Angelis M, Lendahl U, Edlund H. Notch signalling controls pancreatic cell differentiation. Nature 1999; 400:877-81.

Atouf F, Park CH, Pechhold K, Ta M, Choi Y, Lumelsky NL. No evidence for mouse pancreatic beta-cell epithelial-mesenchymal transition in vitro. Diabetes 2007; 56:699-702.

Baeyens L, De Breuck S, Lardon J, Mfopou JK, Rooman I, Bouwens L. *In vitro* generation of insulin-producing beta cells from adult exocrine pancreatic cells. Diabetologia 2005; 48:49-57.

Bernard-Kargar C, Ktorza A. Endocrine pancreas plasticity under physiological and pathological conditions. Diabetes 2001; 50 Suppl 1:S30-5.

Bertelli E, Bendayan M. Intermediate endocrine-acinar pancreatic cells in duct ligation conditions. Am J Physiol 1997; 273:C1641-9.

Bonner-Weir S, Trent DF, Weir GC. Partial pancreatectomy in the rat and subsequent defect in glucose-induced insulin release. J Clin Invest 1983; 71:1544-53.

Bonner-Weir S, Baxter LA, Schuppin GT, Smith FE. A second pathway for regeneration of adult exocrine and endocrine pancreas. A possible recapitulation of embryonic development. Diabetes 1993; 42:1715-20.

Bonner-Weir S. Regulation of pancreatic beta-cell mass in vivo. Recent Prog Horm Res 1994; 49:91-104.

Bonner-Weir S, Taneja M, Weir GC, Tatarkiewicz K, Song KH, Sharma A, O ' Neil JJ. In vitro cultivation of human islets from expanded ductal tissue. Proc Natl Acad Sci USA 2000; 97:7999-8004.

Bonner-Weir S, Inada A, Yatoh S, Li WC, Aye T, Toschi E, Sharma A. Transdifferentiation of pancreatic ductal cells to endocrine beta-cells. Biochem Soc Trans 2008; 36:353-6.

Bottino R, Criscimanna A, Casu A, He J, Van der Windt DJ, Rudert WA, Giordano C, Trucco M. Recovery of endogenous beta-cell function in nonhuman primates after chemical diabetes induction and islet transplantation. Diabetes. 2009 Feb;58(2):442-7.

Brennand K, Huangfu D, Melton D. All beta Cells Contribute Equally to Islet Growth and Maintenance. PLoS Biol 2007; 5(7):e163.

Bresson D, Togher L, Rodrigo E, Chen Y, Bluestone JA, Herold KC, von Herrath M. Anti-CD3 and nasal proinsulin combination therapy enhances remission from recent-onset autoimmune diabetes by inducing Tregs. J Clin Invest 2006; 116:1371-81.

Buch T et al. 2003) , Heppner FL, Tertilt C, Heinen TJ, Kremer M, Wunderlich FT, Jung S, Waisman A. A Cre-inducible diphtheria toxin receptor mediates cell lineage ablation after toxin administration. Nat Methods 2005;2:419-26.

Butler AE, Janson J, Bonner-Weir S, Ritzel R, Rizza RA, Butler PC. Beta-cell deficit and increased beta-cell apoptosis in humans with type 2 diabetes. Diabetes 2003; 52:102-10.

Butler AE, Galasso R, Meier JJ, Basu R, Rizza RA, Butler PC. Modestly increased beta cell apoptosis but no increased beta cell   replication in recent-onset type 1 diabetic patients who died of diabetic ketoacidosis. Diabetologia 2007; 50:2323-31.

Cano DA, Rulifson IC, Heiser PW, Swigart LB, Pelengaris S, German M, Evan GI, Bluestone JA, Hebrok M. Regulated beta-cell regeneration in the adult mouse pancreas. Diabetes 2008; 57:958-66.

Chamson-Reig A, Arany EJ, Hill DJ. Lineage tracing and resulting phenotype of haemopoietic-derived cells in the pancreas during beta cell regeneration. Diabetologia. 2010 Oct;53(10):2188-97.

Chase LG, Ulloa-Montoya F, Kidder BL et al. Islet-derived fibroblastlike cells are not derived via epithelial-mesenchymal transition from Pdx-1 or insulin-positive cells. Diabetes 2007; 56:3–7.

Chatenoud L, Thervet E, Primo J, Bach JF. Anti-CD3 antibody induces long-term remission of overt autoimmunity in nonobese diabetic mice. Proc Natl Acad Sci USA 1994; 91:123-7.

Chong AS, Shen J, Tao J, Yin D, Kuznetsov A, Hara M, Philipson LH. Reversal of diabetes in non-obese diabetic mice without spleen cell derived beta cell regeneration. Science 2006; 311:1774-5.

Chung CH, Hao E, Piran R, Keinan E, Levine F. Pancreatic β-cell neogenesis by direct conversion from mature α-cells. Stem Cells. 2010 Sep;28(9):1630-8.

Collombat P, Hecksher-Sorensen J, Krull J, et al. Embryonic endocrine pancreas and mature β-cells acquire alpha and PP cell phenotypes upon Arx misexpression. J Clin Invest 2007; 117:961–970.

Collombat P, Xu X, Ravassard P, Sosa-Pineda B, Dussaud S, Billestrup N, Madsen OD, Serup P, Heimberg H, Mansouri A. The ectopic expression of Pax4 in the mouse pancreas converts progenitor cells into alpha and subsequently β-cells. Cell 2009;138:449–462.

Criscimanna A, Zito G, Taddeo A, Richiusa P, Pitrone M, Morreale D, Lodato G, Pizzolanti G, Citarrella R, Galluzzo A, Giordano C. In vitro generation of pancreatic endocrine cells from human adult fibroblast-like limbal stem cells. Cell Transpl. 2011; in press

Dabeva MD, Hwang SG, Vasa SR, Hurston E, Novikoff PM, Hixson DC, Gupta S, Shafritz DA. Differentiation of pancreatic epithelial progenitor cells into hepatocytes following transplantation into rat liver. Proc Natl Acad Sci U S A 1997; 94:7356-61.

Delacour A, Nepote V, Trumpp A, Herrera PL. Nestin expression in pancreatic exocrine cell lineages. Mech Dev. 2004; 121:3-14

De Leon DD, Deng S, Madani R, Ahima RS, Drucker DJ, Stoffers DA. Role of endogenous glucagon-like peptide-1 in islet regeneration after partial pancreatectomy. Diabetes 2003; 52:365-71.

Desai BM, Oliver-Krasinski J, De Leon DD, Farzad C, Hong N, Leach SD, Stoffers DA. Preexisting pancreatic acinar cells contribute to acinar cell, but not islet beta cell, regeneration. J Clin Invest 2007; 117:971-7.

Demois A, Van Laethem JL, Quertinmont E, Delhaye M, Geerts A, Deviere J. Endogenous interleukin-10 modulates fibrosis and regeneration in experimental chronic pancreatitis Am J Physiol Gastrointest Liver Physiol 2002;282:G1105-12.

Dor Y, Brown J, Martinez OI, and Melton DA. Adult pancreatic beta-cells are formed by self-duplication rather than stem-cell differentiation. Nature 2004; 429:41-6.

Dudek RW, Lawrence Jr IE, Hill RS, Johnson RC. Induction of islet cytodifferentiation by fetal mesenchyme in adult pancreatic ductal epithelium. Diabetes 1991; 40:1041-8.

Edlund H. Pancreatic organogenesis - developmental mechanisms and implications for therapy. Nat Rev Genet 2002; 3:524-32.

Esni F, Stoffers DA, Takeuchi T, Leach SD. Origin of exocrine pancreatic cells from nestin-positive precursors in developing mouse pancreas. Mech Dev. 2004; 121:15-25.

Finegood DT, Weir GC, Bonner-Weir S. Prior streptozotocin treatment does not inhibit pancreas regeneration after 90% pancreatectomy in rats. Am J Physiol 1999; 276:E822-7.

Gittes GK. Developmental biology of the pancreas: a comprehensive review. Dev Biol. 2009 Feb 1;326(1):4-35.

Gao R, Ustinov J, Pulkkinen MA, Lundin K, Korsgren O, Otonkoski T. Characterization of endocrine progenitor cells and critical factors for their differentiation in human adult pancreatic cell culture. Diabetes 2003; 52:2007-15.

Gershengorn MC, Hardikar AA, Wei C, Geras-Raaka E, Marcus-Samuels B, Raaka BM. Epithelial-to-mesenchymal transition generates proliferative human islet precursor cells. Science 2004; 306:2261-4.

Giannoukakis N, Phillips B, Trucco M. Toward a cure for type 1 diabetes mellitus: diabetes-suppressive dendritic cells and beyond. Pediatr Diabetes 2008; 9:4-13.

Gradwohl G, Dierich A, LeMeur M, Guillemot F. Neurogenin3 is required for the development of the four endocrine cell lineages of the pancreas. Proc Natl Acad Sci USA 2000; 97:1607-11.

Gu G, Dubauskaite J, Melton DA. Direct evidence for the pancreatic lineage: NGN3+ cells are islet progenitors and are distinct from duct progenitors. Development 2002; 129:2447-57.

Gu G, Brown JR, Melton DA. Direct lineage tracing reveals the ontogeny of pancreatic cell fates during mouse embryogenesis. Mech Dev. 2003 Jan;120(1):35-43.

Hanley NA, Hanley KP, Miettinen PJ, Otonkoski T.Weighing up beta-cell mass in mice and humans: Self-renewal, progenitors or stem cells? Mol Cell Endocrinol. 2008; 288:79-85.

Hao E, Tyrberg B, Itkin-Ansari P, Lakey JR, Geron I, Monosov EZ, Barcova M, Mercola M, Levine F. Beta-cell differentiation from nonendocrine epithelial cells of the adult human pancreas. Nat Med 2006; 12:310-6.

Herold KC, Hagopian W, Auger JA, Poumian-Ruiz E, Taylor L, Donaldson D, Gitelman SE, Harlan DM, Xu D, Zivin RA, Bluestone JA. Anti-CD3 monoclonal antibody in new-onset type 1 diabetes mellitus. N Engl J Med 2002; 346:1692-8.

Herold KC, Gitelman SE, Masharani U, Hagopian W, Bisikirska B, Donaldson D, Rother K, Diamond B, Harlan DM, Bluestone JA. A single course of anti-CD3 monoclonal antibody hOKT3gamma1(Ala-Ala) results in improvement in C-peptide responses and clinical parameters for at least 2 years after onset of type 1 diabetes. Diabetes 2005; 54:1763-9.

Hess D, Li L, Martin M, Sakano S, Hill D, Strutt B, Thyssen S, Gray DA, Bhatia M. Bone marrow-derived stem cells initiate pancreatic regeneration. Nat Biotechnol 2003; 21:763-70.

Horb ME, Shen CN, Tosh D, Slack JM. Experimental conversion of liver to pancreas. Curr Biol 2003; 13:105-15.

Ianus A, Holz GG, Theise ND, Hussain MA. In vivo derivation of glucosecompetent pancreatic endocrine cells from bone marrow without evidence of cell fusion. J Clin Invest 2003; 111:843-50.

Inada A, Nienaber C, Katsuta H, Fujitani Y, Levine J, Morita R, Sharma A, Bonner-Weir S. Carbonic anhydrase II-positive pancreatic cells are progenitors for both endocrine and exocrine pancreas after birth. Proc Natl Acad Sci U S A. 2008; 105:19915-19.

Karges B, Durinovic-Bello' I, Heinze E, Boehm B, Debatin K-M, Karges W. Complete long-term recovery of beta-cell function in autoimmune type 1 diabetes after insulin treatment. Diabetes Care 2004; 27:1207-8.

Karges B, Durinovic-Bello' I, Heinze E, Debatin K-M, Boehm B, Karges W. Immunological mechanisms associated with long-term remission of human type 1 diabetes. Diabetes Metab Res Rev 2006; 22:184-9.

Kodama S, Kuhtreiber W, Fujimura S, Dale EA, Faustman DL. Islet regeneration during the reversal of autoimmune diabetes in NOD mice. Science 2003; 302:1223-27.

Kodama S, Toyonaga T, Kondo T, Matsumoto K, Tsuruzoe K, Kawashima J, Goto H, Kume K, Kume S, Sakakida M, Araki E. Enhanced expression of PDX-1 and Ngn3 by exendin-4 during beta cell regeneration in STZ-treated mice. Biochem Biophys Res Commun 2005; 327:1170-8.

Kopp JL, Dubois CL, Schaffer AE, Hao E, Shih HP, Seymour PA, Ma J, Sander M. Sox9+ ductal cells are multipotent progenitors throughout development but do not produce new endocrine cells in the normal or injured adult pancreas. Development. 2011; 138:653-665.

Krakowski ML, Kritzik MR, Jones EM, Krahl T, Lee J, Arnush M, Gu D, Sarvetnick N. Pancreatic expression of keratinocyte growth factor leads to differentiation of islet hepatocytes and proliferation of duct cells. Am J Pathol 1999;154:683-91.

Lardon J, Huyens N, Rooman I, Bouwens L. Exocrine cell transdifferentiation in dexamethasone-treated rat pancreas. Virchows Arch 2004; 444:61-5.

Lee RH, Seo MJ, Reger RL, Spees JL, Pulin AA, Olson SD, Prockop DJ. Multipotent stromal cells from human marrow home to and promote repair of pancreatic islets and renal glomeruli in diabetic NOD/scid mice. Proc Natl Acad Sci U S A 2006; 103:17438-43.

Lin G, Wang G, Liu G, Yang LJ, Chang LJ, Lue TF, Lin CS. Treatment of type 1 diabetes with adipose tissue-derived stem cells expressing pancreatic duodenal homeobox 1. Stem Cells Dev. 2009 Dec;18(10):1399-406.

Lipsett MA, Castellarin ML, Rosenberg L. Acinar plasticity: development of a novel in vitro model to study human acinar-to-duct-to-islet differentiation. Pancreas 2007; 34:452-7.

Martin-Pagola A, Sisino G, Allende G, Dominguez-Bendala J, Gianani R, Reijonen H, Nepom GT, Ricordi C, Ruiz P, Sageshima J, Ciancio G, Burke GW, Pugliese A. Insulin protein and proliferation in ductal cells in the transplanted pancreas of patients with type 1 diabetes and recurrence of autoimmunity. Diabetologia. 2008 Oct;51(10):1803-13.

Means AL, Meszoely IM, Suzuki K, Miyamoto Y, Rustgi AK, Coffey RJ Jr, Wright CV, Stoffers DA, Leach SD. Pancreatic epithelial plasticity mediated by acinar cell transdifferentiation and generation of nestin-positive intermediates. Development 2005; 132:3767-76.

Meier JJ, Bhushan A, Butler AE, Rizza RA, Butler PC. Sustained beta cell apoptosis in patients with long-standing type 1 diabetes: indirect evidence for islet regeneration? Diabetologia 2005; 48:2221-8.

Meier JJ, Lin JC, Butler AE, Galasso R, Martinez DS, Butler PC. Direct evidence of attempted beta cell regeneration in an 89-year-old patient with recent-onset type 1 diabetes. Diabetologia 2006a; 49:1838-44.

Meier JJ, Butler AE, Galasso R, Rizza RA, Butler PC. Increased islet beta cell replication adjacent to intrapancreatic gastrinomas in humans. Diabetologia 2006b; 49:2689-96.

Meier JJ, Butler AE, Saisho Y, Monchamp T, Galasso R, Bhushan A, Rizza RA, Butler PC. Beta-cell replication is the primary mechanism subserving the postnatal expansion of beta-cell mass in humans. Diabetes 2008; 57:1584-94.

Minami K, Okuno M, Miyawaki K, Okumachi A, Ishizaki K, Oyama K, Kawaguchi M, Ishizuka N, Iwanaga T, Seino S. Lineage tracing and characterization of insulin-secreting cells generated from adult pancreatic acinar cells. Proc Natl Acad Sci USA 2005; 102:15116-21.

Moriscot C, de Fraipont F, Richard MJ, Marchand M, Savatier P, Bosco D, Favrot M, Benhamou PY. Human bone marrow mesenchymal stem cells can express insulin and key transcription factors of the endocrine pancreas developmental pathway upon genetic and/or microenvironmental manipulation in vitro. Stem Cells 2005; 23:594-603.

Morton RA, Geras-Raaka E, Wilson LM, Raaka BM, Gershengorn MC. Endocrine precursor cells from mouse islets are not generated by epithelial-to-mesenchymal transition of mature beta cells. Mol Cell Endocrinol 2007; 270:87-93.

Nir T, Melton DA, Dor Y. Recovery from diabetes in mice by beta cell regeneration. J Clin Invest 2007; 117:553-61

Nishio J, Gaglia JL, Turvey SE, Campbell C, Benoist C, Mathis D. Islet recovery and reversal of murine type 1 diabetes in the absence of any infused spleen cell contribution. Science 2006; 311:1775-8.

Ogata T, Park KY, Seno M, Kojima I. Reversal of streptozotocin-induced hyperglycemia by transplantation of pseudoislets consisting of beta cells derived from ductal cells . Endocr J 2004; 51:381-6.

Oh SH, Muzzonigro TM, Bae SH, LaPlante JM, Hatch HM, Petersen BE. Adult bone marrow-derived cells trans-differentiating into insulin producing cells for the treatment of type I diabetes. Lab Invest 2004; 84:607-17.

Pearson KW, Scott D, Torrance B. Effects of partial surgical pancreatectomy in rats. I. Pancreatic regeneration. Gastroenterology 1977; 72:469-73.

Piper K, Ball SG, Turnpenny LW, Brickwood S, Wilson DI, Hanley NA. Beta-cell differentiation during human development does not rely on nestin-positive precursors: implications for stem cell-derived replacement therapy. Diabetologia 2002; 45:1045-7.

Phillips JM, O'Reilly L, Bland C, Foulis AK, Cooke A.Patients with chronic pancreatitis have islet progenitor cells in their ducts, but reversal of overt diabetes in NOD mice by anti-CD3 shows no evidence for islet regeneration. Diabetes. 2007 Mar;56(3):634-40.

Ramiya VK, Maraist M, Arfors KE, Schatz DA, Peck AB, Cornelius JG. Reversal of insulin-dependent diabetes using islets generated in vitro from pancreatic stem cells. Nat Med 2000; 6:278-82.

Rao MS, Subbarao V, Reddy J K. Induction of hepatocytes in the pancreas of copper-depleted rats following copper repletion. Cell Differ 1986; 18:109–17.

Rao MS, Reddy J K. Hepatic transdifferentiation in the pancreas. Semin Cell Biol 1995; 6:151-6.

Rood PP, Bottino R, Balamurugan AN, Fan Y, Cooper DK, Trucco M. Facilitating physiologic self-regeneration: a step beyond islet cell replacement. Pharm Res 2006; 23:227-242.

Rooman I, Heremans Y, Heimberg H, Bouwens L. Modulation of rat pancreatic acinoductal transdifferentiation and expression of PDX-1 in vitro. Diabetologia 2000; 43:907-14.

Rooman I, Lardon J, Bouwens L. Gastrin stimulates beta cell neogenesis and increases islet mass from transdifferentiated but not from normal exocrine pancreas tissue. Diabetes 2002; 51:686-90.

Rooman I and Bouwens L. Combined gastrin and epidermal growth factor treatment induces islet regeneration and restores normoglycaemia in C57Bl6/J mice treated with alloxan. Diabetologia 2004; 47:259-65.

Rosenberg L, Rafaeloff R, Clas D, Kakugawa Y, Pittenger G, Vinik AI, Duguid WP. Induction of islet cell differentiation and new islet formation in the hamster— further support for a ductular origin. Pancreas 1996; 13:38-46.

Ryan EA, Korbutt GS, Toth E, Warnock GL, Kneteman NM, Rajotte RV. Islet transplantation in seven patients with type 1 diabetes mellitus using a glucocorticoid-free immunosuppressive regimen. N Engl J Med 2000; 343:230-8.

Ryu S, Kodama S, Ryu K, Schoenfeld DA, Faustman DL. Reversal of established autoimmune diabetes by restoration of endogenous beta cell function. J Clin Invest 2001; 108:63-72.

Shapiro AM, Lakey JR, Ryan EA, Korbutt GS, Toth E, Warnock GL, Kneteman NM, Rajotte RV. Islet transplantation in seven patients with type 1 diabetes mellitus using a glucocorticoid-free immunosuppressive regimen. N Engl J Med. 2000 Jul 27;343(4):230-8.

Schwitzgebel VM, Scheel DW, Conners JR, Kalamaras J, Lee JE, Anderson DJ, Sussel L, Johnson JD, German MS. Expression of neurogenin3 reveals an islet cell precursor population in the pancreas. Development 2000; 127:3533-42.

Shen CN, Slack JM, Tosh D. Molecular basis of transdifferentiation of pancreas to liver. Nat Cell Biol 2000; 2:879-87.

Stanger BZ, Tanaka AJ, Melton DA. Organ size is limited by the number of embryonic progenitor cells in the pancreas but not the liver. Nature 2007; 445:886-91.

Suarez-Pinzon WL, Yan Y, Power R, Brand SJ, Rabinovitch A. Combination therapy with epidermal growth factor and gastrin increases beta-cell mass and reverses hyperglycemia in diabetic NOD mice. Diabetes 2005a; 54:2596-601.

Suarez-Pinzon WL, Lakey JR, Brand SJ, Rabinovitch A. Combination therapy with epidermal growth factor and gastrin induces neogenesis of human islet {beta}-cells from pancreatic duct cells and an increase in functional {beta}-cell mass. J Clin Endocrinol Metab 2005b; 90:3401-9

Suri A, Calderon B, Esparza TJ, Frederick K, Bittner P, Unanue ER. Immunological reversal of autoimmune diabetes without hematopoietic replacement of beta cells. Science 2006; 311:1778-80.

Szkudelski T. The mechanism of alloxan and streptozotocin action in B cells of the rat pancreas. Physiol Res 2001; 50:537-46.

Thorel F, Népote V, Avril I, Kohno K, Desgraz R, Chera S, Herrera PL Conversion of adult pancreatic alpha-cells to beta-cells after extreme beta-cell loss. Nature. 2010 Apr 22;464(7292):1149-54.

Tourrel C, Bailbe′ D, Meile M, Kergoat M, and Portha B. Glucagon-like peptide-1 and its long-acting analog exendin-4 stimulate β-cell neogenesis in streptozotocin-treated newborn rats resulting in persistently improved glucose homeostasis at adult age. Diabetes 2001; 50:1562-70.

Treutelaar MK, Skidmore JM, Dias-Leme CL, Hara M, Zhang L, Simeone D, Martin DM, Burant CF. Nestin-lineage cells contribute to the microvasculature but not endocrine cells of the islet. Diabetes 2003; 52:2503-12.

Trivedi HL, Vanikar AV, Thakker U, Firoze A, Dave SD, Patel CN, Patel JV, Bhargava AB, Shankar V. Human adipose tissue-derived mesenchymal stem cells combined with hematopoietic stem cell transplantation synthesize insulin. Transplant Proc. 2008 May;40(4):1135-9.

Trucco M. Regeneration of the pancreatic beta cell. J Clin Invest 2005; 115:5-12.

Voltarelli JC, Couri CE, Stracieri AB, Oliveira MC, Moraes DA, Pieroni F, Coutinho M, Malmegrim KC, Foss-Freitas MC, Simões BP, Foss MC, Squiers E, Burt RK. Autologous nonmyeloablative hematopoietic stem cell transplantation in newly diagnosed type 1 diabetes mellitus. JAMA 2007; 297:1568-76.

Wang RN, Kloppel G, Bouwens L. Duct- to islet-cell differentiation and islet growth in the pancreas of duct-ligated adult rats. Diabetologia 1995; 38:1405-11.

Wang RN, Bouwens L, Kloppel G. β-Cell growth in adolescent and adult rats treated with streptozotocin during the neonatal period. Diabetologia 1996; 39:548–57.

Wang S, Jensen JN, Seymour PA, et al. Sustained Neurog3 expression in hormone-expressing islet cells is required for endocrine maturation and function. Proc Natl Acad Sci USA 2009; 106:9715–9720.

White P, May CL, Lamounier RN, Brestelli JE, Kaestner KH. Defining pancreatic endocrine precursors and their descendants. Diabetes 2008; 57:654-68.

Yang L, Li S, Hatch H, Ahrens K, Cornelius JG, Petersen BE, Peck AB. In vitro trans-differentiation of adult hepatic stem cells into pancreatic endocrine hormone-producing cells. Proc Natl Acad Sci USA 2002; 99:8078-83.

Yatoh S, Dodge R, Akashi T, Omer A, Sharma A, Weir GC, Bonner-Weir S. Differentiation of affinity-purified human pancreatic duct cells to beta-cells. Diabetes. 2007 Jul;56(7):1802-9. Epub 2007 May 1.

Xu X, D'Hoker J, Stange G, Bonne S, De Leu N, Xiao X, Van de Casteele M, Mellitzer G, Ling Z, Pipeleers D, Bouwens L, Scharfmann R, Gradwohl G, Heimberg H. Beta cells can be generated from endogenous progenitors in injured adult mouse pancreas. Cell 2008; 132:197–207.

Yin D, Tao J, Lee DD, Shen J, Hara M, Lopez J, Kuznetsov A, Philipson LH, Chong AS. Recovery of islet beta-cell function in streptozotocin-induced diabetic mice: an indirect role for the spleen. Diabetes 2006; 55:3256-63.

Zalzman M, Gupta S, Giri RK, Berkovich I, Sappal BS, Karnieli O, Zern MA, Fleischer N, Efrat S. Reversal of hyperglycemia in mice by using human expandable insulin-producing cells differentiated from fetal liver progenitor cells. Proc Natl Acad Sci USA 2003; 100:7253-8.

Zaret KS. Liver specification and early morphogenesis. Mech Dev 2000; 92:83-88.

Zorina TD, Subbotin VM, Bertera S, Alexander AM, Haluszczak C, Gambrell B, Bottino R, Styche AJ, Trucco M. Recovery of the endogenous beta cell function in the NOD model of autoimmune diabetes. Stem Cells 2003; 21:377-88.

Zulewski H, Abraham EJ, Gerlach MJ, Daniel PB, Moritz W, Muller B, Vallejo M, Thomas MK, Habener JF. Multipotential nestin-positive stem cells isolated from adult pancreatic islets differentiate ex vivo into pancreatic endocrine, exocrine and hepatic phenotypes. Diabetes 2001; 50:521-33.

6

Cell Replacement Therapy: The Rationale for Encapsulated Porcine Islet Transplantation

Stephen J. M. Skinner, Paul L. J. Tan, Olga Garkavenko,
Marija Muzina, Livia Escobar and Robert B. Elliott
Living Cell Technologies (NZ) Ltd
New Zealand

1. Introduction

Among the problems posed by chronic diseases today, one of the most daunting is that posed by diabetes mellitus, which is a very significant public health problem resulting in substantial morbidity and mortality (American Diabetes Association, 2011). With the increasing life-expectancy of the world's population, increasing exposure to environmental trigger factors, the rising incidence of obesity, and lifestyle changes such as unhealthy diets and decreased physical activity, the prevalence of diabetes has risen dramatically over recent years and is now reaching epidemic proportions globally. This rapid increase is a significant cause for concern, with an additional 7 million diagnosed each year (International Diabetes Federation, 2011). Diabetes is now the fourth or fifth leading cause of death in most developed countries (International Diabetes Federation 2000). Globally, it is estimated that more than 200 million adults now have diabetes and this number is expected to increase alarmingly in the coming decades. By the year 2025, it is estimated that almost 333 million people will have the disease (International Diabetes Federation 2006).

Type 1 (insulin-dependent) diabetes accounts for 5% to 10% of all diagnosed cases. In 2003, approximately 4.9 million people (0.09% of the world's population) were estimated to have type 1 disease, with Europe having the highest number of sufferers (1.27 million) followed by North America (1.04 million) and Southeast Asia (0.91 million). The highest prevalence of type 1 diabetes was in North America (0.25%) followed by Europe (0.19%) (International Diabetes Federation 2006). In 2002, there were an estimated 0.9 to 1.2 million people with type 1 diabetes in the USA (American Diabetes Association 2006). The incidence in recent years may have accelerated alarmingly as shown in a recent study from Finland where the rate increased from 31.4 per 100,000 per year in 1980 to 64.2 per 100,000 per year in 2005 (Harjutsalo et al, 2008).

In New Zealand, the incidence of type 1 diabetes has doubled in the last 15 years, reflecting international trends. In 2003, the estimated prevalence of type 1 disease among the population aged <25 years was 0.18%, with the total number of sufferers in this age range numbering 2540. The majority, 85% (2158 people), were of European descent, while 9% were Maori, 2.9% were Pacific peoples, and 3.0% were Asian (Wu et al. 2005).

Although the life-expectancy of patients with type 1 (insulin-dependent) diabetes mellitus has vastly improved since the introduction of insulin, the ability of insulin injections to reliably prevent wide fluctuations in blood glucose levels is often inadequate and many patients develop complications of the disease. These complications cause considerable disability and suffering, and their management has major morbidity and cost consequences. High blood glucose concentrations not only cause acute metabolic problems but also lasting and accumulative damage by chemical reaction (glycation, e.g. Haemoglobin A1c) with a host of physiologically critical proteins. Hence the long term damage to the cardiovascular system, eye, kidney, heart and nervous system. On the other hand, low blood glucose levels, known as hypoglycaemic episodes, are usually perceived by the patient and treated by ingesting glucose or food. But in a significant minority of patients, hypoglycaemic episodes are not perceived and may cause loss of consciousness. These can lead to fatal outcomes for the patient and sometimes for others, such as in situations where the patient is in control of a moving vehicle.

For these reasons, the investment in, and search for, newer treatments that can provide a 'cure' for the disease with normoglycaemic control, or that at least minimizes the damaging effects of extremely high and low blood glucose excursions with markedly better control of metabolic disturbances, has been energetically pursued. In terms of health economics, the benefits in preventing eye, heart and kidney diseases would more than justify a substantial investment in such research and development (Beckwith et al. 2010).

1.1 Background and rationale for cell transplantation

Insulin is essential for normal glucose metabolism. It is released by the beta-islet cells of the pancreas in response to rising blood glucose levels. The feedback mechanisms involved provide a precise, finely tuned response, keeping blood glucose at a concentration of around 4.5mM. Type 1 diabetes is an endocrine disorder caused by autoimmune destruction of the beta-islet cells leading to insulin deficiency. Treatment by injecting various commercially produced insulins subcutaneously, while life-sustaining, can not provide the control of blood glucose provided by a full complement of functional islets.

In order to optimize the control of blood sugar and thus prevent the acute and chronic damage, the most likely way to improve these outcomes is to replace the patient's pancreatic islets with a new pancreas or new islets. Transplanting a whole new pancreas is a very demanding procedure that requires many resources and is found to be less than practical.

1.1.1 Porcine islet cell transplants

Among the newer treatment strategies that have been proposed, transplantation of pancreatic islets, obtained either from other human or animal donors, has received considerable attention worldwide. This is because islet transplantation can restore not only the insulin-secreting unit, but also the precise insulin release in response to rising blood glucose and multiple signals arising within and beyond the islets.

Because human islet transplantation is limited by the shortage of human islet tissue, human embryonic stem cells or induced pluripotent stem (iPS) cells from the patient are being developed into transplantable insulin producing cells. Recent reports indicate that iPS cells may not be transplantable into mice of the same strain without immune rejection (Zhao et al, 2011). The US FDA guidelines highlight concerns that stem cell derived lines may undergo malignant transformation or develop into teratomas after transplantation (Fink et al 2009).

While stem cell line-derived insulin producing cells are still at an early stage of research, pig islets are viewed as a promising alternative since: (a) the supply of pig pancreatic cells can be increased by breeding more donor animals; (b) pig and human insulins have close structural and biological similarities; and (c) physiological glucose levels in pigs are similar to those in humans (Elliott, 2011). The rationale for this treatment approach (termed 'xenotransplantation') is that the implanted pig islets have the potential to mimic the normal physiological insulin response in type 1 diabetics, such that near-normal blood glucose levels may be achievable without insulin injections or with reduced requirements. As a consequence, long-term diabetes complications may be prevented and patients should experience less hypoglycaemia than they do with the currently recommended 'intensive' insulin regimens. Thus the need and rationale for improved diabetes control is clear but the effectiveness and practicality of islet transplants, whether from human, porcine or other sources, has yet to be firmly established. As with any transplanted tissue, organ or cells, whether from human or animal, the host immune system must be considered. Immunosuppression has been studied and used extensively in islet transplant patients. An increasingly successful alternative is immune-isolation, that is to isolate the transplanted cells in capsules or devices that exclude immune cells and antibodies, but allow the free diffusion of glucose, insulin, nutrients and dissolved oxygen and carbon dioxide. The latter approach eliminates the risks associated with immunosuppression.

Some of the **key issues** in implementing **porcine islet xenotransplantation** in the treatment of patients with Type 1 diabetes are:

1.1.1.1 Have 'proof of concept' pre-clinical experiments demonstrated sufficiently effective improvement in the control of Type 1 diabetes in experimental animals?

1.1.1.2 Have the risks to the patient's safety been sufficiently evaluated, including: (a) the risk of transmission of infectious diseases; and (b) risks to the individual from the transplant procedure itself, including allergic reactions and other immunological responses that might compromise the success of the procedure.

1.1.1.3 How rejection of the cells by the recipient's immune system can be effectively prevented.

1.1.1.4 Whether porcine islet xenotransplants can restore, at least partially, the normal regulation of blood glucose (as reflected in decreased insulin requirements and decrease in HbA1c), and the number of islets needed to achieve this.

1.1.1.5 The duration of effectiveness of the transplanted islets (i.e. whether they remain effective over a sufficiently prolonged period to justify the inconvenience and cost of the procedure), and the extent to which the patient's well-being is enhanced and long-term diabetes complications are prevented.

1.1.1.6 Ethical considerations, including cultural, ethical and spiritual dimensions, informed consent issues, and measures to ensure animal welfare.

1.1.1.7 If clinical trials are judged successful by rigorous independent review, will resources to expand the availability of the treatment be provided by commercial and/or government investment?

2. Pre-clinical studies of porcine islet xenotransplantation in non-human primates and rodents

The main body of information from our laboratory on the efficacy and safety of current preparations of porcine islets is derived from studies with islets sourced from Auckland

Islands Pigs. The Auckland Islands (AI) strain is unique due to its isolation for more than 150 years on a sub-antarctic island and is free of pathogens commonly found in other pig herds. These animals are being bred in custom-constructed pathogen-free facilities for transplant purposes and are discussed in detail later in this chapter.

2.1 Studies in non-human primates

The first exploration of primate diabetes treatments with encapsulated porcine islets was undertaken by Sun Y et al (1996) in Toronto, Canada. This pioneering group prepared islets and enclosed them in alginate-polylysine capsules in the early 1980s (Sun AM et al, 1984; Sun Y et al, 1993). They were able to find a number of diabetic cynomolgus monkeys that were ideal for testing these encapsulated porcine islets. These animals responded very well to their encapsulated porcine islets transplant, with significant improvement of their diabetes for 120-800 days. This remarkable achievement was based on decades of research by AM Sun, Y Sun and their colleagues that began in the early 1970s.

In a later non-human primate study the clinical efficacy and safety of an encapsulated neonatal porcine islet preparation was investigated in cynomolgus monkeys with streptozotocin (STZ)-induced diabetes. The islet toxin streptozotocin is injected into the monkeys and causes insulin deficiency. Sixteen monkeys with the disease established were separated into two groups of 8: one group was given microcapsules containing living porcine islets and the other was given the same microcapsules but without islets in them. They received the microcapsule transplants in two doses three months apart by injection into the peritoneal cavity (Elliott et al, 2005). No immunosuppressive drugs were administered.

In the group that received capsules containing islets, evidence of clinical activity was noted at 12 and 24 weeks after the first transplant; the reduction of the mean weekly insulin requirement relative to the control was 36% (p=.02) and 43% (p=.01), respectively at these time points. Blood glucose in the two groups were maintained to similar levels indicating that the reduced requirement for insulin injections in the treated group was significant. Both the islet-treated and control groups tolerated the transplant procedures well. No hypoglycaemic episodes or other adverse events were observed in the islet-treated group. There were no differences between the two groups of monkeys in body weight or hematology and liver enzyme parameters. Two deaths occurred, one in the islet-treated group from lobar pneumonia with disseminated lung abscesses at 13 weeks after the first transplant (despite systemic antibiotic therapy), and the other in the control (empty microcapsules) group as a result of a stroke that followed the development of hypoglycaemia due to failure to consume food after regular insulin therapy.

At terminal autopsy of these monkeys (Figure 1), no gross inflammatory reactions to either encapsulated islets or the empty microcapsules were noted in the animals' peritoneal cavities. The organs (liver, spleen, stomach, intestines, kidney, heart, lungs and brain) appeared normal .

In another streptozotocin diabetic monkey study, where encapsulated adult porcine islets were used, and thus more similar to the adult human islet isolations, diabetes was successfully treated without immunosuppression (Dufrane et al, 2010). However, although efficacy was demonstrated with encapsulated islets, they lost their function after 2 weeks. Successful glucose control was achieved for 6 months using 'monolayer cellular devices' containing up to 30,000 Islet Equivalents (IEQ)/Kg of monkey weight, implanted in the abdominal subcutaneous tissue.

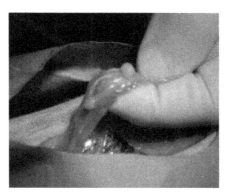

Fig. 1. Clusters of encapsulated porcine islets attached to the mesentery of a cynomolgus monkey.

In contrast, Hering et al (2006) demonstrated that unencapsulated naked porcine islets, injected into the portal vein of the liver, could be used to reverse diabetes for 100 days in cynomolgus monkeys provided comprehensive immunosuppression was given.

2.2 Studies in small animal models of diabetes

The biocompatibility of encapsulated porcine islets and a dose-dependent effect on glycaemic control have been demonstrated in STZ-diabetic rats. Those that developed diabetes were separated into four groups that received intraperitoneal transplants of encapsulated neonatal porcine islets at increasing dosage. The doses, measured in IEQs, were 3000 IEQ (n = 7), 6000 IEQ (n = 6), 12,000 IEQ (n = 6) or 18,000 IEQ (n = 6) of the standard preparation or empty alginate microcapsules (n = 12), insulin requirements were significantly reduced in rats given the higher doses. Prior to transplantation, all rats had comparable blood glucose control with daily isophane insulin injections. At week 12 after transplantation, the reduction in the weekly average daily insulin dose was significantly greater in rats given doses of 18,000 IEQs ($p < 0.01$) or 12,000 IEQs ($p < 0.05$) compared with control animals that received empty alginate microcapsules. Insulin independence was attained in 3 of 6 rats given 18,000 IEQs, 3 of 6 given 12,000 IEQs, 2 of 6 given 6000 IEQs. 1 of the 12 diabetic rats given empty alginate microcapsules did recover, a case of spontaneous islet regeneration which is a known confounding factor in small animal studies (Figure 2).

Similar encouraging results were seen when streptozotocin-induced diabetic mice and genetically predisposed diabetic NOD mice were treated with encapsulated islets.

Thus, immunosuppression may not be necessary when treating diabetes if the islets are efficiently sealed inside capsules or devices with semipermeable membranes. The capsule or device outer membranes exclude immune cells and immunoglobulins but must allow efficient diffusion of glucose, insulin, all nutrients and gases (oxygen, CO_2) necessary for cell nutrition.

This information about the efficacy of encapsulated islets and their tolerance by animal recipients, including some earlier human clinical studies, were assembled in great detail for the submission of applications to the National Regulatory Clinical Trial Agencies of several countries including New Zealand, Russia and Argentina, where the applications were successful, albeit with stringent conditions attached.

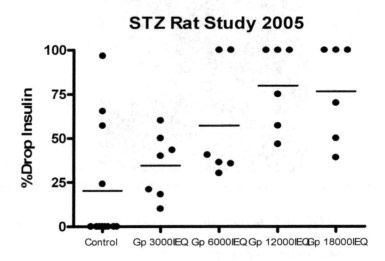

Fig. 2. **Percentage reductions in weekly averages of daily insulin doses 12 weeks after transplantation.** Each point represents individual rats. Reduction of the insulin dose is calculated as the percentage of the baseline average daily insulin dose in the week prior to transplantation. In the three higher doses eight animals were insulin-independent at 12 weeks. The bars represent the average % reduction in insulin dose for the respective groups.

3. Xenotransplantation: Minimizing risks to patient's safety

The introduction of porcine islet transplantation has been delayed by concerns relating to the possible transmission of pig diseases to humans via the transplanted cells and the risk of introducing micro-organisms during cell processing and encapsulation. There is also a potential risk of transmitting porcine disease to close contacts of the human recipient and to the wider community. The risks of infection from the donor animal can be minimized by controlling the breed, source of and health status of the donor animals, with ongoing screening and quarantining. The risk of introducing micro-organisms during cell processing can be minimized by ensuring strict aseptic technique when isolating and encapsulating the islets.

3.1 Risk of infections ('xenoses') resulting from transfer of pig micro-organisms to human recipients

The risk of bacterial, fungal and parasitic infections can be minimized by the use of Designated Pathogen-Free pig herds and by monitoring and treating sows for such infections before pancreatic islets are extracted from their progeny (Garkavenko et al. 2008a). However, this approach will not eliminate porcine endogenous retrovirus sequences (PERVs), which are present in the germline of all pigs (including common New Zealand pig breeds) but cause no known infection in the species. The possible transmission of these retroviruses to humans, and their as yet unknown consequences in recipients, have given rise to some concerns over the safety of xenotransplantation, particularly in view of reports that PERVs from certain pig strains can infect human cells in vitro (Patience et al. 1997;

Martin et al. 1998a) and that immune-incompetent SCID (severe combined immunodeficiency) mice may develop either microchimerism or infection in vivo (van der Laan et al. 2000). The in vitro findings have, however, been shown to be strain-specific (Patience 2001; Clemenceau et al. 2001; Oldmixon et al. 2002) and cells from animals studied by LCT have not shown retrovirus infectivity. Moreover, no evidence of PERV transmission has been detected over 200 patients who have been exposed to pig cells or tissues and tested for evidence of PERV infection using sensitive detection methods (Wynyard et al. 2011; Garkavenko et al. 2008b; Denner 2003; Dinsmore et al. 2000; Heneine et al. 1998; Heneine et al. 2001; Irgang et al. 2003; Martin et al. 1998b; Paradis et al. 1999; Patience et al. 1998; Tacke et al. 2001). In 2 New Zealand diabetic patients who received encapsulated porcine islet xenotransplants, no evidence of PERV proviral DNA or RNA was detectable in white blood cells and plasma up to 6 years after the transplant, and neither patient was found to have suffered any ill health as a result of the procedure (Elliott et al. 2000; Garkavenko et al. 2004a). Similarly, in 4 other patients who received unencapsulated islets in similar studies in NZ, no infection has been found in a follow-up time of up to 9 years (Garkavenko et al. 2004a). More recently one patient shown to have some functional transplanted porcine islets after 9.5 years was shown to be free of PERV.

3.2 Porcine endogenous retrovirus
In several other studies, no evidence of PERV transmission was found among recipients of porcine clotting factor VIII (Hyate:C) in a study of 88 haemophiliacs, despite the fact that all manufactured batches of porcine factor VIII concentrate used by patients were subsequently tested and shown to contain PERV RNA (Heneine et al. 2001). Similarly, no evidence of PERV DNA was found in 2 renal dialysis patients whose circulation had been linked extracorporeally to pig kidneys (Patience et al. 1998).

3.3 Auckland Islands pigs
A further refinement of the source herd has been obtained by the use of pigs derived from a colony abandoned on the Auckland Islands about 150 years ago. These animals are free of all measured viruses except the retrovirus (PERV), and are being bred for xenotransplant purposes in a purpose-built facility. Although PERV cannot be removed from the porcine genome, there is strong evidence that it is not functional in the Auckland Island Pig strain and is not expressed under any of the recommended testing conditions. This strain is now termed a "Null Pig Strain" suitable as a source of tissues for xenotransplantation (Wynyard et al, 2011).

3.4 Neonatal pigs
Nevertheless, the selection of donor animals that do not transmit infectious PERV continues to be important and has to be linked with the selection of donor animals bred in isolation and screened to exclude infection with other exogenous microbes. The use of donor neonatal piglets rather than adult pigs also has the advantage of limiting the exposure time of donor newborn animals to acquired infections as they age.

3.5 No genetic modification
The selection of piglets without genetic modification as a source of tissue offers another advantage. In attempting to prevent immune rejection of porcine tissue, genetically-modified

pigs with the gene for the xeno-antigen alpha-gal eliminated have been developed. However, with the use of alpha-gal gene knock-out pig donor cells, PERV-exiting cells are not enveloped (coated) with the alpha-gal antigen and hence are not recognised as 'foreign' by the recipient's blood complement system (Fujita et al. 2003). It is known that normal human serum contains natural anti-alpha-gal antibodies that inactivate retrovirus (Rother et al. 1995).

3.6 Intact immune system
The maintenance of an intact immune system is an important safety factor. Immunosuppressive drugs are commonly used to prevent immune rejection of transplanted organs and cells. However, the use of alginate-encapsulated islets is intended to allow the survival of transplanted islets and their continued secretion of insulin in the recipient, without the need for life-long immunosuppressive drugs.

3.7 Surveillance
Long-term surveillance of recipients of porcine islet xenotransplants and testing of the transplant material for the presence of PERVs, using highly specific and highly sensitive assays developed for this purpose will always be an integral part of strategies proposed for future clinical trials. This safeguard, which is a necessary precaution recommended for clinical trials of xenotransplantation by authorities in various countries including the USA (US Department of Health & Human Services 2002, 2003), Australia (National Health & Medical Research Council 2002), UK (United Kingdom Xenotransplantation Interim Regulatory Authority 1998, 1999), and Canada (Therapeutic Products Programme, Health Protection Branch, Health Canada 1999), is designed to allow early detection of infectious disease transmission, and includes standard hospital infection control measures to limit the spread of such an infection should one be detected. These carefully structured and independently monitored precautionary measures are now mandatory for all patients enrolled in clinical trials of porcine islet (or other cells) xeno-transplantation and are put in place before the trials begin.

4. Minimizing risks of contaminating with infective agents during product preparation

After the pancreas is removed from the donor animal it must be treated with a series of procedures to isolate the insulin-producing islets, substantially free of the proteolytic exocrine tissue which makes up the majority of the pancreas. It is then kept in cell culture medium and tested for microbiological contamination and for its ability to produce insulin in response to stimulation by exposure to a glucose challenge. This must be done with every batch of islets produced for clinical use. The manufacturing facility, records and staff training need to be regularly inspected by expert teams from government health agencies. Samples of islets from every batch and biopsies of pancreas, heart, lung, spleen, kidney and brain tissues, also blood samples, from every donor animal must also be stored frozen at -80 Centigrade as historical resources that can be retrospectively analyzed, in case of later complications in patients.

5. Preventing rejection of islets by the recipient's immune system

The vulnerability of transplanted islets to the recipient's immune system has been a major scientific challenge and a barrier to successful islet transplantation. The transplanted cells face not only Immediate Blood Mediated Immune Rejection (IBMIR) but also immune attack from a variety of cells which may result in loss of function and cell death. Two approaches are currently used to overcome this:

5.1 Immunosuppressive drugs

The administration of immunosuppressive drugs before a cell transplant and for the rest of the life of the patient. These procedures to manage the immune competence of the patient are essential in greater or lesser forms for all transplants of naked cells except perhaps those that are sourced from the patient (autotransplantation) or from a perfectly matched donor. Even then, any patient-derived cells (e.g. endogenous adult stem cells) that may be induced to mature into functional islet cells may be attacked by auto-immune processes engendered during the auto-immune destruction of the patient's original pancreatic islets, since the newly matured islet cells carry essentially the same antigens (Zhao et al, 2011).

A suppressed immune system, with lower surveillance of foreign antigens, can provide an opportunity for infection. Immunosuppressive agents may also prevent the essential immune surveillance that detects and destroys most cellular chance mutations that lead to cancer cell growth. This has been a serious concern about stem cell transplants that may contain a small number of viable undifferentiated cells that can exhibit uncontrolled replication and form tumours (Bauer SR, 2010).

5.2 Immunoisolation

Immunoprotection of the transplanted cells via the use of a semipermeable membrane that acts as a protective barrier (Figures 3a and 3b). The latter technique appears to be a viable approach, the principle being that the permeability of the outer capsule membrane allows smaller molecules such as glucose, dissolved oxygen and carbon dioxide and all nutrients to penetrate into the capsule and reach the islets. The membrane is constructed to allow insulin and most small proteins to be released out into the bloodstream, but it does not allow the passage of large immune cells or antibodies that would cause rejection of the islets. Indeed, the islets can survive well inside such systems. There are several approaches to providing this immunoprotection which are:

- Encapsulation of the islets within a bead of alginate gel, which is then coated with poly-L-ornithine, poly-L-lysine or some other material to provide perm-selectivity and strength (Calafiore 2006; Weir & Bonner-Weir 1997).
- Tubular diffusion chambers which consist of long (up to 20mm) tubular membranes of 5-6mm inner diameter.
- Perfusion devices (also known as vascularised artificial pancreases) which consist of an outer housing 90 mm in diameter and 20 mm in width that is connected surgically to the patient's vascular system so that it is fed by an artery and drained by a vein. Islets in both perfusion devices and diffusion chambers are usually immobilised with alginate or agar to prevent settling and to provide uniform distribution of nutrients and dissolved oxygen and carbob-dioxide (Maki et al. 1995).
- Co-transplantation with 'nursery' cells such as testicular Sertoli cells which have been claimed to protect against immune-mediated rejection via the production of the immunomodulator TGF-beta1 (transforming growth factor-beta 1) (Suarez-Pinzon et al. 2000; Valdes-Gonzalez, 2005).

Of these approaches, the strategy selected by Living Cell Technologies for intensive investigation is encapsulation of the islets in 'minimal volume' alginate microcapsules developed at the Department of Internal Medicine and Endocrine & Metabolic Services, University of Perugia in Italy (Calafiore 1997; Calafiore et al. 1999). Alginate-encapsulated porcine islets have been extensively investigated in experimental animals both with and without diabetes, and in a small number of human diabetic subjects.

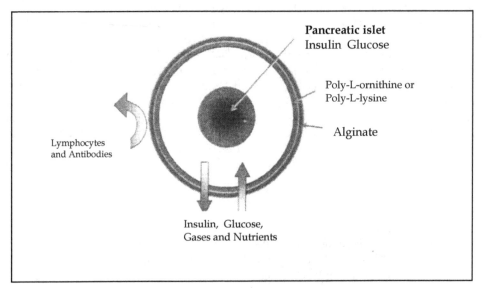

Fig. 3a. **The concept of encapsulation:** enclosure of the islet in an alginate/poly-L-ornithine or poly-L-lysine membrane that is permeable to glucose, nutrients and insulin, but not to lymphocytes and antibodies, provides protection against immune destruction of the cells.

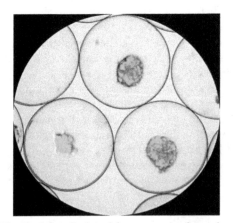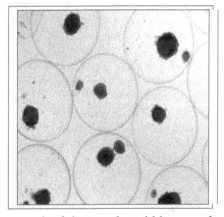

Fig. 3b. **Islets isolated from neonatal porcine pancreas in alginate-polyornithine capsules.** Green fluorescent stain (acridine orange) demonstrating viable cells and red tetra-methyl-rhodamine-ethyl ester (TMRE) stain for mitochodria of viable cells.

6. Alginate-poly-l-ornithine capsules

These capsules, as shown in **Figure 3**, have been the method of choice for many laboratories including our own (Opara & Kendall, 2002; Hernandez et al, 2010; Elliott, 2011). Their biocompatibility is critical to their in vivo efficacy and durability. Alginate is derived from seaweed and has to be highly purified to remove contaminating heavy metals, proteins and endotoxins. Different sources of alginate vary in their chemical composition with different ratios of their main constituents of mannuronic acid and guluronic acids and hence their physical gel properties. The consistency of the microcapsules with respect to their size, wall thickness, compressibility and cell occupancy has to be ensured from batch to batch. The central core containing the islets is liquefied alginate and the outer surface is a membrane formed by ionic interaction between positively charged poly-L-ornithine (or poly-L-lysine) and negatively charged alginate. Properly made, the membrane is remarkably robust (Skinner et al, 2009).

Since up to a million capsules may be required for treatment, the production must be reproducible, using durable equipment to Good Manufacturing Practice (GMP) standards. The main components are carefully engineered flow-through needles which generate reproducible sized droplets impelled by air 'knife' flows or electrostatic mechanisms (Hernandez et al, 2010).

7. Ethical considerations

Embodied in the wider concepts of informed consent are considerations that young people and the old or infirm are not exploited. Peoples with poor understanding of the language and scientific concepts involved are not to be misled. Religious and cultural feelings are not to be disregarded in potential recipients who find it difficult to express their reluctance to participate in the presence of those whom they perceive as medical authorities.

The ethical issues of xenotransplantation include concerns over the cultural, ethical and spiritual dimensions of xenotransplantation; the ethical acceptability of using animals to provide tissue for human transplantation; how the welfare of donor animals can be adequately protected and their suffering reduced; and how the welfare and interests of patients in early clinical xenotransplantation trials can be protected. These issues have been addressed by the Nuffield Council on Bioethics in the United Kingdom (1996) and, in New Zealand, the Bioethics Council, Toi te Taiao (2005). The latter body concluded that prohibition of xenotransplantation could not be justified, given the compelling human need argument, and that it should be allowed to develop in New Zealand, with that development being demonstrably shaped by the resolution and management of safety issues by a competent authority; the relationship between the majority European culture and indigenous Maori people and the cultural, ethical and spiritual factors that matter to most New Zealanders.

In recent years, a number of recommendations to protect the ethical integrity of future human research have been made by various regulatory authorities. Key issues in the conduct of clinical trials of xenotransplantation include the requirement to provide patients with an explanation of the likely success, its attendant risks, and the subsequent quality-of-life that can be expected when obtaining their informed consent, and informing patients that their consent to the procedure includes consent to ongoing post-transplantation microbiological monitoring.

Other international spiritual organisations have given their opinions about xenotransplantation. The Vatican in Rome, Italy have considered xenotransplantation in some depth and suggest it is worthy of serious consideration (Vatican, 2011). Jewish organisations have given qualified support to xenotransplantation as a life enhancing procedure while Muslim opinion is unclear but has generally been negative because of the status of pigs in the religious context.

8. Clinical experiences with xenotransplantation in treating type 1 diabetes

Many of the considerations in the preceding part of this chapter have been opinion and experiment seeking to determine the safety and efficacy of xenotransplantation for Type 1 diabetes in animal models. These animal models are perhaps more or less imperfect as true reflections of the human condition of Type 1 diabetes. It is therefore of critical relevance to review all data and experiences relating to the small number of human exposures to xenotransplanted porcine islets and other cells.

Six patients were treated in 1995-6 with either encapsulated or unencapsulated neonatal porcine islets. One of these, a 41-yr-old Caucasian male with type 1 diabetes for 18 years was given an intraperitoneal transplant of alginate-encapsulated porcine islets at the dose of 15,000 islet equivalents (IEQs)/kg bodyweight (total dose 1,305,000 IEQs) via laparoscopy. By 12 weeks following the transplant, his insulin dose was significantly reduced by 30% (p = 0.0001). The insulin dose returned to the pre-transplant level at week 49. Improvement in glycaemic control continued as reflected by total glycated haemoglobin of 7.8% at 14 months from a pre-transplant level of 9.3%. Urinary porcine C-peptide, derived from the porcine pro-insulin precursor, peaked at 4 months (9.5 ng/ml) and remained detectable for 11 months (0.6 ng/ml). The patient was followed as part of a long-term microbiologic monitoring program which subsequently showed no evidence of porcine viral or retroviral infection.

The patient opted for elective laparoscopy 9.5 yr after transplantation. Abundant nodules were seen throughout the peritoneum. Biopsies of the nodules showed they contained capsules still protecting living cell clusters. Immunohistology noted sparse insulin and moderate glucagon staining cells. The retrieved capsules produced a small amount of insulin when placed in high glucose concentrations in vitro. An oral glucose tolerance test induced a small rise in serum of immuno-reactive insulin, identified as porcine by reversed phase high pressure liquid chromatography (Elliott et al, 2007).

With this demonstration it was clear that this form of xenotransplantation treatment has the potential for sustained benefit in human type 1 diabetics.

Since then two further human studies have started using porcine islets in microcapsules and without immunosuppressive drugs. In 2007, a pilot study with 8 patients was approved by the Scientific and Ethics Committees of the Sklifosovsky Institute, Moscow where islets were obtained from biocertified designated pathogen free pigs and encapsulated under GMP conditions in New Zealand. Adult patients were aged 23-63 with type 1 diabetes as defined by the American Diabetes Association criteria. They were insulin dependent for 5 -15 years. Before the implants, patients had to have stimulated plasma c-peptide levels < 0.2 ng/ml to confirm insulin deficiency. Their diabetes had to be inadequately controlled with HbA1c of > 7% pre-implant. Patients were administered 5,000 or 10,000 islet equivalents per kilogram body weight (IEQ/kg). There were no significant adverse events and no evidence of zoonosis. Patients were also given repeat implants with no untoward effects. Preliminary data shows a reduction in daily insulin dose and reduction in HbA1c compared with pre-implant values following the first implant (Tables 1 and 2) in the majority of patients. Two patients became insulin independent for a period, the maximum being 32 weeks. At the repeat implant, 6 months after the first implant, intact microcapsules were retrieved and subsequently found to contain viable cells. Porcine insulin was also detected in the circulation following glucagon stimulation.

Patient ID	Dose 1st Tx (IEQ/kg)	Insulin Dose	% Dose Reduction	
		Pre 1st Tx	Post-1st Tx	
			3-month	6-month
1	5,000	113	32	34
2	5,000	22	100	32
3	5,000	60	-7	5
4	5,000	30	13	13
5	5,000	68	15	16
6	10,000	41	?	0
7	10,000	37	73	100
8	10,000	83	0	0
Mean		57	32	25

Table 1. **Reduction in daily insulin dose after first implant (Tx) in 8-patient pilot study.** Patient 2 was insulin-independent at 3 months but subsequently needed insulin support. Patient 7 became insulin-independent at 6 months.

Patient ID	Dose 1st Tx (IEQ/kg)	HbA1c (%)		
		Pre-1st Tx	Post-1st Tx	
			3-month	6-month
1	5,000	7.1	6.3	6.9
2	5,000	8.2	7.3	7.0
3	5,000	10.0	7.8	7.3
4	5,000	7.6	7.9	7.6
5	5,000	9.8	6.2	7.2
6	10,000	8.5	-	-
7	10,000	8.3	4.9	6.5
8	10,000	11.3	8.2	8.6
Mean:		8.9	6.9	7.3

Table 2. Reduction in Haemoglobin A1c (HbA1c) after first implant (Tx) in 8-patient pilot study.

In 2009, a Phase I/IIa study approved by the New Zealand government following international peer review and Ethics Committee Approval was commenced. It will include 14 adult patients. Unlike the preceding clinical studies, these patients were required to have unstable type 1 diabetes accompanied with hypoglycemic episodes. The patients are to be administered a single intra-abdominal implant of 5,000, 10,000, 15,000 or 20,000 IEQ/kg. To date no significant adverse events have been attributable to the treatment. At this early stage of the open label study, episodes of hypoglycemic unawareness (Figure 4) and hypoglycemic convulsions have been eliminated in the first patient. This was associated with significant reduction in the severity of hypoglycemic scores. A full one year follow-up of all patients is expected to be completed at the end of 2011. A third trial will be conducted in Argentina in 2011/2. The clinical studies are thus still at the stage of dose finding to determine the optimum dose and dosing regimen.

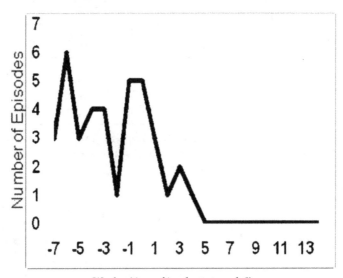

Weeks (time of implant at week 0)

Fig. 4. Example of Elimination of Episodes of Unaware Hypoglycemia (Patient #1, Phase I/IIa Auckland, New Zealand)

9. Conclusion

Xenotransplantation is not yet standard treatment. There is current research into the feasibility of using donor animal organs such a kidney and liver. However, unlike cells, organs are difficult to screen against potential infectious agents. If clinical trials with cell transplants for diabetes are successful, porcine islet transplants will lead the way for the use of other cells for the treatment of nervous system disorders and enzyme deficiencies (Skinner et al, 2009).

Porcine islet xenotransplantation has the potential to be beneficial for those with absolute insulin deficiency. There is now a consensus that the procedure is relatively safe from xenotic infections. The results of several non-human primate and rodent studies indicate significant efficacy may be achieved. The early results of human clinical trials also suggest that this form of treatment for Type 1 diabetes, without immunosuppression, is worthwhile. There is the concern that the treatment may be too expensive to be a practical treatment for the large numbers of patients who are expected to benefit from porcine islet implants. However, a health economic analysis of quality adjusted life years suggests that this approach may be cost effective taking into account the current cost of treating the disease and complications of cardiovascular disease, blindness, limb amputation, end-stage kidney disease and neuropathy (Beckwith et al, 2010).

10. Acknowledgements

The work embodied in this chapter could not have been possible without the integrated energy and persistence of all staff at Living Cell Technologies. Leaders in support are Isobel Cooper, Sandy Ferguson, Peter Hosking and Colleen Pilcher. Previous contributors were Trevor Speight and Michelle Tatnell.

11. References

American Diabetes Association (2011) Diabetes statistics. Available from:
        http://www.diabetes.org/diabetes-basics/diabetes-statistics/ Accessed June 2011.
American Diabetes Association (2011) Food and fitness. Available from:
        http://www.diabetes.org/food-and-fitness/ Accessed June 2011.
American Diabetes Association (2011) Economic consequences of diabetes mellitus in the USA. http://www.diabetes.org/diabetes-basics/diabetes-statistics/ Accessed June 2011.
Bauer SR (2010) Assuring safety and efficacy of Stem-Cell Based products. http://www.fda.gov/BiologicsBloodVaccines/ScienceResearch/BiologicsResearch Areas/ucm127182.htm
Beckwith J, Nyman JA, Flanagan B, Schrover R, Schuurman H-J.(2010) A health-economic analysis of porcine islet xenotransplantation. Xenotransplantation 17: 233-242.
Calafiore R. Perspectives in pancreatic and islet cell transplantation for the therapy of IDDM. Diabetes Care 1997;20:889-96.
Calafiore R, Basta G, Luca G, Lemmi A, Racanicchi L, Mancuso F, Montanucci MP, Brunetti P. (2006) Standard technical procedures for microencapsulation of human islets for graft into nonimmunosuppressed patients with type 1 diabetes mellitus. Transplant Proc. 38(4):1156-7
Calafiore R, Basta G, Luca G, et al.(1999) Transplantation of pancreatic islets contained in minimal volume microcapsules in diabetic high mammalians. Ann N Y Acad Sci 875:219-32.
Clemenceau B, Jegou D, Martignat L, Saï P. (2001) Long-term follow-up failed to detect in vitro transmission of full-length porcine endogenous retroviruses from specific pathogen-free pig islets to human cells. Diabetologia 44:2044-55.
Denner J. (2003) Porcine endogenous retroviruses (PERVs) and xenotransplantation: screening for transmission in several clinical trials and in experimental models using non-human primates. Ann Transplant 8(3):39-48.
Dinsmore JH, Manhart C, Raineri R, Jacoby DB, Moore A.(2000) No evidence of infection of human cells with porcine endogenous retrovirus (PERV) after exposure to porcine fetal neuronal cells. Transplantation 70:1382-9.

Dufrane D, Goebbels RM, Gianello P. (2010) Alginate macroencapsulation of pig islets allows correction of streptozotocin-induced diabetes in primates up to 6 months without immunosuppression. Transplantation. 90(10):1054-62.

Elliott RB (2011) Toward xenotransplantation of pig islets in the clinic. Curr Opin Organ Transplant. 16(2):195-200.

Elliott RB, Escobar L, Garkavenko O, Croxson MC, Schroeder BA, McGregor M, et al.(2000) No evidence of infection with porcine endogenous retrovirus in recipients of encapsulated porcine islet-cell xenograft. Cell Transplant 9(6):895-901.

Elliott RB, Escobar L, Tan PL, Garkavenko O, Calafiore R, Basta P, et al. (2005) Intraperitoneal alginate-encapsulated neonatal porcine islets in a placebo-controlled study with 16 diabetic cynomolgus primates. Transplant Proc 37: 3505-8.

Elliott RB, Escobar L, Tan PL, Muzina M, Zwain S, Buchanan C. (2007) Live encapsulated porcine islets from a type 1 diabetic patient 9.5 yr after xenotransplantation. Xenotransplantation. 14(2):157-61

Fink DW Jr (2009) FDA regulation of stem cell based products. Science 324 (5933) 1662-1663

Fujita F, Yamashita-Futsuki I, Eguchi S, Kamohara Y, Fujioka H, Yanaga K, et al.(2003) Inactivation of porcine endogenous retrovirus by human serum as a function of complement activated through the classical pathway. Hepatol Res 2003;26(2):106-113.

Garkavenko O, Croxson MC, Irgang M, Karlas A, Denner J, Elliott RB. (2004a) Monitoring for presence of potentially xenotic viruses in recipients of pig islet xenotransplantation. J Clin Microbiol 2004;42(11):5353-6.

Garkavenko O, Dieckhoff B, Wynyard S, Denner J, Elliott RB, Tan PL, Croxson MC. (2008) Absence of transmission of potentially xenotic viruses in a prospective pig to primate islet xenotransplantation study. J Med Virol. 80(11):2046-52.

Garkavenko O, Wynyard S, Nathu D, Simond D, Muzina M, Muzina Z, Scobie L, Hector RD, Croxson MC, Tan P, Elliott BR. (2008) Porcine endogenous retrovirus (PERV) and its transmission characteristics: a study of the New Zealand designated pathogen-free herd. Cell Transplant. 17(12):1381-8.

Harjutsalo V, Sjöberg L, Tuomilehto J (2008) Time trends in the incidence of type 1 diabetes in Finnish children: a cohort study. Lancet. 371(9626):1777-82.

Heneine W, Switzer WM, Soucie JM, Evatt BL, Shanmugam V, Rosales GV, et al. (2001) Evidence of porcine endogenous retroviruses in porcine factor VIII and evaluation of transmission to recipients with hemophilia. J Inf Dis 183:648-52.

Heneine W, Tibell A, Switzer WM, Sandstrom P, Rosales GV, Mathews A, et al.(1998) No evidence of infection with porcine endogenous retrovirus in recipients of porcine islet-cell xenografts. Lancet 352(9129):695-9.

Hering BJ, Cooper DK, Cozzi E, Schuurman HJ, Korbutt GS, Denner J, O'Connell PJ, Vanderpool HY, Pierson RN 3rd (2009) The International Xenotransplantation Association consensus statement on conditions for undertaking clinical trials of porcine islet products in type 1 diabetes--executive summary. Xenotransplantation.16: 196-202.

Hering BJ, Wijkstrom M, Graham ML, Hardstedt M, Aasheim TC, Jie T, et al (2006) Prolonged diabetes reversal after intraportal xenotransplantation of wild-type porcine islets in immunosuppressed nonhuman primates. Nat Med 12: 301-3.

Hernández RM, Orive G, Murua A, Pedraz JL.(2010) Microcapsules and microcarriers for in situ cell delivery. Adv Drug Deliv Rev. 2010 Jun 15;62(7-8):711-30

International Diabetes Federation (2011) Available at: http://www.idf.org Accessed June, 2011.

Irgang M, Sauer IM, Karlas A, Zeilinger K, Gerlach JC, Kurth R, et al. (2003) Porcine endogenous retroviruses: no infection in patients treated with a bioreactor based on porcine liver cells. J Clin Virol 28(2):141-54.

Maki T, Mullon CJP, Soloman BA, et al.(1995) Novel delivery of pancreatic islet cells to treat insulin-dependent diabetes mellitus. Clinical Pharmacokinetics 28(6):471-82.

Martin U, Kiessig V, Blusch JH, et al. (1998a) Expression of pig endogenous retrovirus by primary porcine endothelial cells and infection of human cells. Lancet 352(9129):692-4.

Martin U, Steinhoff G, Kiessig V, et al. (1998b) Porcine endogenous retrovirus (PERV) was not transmitted from transplanted porcine endothelial cells to baboons in vivo. Transpl Int 1998;11:247-51.

National Health & Medical Research Council (NHMRC) [Australia]. Xenotransplantation Working Party. Draft guidelines and discussion paper on xenotransplantation. Canberra: Commonwealth of Australia, 2002. Available from: http://www.nhmrc.gov.au.

Nuffield Council on Bioethics. Animal-to-human transplants: the ethics of xenotransplantation. London: Nuffield Council on Bioethics, 1996: 109-17.

Oldmixon BA, Wood JC, Ericsson TA, et al.(2002) Porcine endogenous retrovirus transmission characteristics of an inbred herd of miniature swine. J Virol 76:3045-8.

Opara EC, Kendall WF Jr.(2002) Immunoisolation techniques for islet cell transplantation. Expert Opin Biol Ther. 2(5):503-11.

Paradis K, Langford G, Long Z, Heneine W, Sandstrom P, Switzer WM, et al.(1999) Search for cross-species transmission of porcine endogenous retrovirus in patients treated with living pig tissue. Science 1999;285:1236-41.

Patience C. (2001) Swine defective for transmission of porcine endogenous retrovirus and uses thereof. Patent WO 01/53825 A1, .

Patience C, Patton GS, Takeuchi Y, Weiss RA, McClure MO, Rydberg L, et al. (1998) No evidence of pig DNA or retroviral infection in patients with short-term extracorporeal connection to pig kidneys. Lancet 352:699-701.

Rother RP, Fodor WL, Springhorn JP, Birks CW, Setter E, Sandrin S, et al. (1995) A novel mechanism of retrovirus inactivation in human serum mediated by anti-alpha-galactosyl natural antibody. J Exp Med 182(5):1345-55.

Skinner SJ, Geaney MS, Lin H, Muzina M, Anal AK, Elliott RB, Tan PL. (2009) Encapsulated living choroid plexus cells: potential long-term treatments for central nervous system disease and trauma.J Neural Eng. 6; 319-26

Suarez-Pinzon W, Korbutt GS, Power R, et al. (2000) Testicular sertoli cells protect islet beta-cells from autoimmune destruction in NOD mice by a transforming growth factor-beta1-dependent mechanism. Diabetes 49:1810-8.

Sun YL, Ma X, Zhou D, et al. (1993) Porcine pancreatic islets: isolation, microencapsulation, and xenotransplantation. Artif Organs 17(8):727-33.

Sun AM, O'Shea GM, Goosen MF. (1984) Injectable microencapsulated islet cells as a bioartificial pancreas. Appl Biochem Biotechnol. 10:87-99

Sun Y, Ma X, Zhou D, et al. (1996) Normalization of diabetes in spontaneously diabetic cynomolgus monkeys by xenografts of microencapsulated porcine islets without immunosuppression. J Clin Invest 98:1417-22.

Tacke SJ, Bodusch K, Berg A, Denner J. (2001) Sensitive and specific immunological detection methods for porcine endogenous retroviruses applicable to experimental and clinical xenotransplantation. Xenotransplantation 8(2):125-35.

Therapeutic Products Programme, Health Protection Branch, Health Canada.(1999) Proposed Canadian Standard for Xenotransplantation. Ottawa, ON, Canada, Jul 1999.

Toi te Taiao: the Bioethics Council (New Zealand).(2005) The cultural, ethical and spiritual aspects of animal-to-human transplantation. A report on xenotransplantation (August 2005). Available at:
http://ndhadeliver.natlib.govt.nz/ArcAggregator/arcView/IE1074184/
http://www.bioethics.org.nz/publications/xeno-final-report-aug05/index.htm
Accessed July 2011

United Kingdom Xenotransplantation Interim Regulatory Authority.(1998) Guidance on making proposals to conduct xenotransplantation on human subjects.

United Kingdom Xenotransplantation Interim Regulatory Authority. (1999) Draft report of the infectious surveillance steering group of the UKXIRA.

US Department of Health & Human Services. Public Health Service (PHS) (2002) Guidelines on infectious disease issues in xenotransplantation. Available from: http://www.fda.gov/cber/gdlns/xenophs0101.htm

US Department of Health & Human Services, Food and Drug Administration, Center for Biologics Evaluation and Research (CBER).(2003) Guidance for industry. Source animal, product, preclinical, and clinical issues concerning the use of xenotransplantation products in humans. Final guidance, April 2003. Available from: http://www.fda.gov/cber/gdlns/clinxeno.htm.

Valdes-Gonzalez RA, Dorantes LM, Garibay GN, Bracho-Blanchet E, Mendez AJ, Davila-Perez R, et al. (2005) Xenotransplantation of porcine neonatal islets of Langerhans and Sertoli cells: a 4-year study. Eur J Endocrinol 153(3):419-27.

van der Laan LJW, Lockey C, Griffeth BC, et al.(2000) Infection by porcine endogenous retrovirus after islet xenotransplantation in SCID mice. Nature 407:90-4.

Vatican (2011) Prospects for Xenotransplantation.
http://www.vatican.va/roman_curia/pontifical_academies/acdlife/documents/r c_pa_acdlife_doc_20010926_xenotrapianti_en.html Accessed June 2011.

Weir GC, Bonner-Weir S. (1997) Scientific and political impediments to successful islet transplantation. Diabetes 46(8):1247-56.

Wynyard S, Garkavenko O, Elliot R.(2011) Multiplex high resolution melting assay for estimation of Porcine Endogenous Retrovirus (PERV) relative gene dosage in pigs and detection of PERV infection in xenograft recipients. J Virol Methods. 175(1):95-100.

Zhao T, Zhang ZN, Rong Z, Xu Y. (2011) Immunogenicity of induced pluripotent stem cells. Nature. 474 (May 13. [Epub ahead of print])

Part 3

Diabetes and Oral Health

7

Impact of Hyperglycemia on Xerostomia and Salivary Composition and Flow Rate of Adolescents with Type 1 Diabetes Mellitus

Ivana Maria Saes Busato, Maria Ângela Naval Machado,
João Armando Brancher, Antônio Adilson Soares de Lima,
Carlos Cesar Deantoni, Rosângela Réa and Luciana Reis Azevedo-Alanis
Pontifical Catholic University of Paraná
Brazil

1. Introduction

Xerostomia is defined as a subjective sensation of having a dry mouth (Fox et al., 1987) and is reported by the patient (Guggenheimer & Moore, 2003; Moore et al., 2001). The subjective feeling of dry mouth (xerostomia) is one of the oral manifestations of diabetes (Sreebny et al., 2006; von Bültzingslöwen et al., 2007). Xerostomia results from a reduction in saliva secretion, although it may occur in spite of the presence of a normal salivary flow rate (Guggenheimer & Moore, 2003; Scully, 2003). Altered saliva composition rather than the quantity of saliva may play a role in the induction of xerostomia (Anttila et al., 1998; Fox, 1996).

Type 1 diabetes mellitus (DM1) is a metabolic dysfunction characterized by hyperglycemia resulting from definitive deficiency in insulin secretion caused by autoimmune illness and genetic factors (ADA, 2004). The American Diabetes Association (ADA) reports that 75% of DM1 cases are diagnosed in persons under the age of 18 years (ADA, 2006). Glycemic control is fundamental to the management of diabetes and is associated with sustained decreased rates of microvascular (retinopathy and nephropathy) as well as neuropathic complications (ADA, 2008). Glycemic control has a modifying effect on the relation between dental caries and salivary factors in young patients (Syjälä et al., 2003).

Patients with DM1, particularly those who have poor glycemic control, may have decreased salivary flow rate (Guggenheimer & Moore, 2003). Many clinical problems develop in the presence of xerostomia, such as: difficulty in swallowing and speech, high susceptibility to oral infections (mainly candidiasis and dental caries), gingivitis and mucositis (Anttila et al., 1998). Furthermore, xerostomia was shown to have a negative impact on the quality of life of adolescents with DM1 (Busato et al., 2009).

The relationship among DM1, salivary composition and xerostomia has been widely investigated (Swanljung et al., 1992; Moore et al., 2001; López et al., 2003; Siudikiene et al., 2006; Siudikiene et al., 2008; Orbak et al., 2008). It has been found that most DM1 patients have salivary dysfunction as well as differences in biochemical salivary composition compared with healthy subjects (Swanljung et al., 1992; Moore et al., 2001; López et al., 2003; Siudikiene et al., 2006; Siudikiene et al., 2008; Orbak et al., 2008). Moreover, there is a lack of studies showing the relationship among hyperglycemia, xerostomia and salivary factors, especially in adolescents with DM1. Thus, the aim of this study was to evaluate the association among hyperglycemia, xerostomia, salivary flow and composition of adolescents with DM1.

1.1 Materials and methods

This study was approved by the Research Ethics Committee of the Pontifical Catholic University of Paraná and by the Management of the Paraná Federal University Teaching Hospital. Patients and their parents or guardians were informed about the objective and the other aspects of the study and signed a Term of Independent Informed Consent.

1.1.1 Study groups and study design

A case-control epidemiologic study was performed on adolescents, allocated between two groups: control group, comprised of 51 non-diabetic subjects who were recruited from public high schools, and DM1 group, comprised of 51 adolescents with DM1, who receive follow-up at the Diabetes Outpatients Department of the Paraná Federal University Teaching Hospital. DM1 group and control group were paired regarding gender and age (14 – 19 years). DM1 diagnosis using the ADA (ADA, 2004) classification was established as a criterion for inclusion in DM1 group. The criterion for inclusion in control group was that of non-diabetic adolescents who had not used any medication for at least one month. The exclusion criteria used for both groups were: presence of systemic conditions that could influence salivary gland physiology, psychotropic drugs users, smokers, illicit drugs users or alcohol users (Busato et al., 2009).

1.1.2 Glycemic control

The results of postprandial capillary glucose (CG) tests performed at the time of saliva collection were recorded. Patients with good glycemic control were considered to be those with CG values of ≤ 130 mg/dL (DM1-A group), whereas hyperglycemic patients were considered to be those with CG values of > 130 mg/dL (DM1-B group) (ADA, 2006; 2008).

1.1.3 Xerostomia

Xerostomia was defined as a dry mouth sensation, reported by the subject. The subjects were asked if they had had a dry mouth sensation in the last six months (question A). If the answer was positive to xerostomia, they were also asked if it had occurred constantly during the last six months. Xerostomia was considered to exist if it had occurred daily during the six-month period. This evaluation was completed by the following questions: How would you describe the amount of saliva in your mouth? (question B). Do you have difficulty in swallowing food? (question C). Do you need to have something to drink in order to be able to swallow your food? (question D) (Carda et al., 2006).

Xerostomia was weighted according to three scales of perception: xerostomia 1 (dry mouth), when the answer to question A was "yes"; xerostomia 2, when there was a positive answer for question A and one other question (B, C or D); xerostomia 3, when there was a positive answer to question A and to two or more questions relating to xerostomia (B, C or D).

1.1.4 Saliva collection and treatment

Salivary flow was evaluated by means of stimulated saliva collection. The method used was that of mechanical masticatory stimulation, using a piece of sterile rubber tourniquet of a standardized size (1.5 cm), masticated continuously by the patient for six minutes. Saliva produced during the first minute of stimulation was discarded. During the following five minutes, the patient expelled saliva into a sterilized universal collecting recipient that had been previously weighed using Marte® analytical scales, model AL 500 (São Paulo-SP/Brazil). The saliva was collected between 8 a.m. and 10 a.m. Stimulated saliva flow rate (SSFR) was evaluated by means of the gravimetric method and expressed in mL/min (Banderas-Tarabay et al., 1997).

The remaining saliva samples were centrifuged (3,000 g for 10 min). Total protein and calcium salivary concentrations were determined using a colorimetric method (LABTEST® kits/Vista Alegre-MG/Brazil). Amylase salivary concentrations were determined by a kinetic colorimetric method (LABTEST® kits/Vista Alegre-MG/Brazil). Urea salivary concentrations were determined by an enzymic colorimetric method (LABTEST® kits/Vista Alegre-MG/Brazil). Salivary glucose was analysed by an enzymic colorimetric method (BIOCLIN® kits/Belo Horizonte-MG/Brazil). The determination of the salivary concentrations was performed three times.

1.1.5 Statistical analysis

The data were analysed using SPSS version 15.0 for Windows. Normality analysis was performed using the Kolmogorov-Smirnov Test, and the Levene test was used to analyse variance homogeneity. The other tests used were Mann-Whitney test and Fisher's exact test considering statistically significant values ($p \leq 0.05$ and CI 95%).

2. Results and discussion

A total of 102 subjects were included in this study: 51 patients with DM1 (DM1 group) and 51 subjects without DM1 (control group). Twenty-seven subjects were female (52.9%) and 24 were male (47.1%) in each group (DM1 group and control group). Average age was 17 years (14-19, SD = 1.4) in both groups. In DM1 group, average CG was 200.5 mg/dL (SD = 108.09).

In the present study, hyperglycemia (CG > 130 mg/dL) was observed in 33 (65%) adolescents with DM1 (DM1-B group) while 18 (35%) showed good glycemic control (DM1-A group). DM1, regardless of glycemic control, was a risk factor for higher xerostomia prevalence and increased glucose salivary concentrations. Hyperglycemia was a risk factor for SSFR reduction and increased urea and calcium salivary concentrations.

The presence of xerostomia 1 (dry mouth) was indicated by 27/51 (53%) subjects in DM1 group, and 8/51 (16%) subjects in control group (P < 0.001) (Table 1). A total of 12 subjects (24%) stated the need to drink liquids during meals in DM1 group in contrast to 2 (4%) subjects in control group ($P = 0.004$). There were no significant differences between DM1 group and control group for the following questions: difficulty in swallowing food and amount of saliva perceived (P > 0.05). Only DM1 group subjects presented xerostomia 2 (n=10, 20%) and xerostomia 3 (n=5, 10%). There were significant differences between DM1 group and control group regarding xerostomia 2 ($P = 0.001$) and xerostomia 3 ($P = 0.028$) (Table 1).

Among well-controlled adolescents (DM1-A group), 11/18 (61%) subjects reported xerostomia 1, in contrast to 16/33 (48%) hyperglycemic adolescents (DM1-B group). There were significant differences between DM1-A and control group, and DM1-B and controls for xerostomia 1 ($P < 0.05$) (Table 2). Table 2 shows the mean and the standard deviations of the salivary concentrations of total protein, amylase, urea, calcium and glucose in DM1, DM1-A, DM1-B and control groups. There were significant differences between DM1 and control groups for salivary concentrations of total protein ($P = 0.009$), calcium ($P = 0.001$), and glucose ($P = 0.021$). There were significant differences regarding total proteins ($P = 0.007$) and glucose ($P = 0.024$) salivary concentrations when DM1-A group was compared with control group. DM1-B group (adolescents with hyperglycemia) showed higher urea ($P = 0.042$), calcium ($P < 0.001$), and glucose ($P = 0.038$) salivary concentrations compared with controls.

Variables n (%)		DM1-group n = 51	Control group n = 51	P value
Xerostomia 1 (dry mouth)	Yes	27 (53)	8 (16)	<0.001 †
	No	24 (47)	43 (84)	
Need to drink	Yes	12 (24)	2 (4)	0.004 †
	No	39 (76)	49 (96)	
Amount of saliva perceived	Low	5 (10)	2 (4)	NS
	Normal	46 (90)	49 (96)	
Difficulty in swallowing	Yes	3 (6)	1 (2)	NS
	No	49 (94)	50 (98)	
Xerostomia 2	Yes	10 (20)	0 (0)	0.001 †
	No	41 (80)	51 (100)	
Xerostomia 3	Yes	5 (10)	0 (0)	0.028 †
	No	46 (90)	51 (100)	

DM1-group: adolescents with DM1, Control group: adolescents without DM1

† Fisher's exact test P ≤ 0.05, NS non-significant (P > 0.05)

Table 1. Characteristics of xerostomia of the studied population

Variables N (%) or mean (SD)	DM1-group n = 51	DM1-A n=18	DM1-B n=33	Control group n = 51	P value
Xerostomia 1					
Yes	27 (53)	11 (61)	16 (48)	8 (16)	<0.001[a c] †
No	24 (47)	7 (39)	17 (52)	43 (84)	0.001[b] †
SSFR (mL/min)	0.932 (0.537)	1.140 (0.688)	0.812 (0.361)	1.224 (0.577)	0.003[a] Ŧ NS[b] 0.002[c] Ŧ
Total Protein (mg/dL)	218 (386)	139 (67)	262 (460)	239 (144)	0.009[a] Ŧ 0.007[b] Ŧ NS[c]
Amylase (U/dL)	758 (33)	767 (35)	757 (31)	778 (9)	NS[a b c]
Urea (mmol/L)	5.340 (2.157)	4.662 (1.565)	5.769 (2.140)	4.957 (2.040)	NS[a b] 0.042[c] Ŧ
Calcium (mmol/L)	0.752 (0.496)	0.562 (0.366)	0.803 (0.515)	0.401(0.338)	0.001[a] Ŧ NS[b] <0.001[c] Ŧ
Glucose (mmol/L)	0.174 (0.183)	0.158 (0.154)	0.170 (0.189)	0.098 (0.115)	0.021[a] Ŧ 0.024[b] Ŧ 0.038[c] Ŧ

DM1-group: adolescents with DM1; DM1-A: adolescents with DM1 (CG ≤ 130mg/dL); DM1-B: adolescents with DM1 (CG > 130mg/dL); and Control group: adolescents without DM1
SSFR (stimulated salivary flow rate)
Ŧ Mann-Whitney U test, † Fisher's exact test, NS non-significant (P > 0.05)
[a] p value of DM1-group X control group; [b] p value of DM1-A X control group; and [c] p value of DM1-B X control group

Table 2. Salivary characteristics and xerostomia of the studied population

In the present study, xerostomia 1 prevalence was demonstrated in 27 (53%) adolescents with DM1 (DM1 group): 11 (61%) with good glycemic control and 16 (48%) with hyperglycemia, in contrast to 8 (16%) non-diabetes ones (control group) (Tables 1 and 2). Xerostomia was significantly associated with DM1 (Table 1) regardless of hyperglycemia (Table 2). Xerostomia 2 and xerostomia 3 only occurred in DM1 group, demonstrating that xerostomia is one of the oral manifestations of diabetes (Sreebny et a.l, 2006; von Bültzingslöwen et al., 2007). Xerostomia prevalence in elderly diabetic patients varies from

24.1% in patients with DM1 (Moore *et al* 2001) up to 76.4% in patients with type 2 DM (Carda et al., 2006). Moreover, there are limited accounts in the literature regarding the prevalence of xerostomia in adolescents with DM1, which makes direct comparisons between our study and other studies in adults difficult.

The need to drink liquids during meals was reported by 12 (24%) adolescents with DM1 and by 2 (4%) adolescents without diabetes (P = 0.004, Table 1). Nevertheless, in spite of this relationship between DM1 and "need to drink", it should be emphasized that family and individual habits may be related to this relationship. The habit of drinking juices, soft drinks or even water during meals is very common and frequently does not indicate a real necessity to drink in order to be able to swallow food. The clinical importance of the need to drink during meals among adolescents with DM1 needs to be further investigated in other studies.

In this study, average SSFR was 0.932 mL/min in DM1 group and 1.224 mL/min in control group (P = 0.003). In DM1-A group, average SSFR was 1.140 mL/min, presenting no significant difference compared with controls (P > 0.05) (Table 2). In the hyperglycemic subjects group (DM1-B), average SSFR was 0.812 mL/min. There was significant difference for SSFR between DM1-B and control groups (P = 0.002) (Table 2). Average SSFR values vary from 0.79 mL/min in children and adolescents with DM1 (Belazi et al., 1998) reaching 1.17 mL/min in adolescents with DM1 (Siudikiene et al., 2006). The latter value (Siudikiene et al., 2006) is similar to the average SSFR in well-controlled adolescents in the present study (DM1-A group, 1.140 mL/min, Table 2). The average SSFR value was significantly different between DM1 group (0.932 mL/min) and control group (1.224 mL/min), which is in consonance with previous studies with adolescents with DM1 (Siudikiene et al., 2006, 2008). In the present study, hyperglycemia was associated to a reduction in salivary flow (Table 2). This result agrees with a previous study, where it was suggested that it might be that the overall dehydration associated with hyperglycemia decreased the volume of saliva excreted (Karjalainen et al., 1996). Low salivary flow can influence increased caries experience in DM patients (Siudikiene et al., 2006, Márton et al., 2008). Furthermore, the subjective feeling of dry mouth (xerostomia) may result from a reduction in saliva secretion and was shown to have a negative impact on the quality of life of adolescents with DM1 (Busato et al., 2009).

Saliva contains immunological and non-immunological proteins with antibacterial properties (Humphrey & Williamson, 2001). In this study, good glycemic control (DM1-A group) was associated to a decrease in total proteins salivary concentration compared with controls. Conversely, there was no significant difference for salivary concentration of total proteins in the presence of hyperglycemia (DM1-B group) compared with non-diabetic subjects (control group). Moreover, amylase salivary concentration in adolescents with DM1 did not show significant differences compared with controls. Previous studies (Twetman et al., 2002; Mata et al., 2004; Carda et al., 2006; Moreira et al., 2009) have shown significant differences in total proteins salivary concentrations between subjects with and without DM1. Others studies are needed to further investigate the association of hypoglycemia with total proteins salivary concentrations in adolescents with DM1.

Salivary calcium concentration has a fundamental role in maintaining tooth integrity though the modulation of remineralization and demineralization (Humphrey & Williamson, 2001). In the present study, hyperglycemia was associated to an increase in salivary concentration of calcium (Table 2), and calcium salivary concentration in DM1 group was significantly higher compared with that of control group, in consonance with a previous study (Mata et al., 2004).

3. Conclusion

In this study, the glucose salivary concentration was significantly higher in DM1, DM1-A and DM1-B groups when each one was compared with control group. Some studies (Belazi et al., 1998; López et al., 2003; Moreira et al., 2009) have shown this difference, whereas others studies (Swanljung et al., 1992; Carda et al., 2006) have not found difference in glucose salivary concentrations between subjects with and without DM1. The increased concentrations of glucose in the saliva of adolescents with DM1 may be important for controlling and monitoring the disease. It may possibly be related to blood glucose (Belazi et al., 1998; Iughetti et al., 1999; Mata et al., 2004).

There were no significant differences for urea salivary concentrations between adolescents with DM1 (DM1 group) and without DM1 (control group), which is in accordance with a previous study (Meurman et al., 1998) and contradicts others (López et al., 2003; Carda et al., 2006). Moreover, in the latters (López et al., 2003; Carda et al., 2006), subjects with DM1 showed higher urea salivary concentrations compared with controls.

In the present study, hyperglycemia was associated with an increased urea salivary concentration, with significant difference between DM1-B and control groups (Table 2). Hyperproteic diet and dysfunction of urea excretion due to renal failure may increase urea values in plasma and urine (Searcy et al., 1964). Future studies are needed to further investigate the relationship among the increased values of urea salivary concentration in adolescents with hyperglycemia, renal dysfunction and diet.

The significant difference in salivary composition and SSFR between adolescents with and without DM1 and the significantly higher xerostomia prevalence noted in adolescents who have DM1 may suggest an increased risk of dental caries and oral disease in DM1 patients. Furthermore, xerostomia has been shown to have a negative impact on the quality of life of adolescents with DM1 (Busato et al., 2009).

Moreover, there are limited accounts in the literature regarding the prevalence of hyperglycemia and its association with salivary composition, flow rate and xerostomia in adolescents with DM1, which makes direct comparisons between our study and other studies difficult.

4. Acknowledgment

Authors would like to thank the Director and the employees of the Hospital de Clínicas, Universidade Federal do Paraná. This study was supported by MCT/CNPq grant n° 477932/2007-0.

5. References

American Diabetes Association-ADA. (2004). Diagnosis and classification of diabetes mellitus. *Diabetes Care*, Vol. 27, No. Suppl 1, (jan), pp. (S5-10), ISSN 1935-5548

American Diabetes Association-ADA. (2006). Standards medical care in diabetes-2006. *Diabetes Care*, Vol. 29, No. Suppl 1, (jan), pp. (S4-42), ISSN 1935-5548

American Diabetes Association-ADA. (2008). Standards of Medical Care in Diabetes-2008. *Diabetes Care*, Vol. 31, No. Suppl 1, (jan), pp. (S12-54), ISSN 1935-5548

Anttila SS.; Knuuttila ML. & Sakki TK. (1998). Depressive symptoms as an underlying factor of the sensation of dry mouth. *Psychosom Med*, Vol. 60, No.2, (apr), pp. (215-218), ISSN 1534-7796

Banderas-Tarabay JÁ.; González-Begné M., Sánchez-Garduño M., Millán-Cortéz E., López-Rodrígues A. & Vilchis-Velázquez A. (1997). The flow and concentration of proteins in human whole saliva. *Salud Publica Mex*, Vol. 39, No.5, (Sep-Oct), pp. (433-441), ISSN 1606-7916

Belazi MA.; Galli-Tsinopoulou A., Drakoulakos D., Fleva A. & Papanayiotou PH. (1998). Salivary alterations in insulin-dependent diabetes mellitus. *Int J Paediatr Dent*, Vol. 8, No.1, (mar), pp. (29-33), ISSN 1365-263X

Busato IMS.; Ignácio SA., Brancher JA., Grégio AM., Machado MA. & Azevedo-Alanis LR. (2009). Impact of xerostomia on the quality of life of adolescents with type 1 diabetes mellitus. *Oral Surg Oral Med Oral Pathol Oral Radiol Endod*, Vol. 108, No.3, (sep), pp. (376-382), ISSN 1528-395X

Carda C.; Mosquera-Lloreda N., Salom L., Gomez de Ferraris ME. & Peydró A. (2006). Structural and functional salivary disorders in type 2 diabetic patients. *Med Oral Patol Oral Cir Bucal*, Vol. 11, No.4, (jul 1), pp. (E309-314), ISSN 1698-6946

Fox PC. (1996). Differentiation of dry mouth etiology. *Adv Dent Res*, Vol. 10, No.1, (apr), pp. (13-16), ISSN1544-0737

Fox PC.; Busch KA. & Baum BJ. (1987). Subjective reports of xerostomia and objective measures of salivary gland performance. *J Am Dent Assoc*, Vol. 115, No.4, (oct), pp. (581-584), ISSN 1943-4723

Guggenheimer J. & Moore PA. (2003). Xerostomia: etiology, recognition and 1. treatment. *J Am Dent Assoc*, Vol. 134, No.1, (jan), pp. (61-69), ISSN1943-4723

Humphrey RDH. & Williamson RT. (2001). A review of saliva: normal composition, flow, and function. *J Prosthet Dent*, Vol. 85, No.1, (feb), pp. (162-169), ISSN 1097-6841

Iughetti L., Marino R., Bertolani MF. & Bernasconi S. (1999). Oral health in children and adolescents with IDDM--a review. *J Pediatr Endocrinol Metab*, Vol. 12, No.suppl 2, pp. (603-610), ISSN 0334-018X

Karjalainen KM., Knuuttila MLE. & Käär M-L. (1996). Salivary factors in children and adolescents with insulin-dependent diabetes mellitus. *Pediatr Dent*, Vol. 18, No.4, (Jul-Aug), pp. (306-311), ISSN 0164-1263

López MM., Colloca ME., Páez RG., Schallmach JN., Koss MA. & Chervonagura A. (2003). Salivary characteristics of diabetic children. *Braz Dent J*, Vol. 14, No.1, (jun), pp. (26-31), ISSN 0103-6440

Márton K., Madléna M., Bánóczy J., Varga G., Fejérdy P., Sreebny LM. & Nagy G. (2008). Unstimulated whole saliva flow rate in relation to sicca symptoms in Hungary. *Oral Dis*, Vol. 14, No.5, (jul), pp. (472-477), ISSN 1601-0825

Mata AD., Marques D., Rocha S., Francisco H., Santos C., Mesquita MF. & Singh J. (2004).
    Effects of diabetes mellitus on salivary secretion and its composition in the human.
    Mol Cell Biochem, Vol. 261, No.1-2, (dec), pp. (137-142), ISSN 1573-4919

Meurman JH., Collin HL., Niskanen L., Töyry J., Alakuijala P., Keinänen S. &
    Uusitupa M. (1998). Saliva in non-insulin-dependent diabetic patients
    and control subjects: the role of the autonomic nervous system. *Oral Surg Oral
    Med Oral Pathol Oral Radiol Endod,* Vol. 86, No.1, (jul), pp. (69-76), ISSN 1528-
    395X

Moore PA., Guggenheimer J., Etzel KR., Weyant RJ. & Orchard T. (2001). Type 1 diabetes
    mellitus, xerostomia, and salivary flow rates. *Oral Surg Oral Med Oral Pathol Oral
    Radiol Endod,* Vol. 92, No.3, (sep), pp. (281-291), ISSN 1528-395X

Moreira AR., Passos LA., Sampaio FC., Soares MSM. & Oliveira RJ. (2009). Flow rate, pH
    and calcium concentration of saliva of children and adolescents with type 1
    diabetes mellitus. *Braz J Med Biol Res,* Vol. 42, No.8, (aug), pp. (707-711), ISSN 1414-
    431X

Orbak R., Simsek S., Orbak Z., Kavrut F. & Colak M. (2008). The influence of type-1 diabetes
    mellitus on dentition and oral health in children and adolescents. *Yonsei Med J,* Vol.
    49, No. 3, (jun), pp. (357-765), ISSN 1976-2437

Scully C. (2003). Drugs effects on salivary glands: dry mouth. *Oral Dis,* Vol. 9, No.4, (jul), pp.
    (165-176), ISSN 1601-0825

Searcy RL., Korotzer JL., Douglas GL. & Bergquist LM. (1964). Quantitation of serum urea as
    microcapillary columns of dixanthylurea. *Clin Chem,* Vol. 10,(feb), pp. (128-135),
    ISSN 0009-9147

Siudikiene J., Machiulskiene V., Nyvad B., Tenovuo J. & Nedzelskiene I. (2006). Dental
    caries and salivary status in children with type 1 diabetes mellitus, related to
    metabolic control of the disease. *Eur J Oral Sci,* Vol. 114, No.1, (feb), pp. (8-14),
    ISSN 1600-0722

Siudikiene J., Machiulskiene V., Nyvad B., Tenovuo J. & Nedzelskiene I. (2008). Dental caries
    increments and related factors in children with type 1 diabetes mellitus. *Caries Res,*
    Vol. 42, No.5, (aug), pp. (354-362), ISSN 1421-976X

Sreebny LM., Yu A., Green A. & Valdini A. (1992). Xerostomia in diabetes mellitus. *Diabetes
    Care,* Vol. 15, No.5, (jul), pp. (900-904), ISSN 1935-5548

Swanljung O.; Meurman JH.; Torkko H.; Sandholm L.; Kaprio E. & Maenpaa J. (1992). Caries
    and saliva in 12-18-year-old diabetics and controls. *Scand J Dent Res,* Vol. 100, No.6,
    (dec), pp. (310-313), ISSN 0029-845X

Syjälä A-M H., Niskanen MC., Ylöstalo P. & Knuuttila MLE. (2003). Metabolic control
    as a modifier of the association between salivary factors and dental caries
    among diabetic patients. *Caries Res,* Vol. 37, No.2, (apr), pp. (142-147), ISSN
    1421-976X

Twetman S., Johansson I., Birkhed D. & Nederfors T. (2002). Caries incidence in young
    type 1 diabetes mellitus patients in relation to metabolic control and caries-
    associated risk factors. *Caries Res,* Vol. 36, No.1, (Jan-Feb), pp. (31-35), ISSN
    1421-976X

von Bültzingslöwen I., Sollecito TP., Fox PC., Daniels T., Jonsson R., Lockhart PB., Wray D., Brennan MT., Carrozzo M., Gandera B., Fujibayashi T., Navazesh M., Rhodus NL. & Schiødt M. (2007). Salivary dysfunction associated with systemic diseases: systematic review and clinical management recommendations. *Oral Surg Oral Med Oral Pathol Oral Radiol Endod,* Vol. 103, No.suppl 1, (mar), pp. (S57.e1-15), ISSN 1528-395X

8

Dental Conditions and Periodontal Disease in Adolescents with Type 1 Diabetes Mellitus

S. Mikó and M. G. Albrecht

Semmelweis University, Department of Conservative Dentistry,
Hungary

1. Introduction

The importance of type 1 (diabetes mellitus) DM lies in the function it plays in dentition and oral health for children and adolescents. The consequences of DM concerning oral health are in connection with the systemic changes[1] caused by the disease, though the results are in certain cases conflicting. Oral manifestations related to DM may have a strong inclination to periodontal disease[23], as well as an increased incidence of dental caries, mucosal lesions and dry mouth (xerostomia). However, as mentioned before, the results are not entirely in accord[456]. Children and adolescents with type 1 DM are more susceptible to infections in the dental connective tissues than those without type 1 DM. The dentist's liablility is to evaluate the dangers and maintain adequate oral hygiene to prevent the occurrence of disfunctional oral effects of type 1 DM.

2. Periodontal disease

Periodontitis is a chronic multifactorial plaque induced Gram-negative anaerobic infection of the periodontium that results in the destruction of periodontal tissues and loss of alveolar bone.[7] Periodontitis is to be treated by the mechanical removal of supra- and subgingival bacterial plaque with scalers, curettes or ultrasonic devices (scaling and root planing [SRP]), and by instructing the parient about oral hygiene. The development of new dental plaque deposits and re-infection of the subgingival tissues can only be prevented in case of a near-ideal oral hygiene. For the improvement of clinical periodontal status the regular use of systemic or local antibiotics as an adjunctive therapy to SRP is still concerned problematic.[8910] Deep residual periodontal lesions can usually be reduced or eliminated by surgery.

2.1 Diabetes and periodontal disease

There is an extensive debate on the influence of DM on the risk of periodontal disease. According to most of the experts, patients suffering from diabetes mellitus are highly susceptible to develop periodontal disease.[111213141516] In 1993, periodontal disease was termed as the sixth complication of diabetes[17], while in the report of the Expert Comittee on the Diagnosis and Classification of Diabetes Mellitus issued in 1997, periodontal disease was mentioned as a disease of very high incidence in case of patients with diabetes.[18] Many papers on the subject have outlined that the inclination, extent, severity and development of periodontal disease are significantly increased in case of patients with diabetes.[19][20] Impaired immune response, different bacterial microflora and collagen metabolism are involved in the pathogenesis of diabetic periodontal disease[21]. This is especially true if the diabetes is poorly controlled[22] and there is a lasting periodontal disease in case of type 1 DM individuals[23].

Gingival bleeding is a sign of inflammation. Vascular changes in diabetes mellitus may result in increased gingival bleeding. If however the diabetes is adequately treated, there are fewer vascular changes.[24] Gingival bleeding is in positive correlation with the accumulation of plaque and calculus.[25] Diabetics showed more plaque and higher calculus index scores than the control groups.[26] Calcium concentration was high in both the parotid and submandibular saliva of patients with type 1 DM.[27] This result may explain the regularly experienced increase in calculus formation in the case of these patients.[28][29] Individuals with a decreased glucose tolerance showed a higher rate of pocket formation, presence of calculus, increased tooth mobility and tooth loss.[30] Variable models have been developed to give reason to this correlation such as periodontal chronic inflammation which results in increased circulating cytokines and inflammatory mediators, autoimmune response to the chronic periodontal infection that gives way to endothelial dysfunction, or the presence of certain factors that leads to increased inclination both to periodontal disease and diabetes vascular diseases at the same time.[31]

Statistically significant relation has been detected between the HbA1C levels of the patients and the biomass, haemolysin activity and proteinase activity. The biofilm formation is likely to have an effect on the pathogenicity of oral candidosis.[32]

There is, however, a minority of experts who are sceptical about the high risk of type 1 DM.[33][34][35][36]

Today Glickman's theory is the most widely accepted one. According to Glickman, the father of modern periodontology, diabetes are not the direct cause, but a predisposing condition for periodontal disease.[37] There is a bidirectional relationship between diabetes and periodontal diseases[38]. Diabetic adolescents have more prevalence and more severe gingival inflammation than healthy control persons of the same age[39], despite similar plaque scores[51]. Metabolic imbalances in the tissues may reduce the resistance of diabetics to infection,[40] and thus affect the initiation, developement and progression of periodontal disease.[41] Adolescents with type 1 DM develop an earlier and higher gingival inflammatory response to a similar bacterial challenge than non diabetics.[34][42] In accordance with this fact, extended studies have shown that severe periodontal disease in diabetic patients is primarily related to poor metabolic control and other diabetes complications occurring during the follow-up process.[43][44] Still, long-duration diabetics resulted in more severe periodontitis than short-duration diabetics.[45] It has been proposed that fine periodontal treatment of diabetic patients may lead to the lowering of diabetic complications.[46][47][48] Chronic Gram-negative infections and chronic endotoxaemia, which arise in case of periodontal disease, may also increase insulin resistance and reduce metabolic control in case of diabetic patients. This entails the hypothesis that elimination or control of periodontal infection may improve the metabolic control of diabetes.[49][50] It has been proposed that a microbiological imbalance in the gut may increase the gram-negative bacterial load, which would also increase the systematic inflammatory burden through the lipopolysaccharides leakage into the circulation. Increased inflammation leads to insulin resistance.[51][52][53] According to a study, insulin requirements were lowered following periodontal treatment and reduction of inflammation in diabetic patients.[54] It has been demonstrated that the interaction of periodontal bacterial byproducts with mononuclear phagocytic cells and fibroblasts induces the chronic release of cytokines (IL-1β, IL-6, TNF-α), PGE2 and CRP.[55]

Recently many studies have proposed that periodontal disease is a substantial aggravating factor in restoring the health of patients with diabetes.[56] It is mainly due to the fact that it maintains a chronic systemic inflammatory process. However, the causality between periodontitis and altered glycaemic control can only be justified epidemiologically with prospective interventional studies.[57] The control of periodontal disease could be an essential part of the overall treatment of diabetic patients: the periodontal therapy may improve glycaemic control, and could lead to a significant lowering of HbA1c values.[40]

Concerning the adolescents, the oral hygiene seems to be better in case of the diabetic patients than in case of the other group of young patients who have shown highly variable work shifts leading to poor oral hygiene. The difference is reflected by a lesser bacterial plaque among the diabetics. This is in conflict with the results of other authors who observed similar oral hygiene status and plaque indexes in the two groups, or even comparatively increased plaque accumulation among the diabetics.[58] The reason for this may be the following: although the diabetics were controlled, they showed a high gingival response to the irritation caused by bacterial plaque retention.[59] Regularly diabetics have a greater incidence regarding periodontal disease than healthy individuals[60][61], though other studies have not detected such relation between periodontal disease and diabetes.[62][63][64] They didn't confirm any association between diabetes and periodontal disease in adolescents. They believe that there is no difference between on the one part type 1 DM adolescents and children, and on the other healthy individuals regarding clinical periodontal status. However Fructosamine value, used to diagnose and monitor diabetes, was observed to be in correlation with the gingival index score in case of type 1 DM adolescents and children, but not in case of healthy control subjects.[65] Bay et al.[34] found no difference in the degree resolution of gingivitis following scaling and root planning between young diabetics and healthy control group. Barnett et al.[35] studied periodontitis prevalence in young diabetics but none of the individuals showed radiographic sign of periodontitis.

Despite the comparatively better control of bacterial plaque among the diabetics, a change in their periodontal response was detected. Therefore it seems that local immune response may possibly change among these patients, and the lesions caused by microbial agents in case of periodontal disease, which can be associated with a lesser tissue repair capacity, might be the reason for the increased deterioration of periodontal structures shown in the diabetic group.[4]

It is possible, that the diversities observed by the different authors result from local health care habits. In an area with a tradition of good oral hygene, the oral hygiene habits of diabetes are not better than those of healthy people. Therefore in case of similar oral hygiene habits, diabetical patients show lower periodontal values than healthy persons because of the above mentioned immune response. In areas where the dental treatment habits of the population are poorer, the greater attention of well-controlled DM patients to oral hygiene results in higher values than those of healthy individuals.

2.2 Prevalence of gingivitis, periodontitis in adolescents with type 1 DM

Since there are conflicting reports in the literature, the aim of this study was analyse the periodontal disease in adolescents with type 1 diabetes mellitus.[66] Characterization of risk factors, local such as oral hygiene-, general (duration of DM, age, degree of metabolic control of DM) and contributory factors-, such as toothbrushing, have been identified that determining the risk factors place people enhanced risk in development and progression of periodontal diseases.

A dental clinical cross-sectional examination was carried out on 259 adolescents of ages 14-19 with type 1 DM in comparison with a non-DM group as control group. Children who had been under the age of eight at the onset of DM were excluded, as where those with any additional disease or taking other chronic medication. The control group comprised of metabollically healthy individuals. The DM patients were classified according to the categories recommended by the World Health Organisation (1999). The Greene-Vermillion OHI-S index was used to determine the level of oral hygiene. Periodontal changes were rated by the Russell's periodontal index (PI), which estimates the degree of periodontal disease occurring in the mouth by measuring both bone loss around the teeth and gingival inflammation. This method is regularly used in the epidemiological investigation of the disease.[67] Alveolar bone loss was tested according to Schei et al (1959), and Hirschman et al (1994) with panoramic radiograph and vertical or posterior bitewings radiographs.

The DM subjects were characterised according to the following criteria: mean postprandial blood glucose level during the period of 6 months prior to the dental examination; glycosylated haemoglobin (HbA1C) level; duration of the DM; the age at the onset of DM. The ADA (2005) criteria were used concerning the DM control. Diabetes mellitus was well-controlled (in 210 cases), if six months before the dental examination the mean postprandial blood glucose level of the patients was normal or near normal (below 7.5 mmol/l), there was no glycosuria HbA1C≤ 6.5%, and severe hypoglicaemia did not occur. Control was taken to be poor when the postprandial blood sugar was ≥ 7.5 mmol/l and/or haemoglobin was > 6.5%, or in case of patients with asymptomatic hypoglicaema.

The incidence of gingivitis and periodontitis was much higher in case of diabetic adolescents than in case of metabolically healthy persons (p< 0. 0001) and especially in case of girls (p< 0. 001). Healthy periodontium was only found in case of 2.6% of the DM adolescents and the rest of DM patients had either gingivitis (61.03%) or periodontitis (39%), while a high rate of metabolically healthy persons (80.5%) has shown a healthy periodontium. Gingivitis and periodontitis was experienced in case of 18.4% and 1.1% of the patients. (Fig.1.)

With the fall of oral hygiene (OHI-S) index (p< 0. 0001) the intensity of gingivitis and periodontitis (PI) has become more severe. (Fig.2.)

An important positive correlation has been shown between the control level of the disease and the intensity of gingivitis and periodontitis. In case of well-controlled 'Type 1' diabetic adolescents the PI mean value was lower than in case of patients with poor glycemic control (p< 0. 001).

In the diabetic group the periodontal disease was detected to be severe in case of those who had a lasting DM (>5 years) (p<0.001).

The majority of the control persons showed no alveolar bone loss (83% had intact alveolar bone) and those who had alveolar bone loss, had primarily that of horizontal type. In case of diabetic adolescents prevalence of intact alveolar bone was lower (61.8%) than in case of the control group. Therefore higher degree of alveolar bone resorption (both horizontal and horizontal+vertical type) was experienced in case of diabetic patients than in case of the control group (p<0.001).

The mean values of alveolar bone resorption were higher in case of diabetic boys than in case of diabetic girls (p<0.0001).

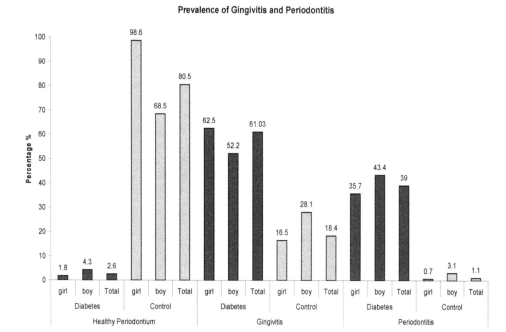

Fig. 1. Prevalence of gingivitis and periodontis

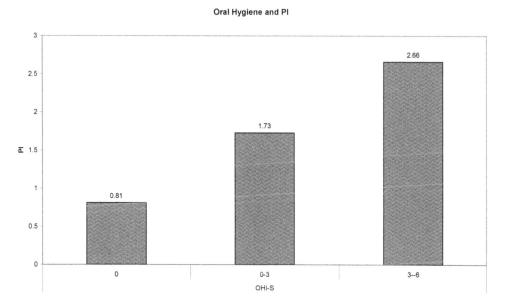

Fig. 2. The mean value of PI according to oral hygiene (OHI-S)

The intensity of gingivitis and periodontitis, as well as the increased alveolare bone loss was more prevalent and more severe in diabetic adolescents than in healthy individuals. Several authors suggested a correlation between diabetes mellitus and periodontal diseases. According to them periodontal disease is one of the most prevalent and rapidly progressive complications[3738] of DM in case of adults.

Sappala et al. (1993) has shown that adults with Type 1 diabetes mellitus have higher degree of attachment loss and bone loss than control subjects under similar dental plaque conditions. The authors received the same results for diabetic adolescents. The oral hygiene (OHI-S), especially the debris index was worse in case of diabetic individuals than in case of the control persons and correlation was found between on the one part the intensity of gingivitis and periodontitis and on the other the oral hygiene. However De Pommereu et al.[57] found more serious gingivitis in diabetics than in control persons, although plaque scores were the same in both groups. Interestingly, according to the present study diabetic adolescents, especially boys have more severe alveolare bone destruction than non-diabetics.

The present study demonstrates that severity of periodontal disease increases with the duration of diabetes mellitus, in agreement with the results in case of adults measured by Pavez[23] and Greene Vermillion (1964), Rosenthal et al. (1988), and Lopey et al. (2002).

This study shows that the poorly controlled type 1 DM with elevated blood glucose and glycosylated hemoglobin (HgA $_{1c}$) levels have more incidental and serious periodontal diseases with alveolare bone loss in case of adolescents with lasting diabetes mellitus. Adequate metabolic control of diabetes mellitus lowers inclination to infection. This is also crucial for the prevention of periodontal disease in case of adolescents with diabetes mellitus. In case of adult diabetic patients with poorly controlled diabetes mellitus, increased metabolic control may improve periodontal condition (Miller et al. 1992, Yki-Jarvinen 1989, Harris 1995, RST/AAP 1999).

Periodontitis is a complex multifactorial disease. It can especially cause a problem for adolescents with DM. Inadequate oral hygiene is responsible for high oral debris in case of diabetic adolescents, being in correlation with the status of periodontium.

Several other charcteristics such as long duration, early onset (under 14 years), and degree of metabolic control, have been determined as factors increasing the risk of disease. In case of diabetic girls the monthly hormonal level alterations of the gingival may play a role in the development and progression of gingivitis, periodontitis and alveolare bone resorption.

Frequent dental treatments may help maintain good oral health. Treatment is especially crucial at the onset of the disease. Dental care at the early stages of the disease, reducing susceptibility to infection, is also significant for the prevention of periodontal disease in case of adolescents with type 1 diabetes mellitus. Children should also be checked regularly for bleeding gums or inflammation for to prevent the alveolare bone loss, which leads to irreversible changes of periodontium.

The education of youngsters on proper home oral care is the basic method for periodontal greatment and prevention. In most cases the gingivitis can be resolved by plaque control.

3. Caries

Dental   caries   is   a chronical   bacterial   disorder where bacterial processes   damage hard tooth structure (enamel, dentin, and cementum).[68] The tissues break down progressively, resulting in dental caries (cavities, holes in the teeth). The basic factors are the causal microorganism, the host (tooth), the substrate (diet), and the immune capacity of the patient.

Two groups of bacteria may cause caries: *Streptococcus mutans*[69] and *Lactobacillus*[2570]. Bacteria gather around the teeth and gum in a sticky, creamy-coloured mass called plaque, which serves as a biofilm. Bacteria in an individual's mouth transform glucose, fructose, and most regularly sucrose into acids such as lactic acid through a glycolytic process called fermentation.[71] In direct relation with the tooth, these acids may lead to demineralization, i.e. the dissolution of its mineral content. However the process is dynamic. If the acid is neutralized by saliva or mouthwash, remineralization may arise. Fluoride toothpaste or dental varnish can help remineralization.[72] If the demineralization process is continuous, enough mineral content could be lost so that the soft organic material left behind disintegrates, forming a cavity or hole. Caries is one of the most common diseases of the world at present.

3.1 Diabetes and caries

Epidemiological studies do not seem to be in accord on the characteristics of diabetes mellitus (DM) concerning the incidence of dental caries in case of both children and adults[73747576777 8]. Although adolescents may be more caries-prevalent than individuals of other ages, only few studies deal with this age group. In case of type 1 diabetics an increased prevalence was detected[79], located particularly in the root or dental neck regions.[70] However studies differ whether control of DM or sucrose-free diet of DM patients is more likely to promote or inhibit the development of dental caries. Opinions do not match concerning the dental condition for patients with DM or the outcome of early DM manifestation regarding the dental condition.

Cross-sectional studies have reported a low prevalence of caries in case of children and adolescents with type 1 DM, and this has mainly been explained by the sucrose-restricted diet, which is a part of the lifelong treatment.[8081] According to Wegner,[82] the frequency of caries in DM childen is at least not lower than in non-DM children. Wegner[83] also observed that, directly after the diagnosed onset of their disease, some young DM patients displayed a higher activity of caries than healthy subjects of the same age, but the frequency of caries gradually diminished in association with dietary restriction and treatment with insulin. Other researchers proposed a relationship between the development of caries and the level of metabolic control.[298485] These researches showed a higher prevalence of caries in case of poorly controlled DM than in case of well-controlled disease. The reason is that higher glucose content in oral fluids adds to bacterial proliferation, enhancing the formation of dental plaque. It has been shown for all concerning age groups that children with DM have less caries than non-diabetic children.[26] However, these experiments also demonstrated that the result was due to an abundance of sites where teeth were lost without replacement. The complications were not symptoms of type 1 DM, they might be caused by poor medical and dental care. Some studies proposed that salivary secretion rates should be substantially lowered in case of children with type 1 DM when compared to healthy children.[86] Reduced salivary secretion increases the probability of caries, although adequate metabolic control prevents the most dangerous salivary alterations such as high glucose content and low pH, while a fine diabetic diet, rich in fiber and poor in simple carbohydrates, can decelerate the development of plaque and the proliferation of acidogenic bacterial microflora.[2987] Individuals at ages of adolescence generally clean their teeth less frequently than persons at ages after adolescence.[88] Behavioral factors such as dental self-efficacy are in relation with DM self-efficacy and adherence.[71] Adequate oral health habits may lead to lower incidence of caries. On the other hand, Moore et al. observed similar regularities concerning the use of dentifrice and dental floss between diabetics and non-diabetics[89]. However other studies demonsrtated that diabetic patients used dental floss more frequently than non-diabetics.[90] It seems that there are contradicting studies on the dental condition in case of patients with DM as well as on the effect of early DM manifestation on the dental condition.

3.2 Dental caries in adolescent with type 1 DM

Since there are conflicting reports regarding the dental condition in patients with DM or the effect of early DM manifestation on dental condition, the aim was to analyse the dental status DMF-T and the   prevalence of dental caries in adolescents with type 1 DM   and compare the findings with those from metabolically healthy individuals, in an effort to determine the risk factors play a role in the development of dental caries in DM adolescents.[91]

A dental clinical cross-sectional examination was carried out on 259 adolescents aged 14-19 years with type 1 DM in comparison with a non-DM group as control. Children who had been under the age of eight at he onset of DM were excluded, as where those with any additional disease or taking other chronic medication. The control group comprised metabollically healthy individuals. The DM patients were classified according to the categories recommended by the World Health Organisation (WHO). Caries was assessed by the DMF-T index. Within this index, F was used for the filled teeth, D denoted the number of untreated carious teeth without regard to whether the lesion was enamel or of root. Extractions for orthodontics or periodontal reasons were excluded. The Greene-Vermillion OHI-S index was used to determine the level of oral hygiene. The DM subjects were characterised according to the following criteria: mean postprandial blood glucose level and during the period of 6 months prior to the dental examination; glycosylated haemoglobin (HbA1C) level; the duration of the DM; and the age at the onset of DM: Concerns by DM control, the ADA (2005) criteria were offered. Diabetes mellitus was well-controlled (210 cases) if six months before the dental examination the mean postprandial blood glucose level of the patients was normal or near normal (below 7.5 mmol/l) there was no glycosuria HbA1C$\leq$ 6.5% and severe hypoglicaemia is did not occur. Control was taken as poor when the postprandial blood sugar was $\geq$ 7.5 mmol/1 and/ or haemoglobin was > 6.5%, or in cases of patients with asymptomatic hypoglicaema.

The DM adolescents had a slightly higher mean DMF-T score than the control subjects. The difference was found to be statistically significant ($p < 0.001$).

When the components of DMFT were considered, there were more filled (F) ($p < 0.001$) and fewer decayed teeth (D) ($p < 0.0001$) among the DM adolescents than in the healthy controls. When the number of missing teeth was considered, there were no significant differences between the DM patients and the healthy controls.

The DM boys had a slightly higher mean DMFT score than the DM girls ($p < 0.001$). More decayed (D) ($p < 0.001$) and filled (F) teeth were found among the DM boys than among the DM girls ($p < 0.001$). As regard the number of extracted (M) teeth, there were no significant differences between the boys and the girls.

The age of the patient at the onset of DM was correlated to the caries condition (D). This suggested that the early onset of DM (before the age of 14) was related to significantly fewer decayed and filled teeth compared with the patients in whom the DM had developed after age 14 years ($p < 0.01$). (Fig.3.)

However the adolescents with good oral hygiene (OHI-S=0), there was a significant differences ($P < 0.0001$). (Fig.4.) A positive correlation was found between of the level of control of the DM and the dental condition. In the well-controlled DM adolescents the mean number of decayed (D) teeth was lower ($p < 0.0001$), but the numbert of filled (F) teeth was higher than in patients with poorer glycemic control($P < 0.001$). (Fig.5.)

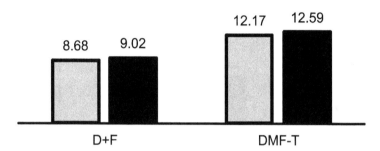

Fig. 3. The mean number of the DMF-T and D+F according to the age of the patient at the onset of type 1 DM

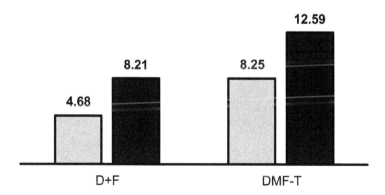

Fig. 4. The mean number of the DMF-T and D+F according to the age of the patient at the onset of type 1 DM in patients with good oral hygiene (OHI-S=0)

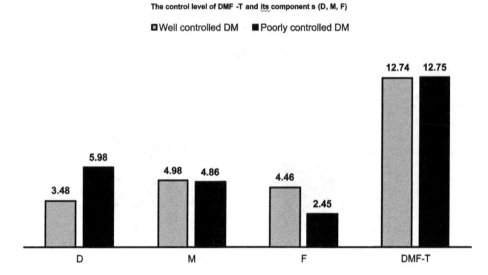

Fig. 5. The control level of DMF-T and its components (D, M, F)

This study of adolescents with type 1 DM demonstrated that none of the subjects has intact dentitions. Poor glicaemic control and the early onset of DM may increase the risk of dental caries but appropriate oral hygiene together with satisfactory metabolic control may prevent the development of dental caries in adolescents with type 1 DM.

4. Tooth eruption

Eruption is the phisiological process of tooth development and growth during which the teeth enter the mouth and become visible. Normally they cut themselves throught the oral mucosa without any inflammation.

Mixed dentition starts when the first permanent molar appears in the mouth, usually at five or six years, and ends when the last primamry tooth is lost, usually at ten, eleven, or twelve years.[92] Afterwards the permanent dentition begins and lasts as long as the person lives or until all of the teeth are lost (edentulism).

4.1 Diabetes mellitus and accelerated eruption

It has been demonstrated that diseases containing metabolic instabilities, such as diabetics, weaken the resistance to inflammation[93]. As a result, the gingival inflammation accompanies eruption in the diabetic patients at an increased rate as compared to the non-diabetic individuals.

Information on dentition concerning the age group from 5 to 9 is limited to about 60 type 1 DM children. Ziskin[94] et al. detected a small and insubstantial affect of diabetes on dental development. Studies concerning accelerated dental development in case of diabetic children who are less than 11.5 years old are not in accord. Older diabetic children manifested delayed dental development.[95] The edentulous interval was longer in case of diabetic children than in case of the control population.

Adler et al.[96] proposed that metabolic disorders cause the acceleration and delay experienced in dentition. A biphasic effect of the diabetic state on dental development was detected: on the one hand acceleration in the early diabetes, and on the other retardation in lasting diabetes.[92] The result conflicted with common knowledge: acceleration was observed in dentition until the age of 10 and delay after the age of 10 (especially for the eruption of canine and the premolars).[26] This may be in correlation with diseases containing metabolical instabilities, such as diabetes.

Other studies showed that children with diabetes in the late mixed dentition period (ages 10-14) had a higher inclination for advanced tooth eruption than those without diabetes. Alterations in tooth eruption were not detected in the early mixed dentition group (ages 6-10). Individuals with higher height showed higher propensity for expedited tooth eruption. The expetited eruption among patients with higher height was more characteristic in the older group than in the younger one.[97]

5. Diabetes and dental, periodontal prevention in adolescents

Diabetes is a chronic metabolic disease which affects the entire organism, disturbing especially the oral health. Health habits are substantial for preventing dental and periodontal diseases and maintaining oral health in a population of patients with type 1 DM.

It is a vital task for dentists to foster good oral health habits, executing periodic dental examinations and ensuring sufficient oral hygiene. These conditions significantly affect the diabetic patients' oral health. Dentists must minimize the risk factors of periodontal disease, caries and oral soft tissue pathologies.[88] Dentists should continually instruct and motivate the patient concerning oral hygiene.

Dental practice showed that health promoting methods reduce the patient's smoking habits.[98] It is possible to use pharmacological and behavioral strategies in a private practitioner's office to help patients quit smoking.[99] However inadequate undergraduate dental education and practitioner continuing education threaten to be an obstacle for the daily use of these practices.[100] There are positive signs conserning the improvement of educational opportunities, nevertheless the incorporation of these technics in the clinical practice must still be highlighted.[101]

There are two kinds of professional oral hygiene promotion: active and sustaining procedure. The initial or causal promotion is to eliminate the plaque and the plaque retentional factors and to remove the supra- and subgingival calculus, as well as the root planing and the curettage and to eliminate the carious lesions. The goal of these procedures is to terminate the inflamation of the gingiva and to stop further development of the gingival recession, thus eliminating the bacterial elements responsible for inflammation. The most important condition of efficient private oral hygiene is the smooth cleanable tooth surface. For it is useless to instruct the patient even on the most refined tooth brushing technique or on the use of dental floss if the teeth are covered with calculus or there are overfilled interdental spaces. Dental practice should include dental check within one or two months, oral hygiene treatment, repeated fixing of gingival and periodontal indexes, as well as their comparison with the initial values, and in certain cases causal surgical periodontal interventions. Nontheless, further instructions and motivations are also essential.

6. References

[1] Hanssen KF. Blood glucose control and microvascular and macrovascular complications in diabetes. *Diabetes.* 1997;46:S101-S103.

[2] Seppal B, Seppala M, Ainamo J. A longitudinal study on insulindependent diabetes mellitus and periodontal disease. *J Clin Periodontol* 1993;20:161-5.

[3] Mattson JS, Cerulis DR. Diabetes mellitus: A review of the literature and dental implications Compendium 2001;22:757-72.

[4] Miralles-Jorda L, Silvestre-Donat FJ, Grau Garcia-Moreno DM, Hernandez-Mijares A. Buccodental pathology in patients with insulin-dependent diabetes mellitus: a clinical study. *Med Oral.* 2002 Jul-Oct;7(4):298-302.

[5] Sreebny LM, Yu A, Green A, Valdini A. Xerostomia in diabetes mellitus. *Diabetes Care.* 15:900-904, 1992

[6] Swanljung O, Meurman JH, Torkko H, Sandholm L, Kaprio E, Mäenpää J. Caries and saliva in 12-18-year-old diabetics and controls. *Scand J Dent Res* 100:310-313,1992

[7] Page RC; Schroeder HE. Pathogenesis of Inflammatory Periodontal Disease: A Summary of Current Work. *Lab Invest.* 1976;34(3):235-249.

[8] Darré L, Vergnes JN, Gourdy P, Sixou M. Efficacy of periodontal treatment on glycaemic control in diabetic patients: a meta-analysis of interventional studies. *Diabetes Metab* 2008; 34: 497– 506.

[9] Llambés F, Silvestre FJ, Hernández- Mijares A, Guiha R, Caffesse R. Effect of non-surgical periodontal treatment with or without doxycycline on the periodontium of type 1 diabetic patients. *J Clin Periodontol* 2005; 32: 915– 920.

[10] Martorelli de Lima AF, Cury CC, Palioto DB, Duro AM, da Silva RC, Wolff LF. Therapy with adjunctive doxycycline local delivery in patients with type 1 diabetes mellitus and periodontitis. *J Clin Periodontol*2004; 31: 648– 653.

[11] Miotti F, Ferro R, Saran G. Diabetes in oral medicine (Current status of knowledge, diagnosis, therapy and dental prevention) *G Stomatol Ortognatodonzia.* 1985;4:3-14.

[12] Finestone AJ, Boorujy SR. Diabetes mellitus and periodontal disease. *Diabetes.* 1967;16:336-340.

[13] Sznajder N, Carraro JJ, Rugna S, Sereday M. Periodontal findings in diabetic and nondiabetics patients. *J Periodontol.* 1978;49:445-448.

[14] Cianciola LJ, Park BH, Bruck E, Mosovich L, Genco RJ. Prevalence of periodontal disease in insulin-dependent diabetes mellitus (juvenile diabetes). *J Am Dent Assoc.* 1982;104:653-660.

[15] Hugoson A, Thorstensson H, Falk H, Kuylenstierna J. Periodontal conditions in insulin-dependent diabetics. *J Clin Periodontol.* 1989;16:215-223.

[16] Tervonen T, Karjalainen K. Periodontal disease related to diabetic status. A pilot study of the response to periodontal therapy in type 1 diabetes. *J Clin Periodontol.* 1997;24:505-10.

[17] Löe H:Periodontal disease: the sixth complication of diabets mellitus. *Diabetes Care.* 1993; 16:329-334.

[18] Expert Comittee on the Diagnosis and Classification of Diabetes Mellitus: Report of the Expert Comittee on the Diagnosis and Classification of Diabetes Mellitus. *Diabetes Care* 1997;20:1183-1187.

[19] Taylor G: Bi-directional interrelationships between diabetes and periodontal diseases: epidemiologic perspective. *Ann Periodontol* 2001;6:99-112

[20] Mealey BL, Oates TW; American Academy of Periodontology. Diabetes mellitus and periodontal diseases. *J Periodontol.* 2006;77:1289-303.

[21] Hirschmann PN, Horner K, Rushnton VE. Selection criteria for periodontal radiograph. *Br Dent J* 1994:176:324-325

[22] Iughetti L, Marino R, Bertolani MF, Bernasconi S. Oral health in children and adolescents with IDDM--a review. *J Pediatric Endocrinol* 1999:12:603-610.

[23] Karjalainen KM, Knuuttila ML. The onset of diabetes and poor metabolic control increases gingival bleeding in children and adolescents with insulin-dependent diabetes mellitus. *J Clin Periodontol* 1996:23:1060-1067.

[24] Tchobroutsky G. Relation of diabetic control to developement of microvascular complications. *Diabetologia*. 1978;15:143-152.

[25] Carranza FA, Newman MG. Clinical periodontology. 8th ed. Philadelphia: WB Saunders Co; 1996. Irving Glickman's *Clinical Periodontology* Glickman; pp.281-297.

[26] Orbak R, Simsek S, Orbak Z, Kavrut F, Colak M.The Influence of Type 1 Diabete Mellitus on Dentition and Oral Health in Children and Adolescents. *Yonsei Med J*. 2008;49(3):357-365.

[27] Goteiner D, Vogel R, Deasy M, Goteiner C. Periodontal and caries experience in children with insulin-dependent diabetes mellitus. *J Am Dent Assoc*. 1986;113:277-279.

[28] Swanljung O, Meurman JH, Torkko H, Sandholm L, Kaprio E, Mäenpää J. Caries and saliva in 12-18 year old-diabetics and controls. Scand J Dent Res. 1992;100:310-313.

[29] Karjalainen KM, Knuuttila ML, Käär ML. Relationship between caries and level of metabolic balance in children and adolescents with insulin-dependent diabetes mellitus. Caries Res. 1997;31:13-18.

[30] Sheridan RC, Cheraskin E, Flyn AC. Epidemiology of diabetes mellitus II. 100 dental patients. J Periodontol. 1959;30:298-323.

[31] Seymour GJ, Ford PJ, Cullinan MP, Leishman S, Yamazaki K. Relationship betweenperiodontal infections and systemic disease. *Clin Microbiol Infect*. 2007;13 4:3-10.

[32] Rajendran R, Robertson D, Hodge PJ, Lappin DF, Ramage G. Hydrolytic Enzyme Production is Associated with Candida Albicans Biofilm Formation From patients with Type 1 Diabetes. *Mycopathologia*. 2010;170:4:229-235.

[33] Benveniste R, Bixler D, Conneally PM. Periodontal disease in diabetics. *J Periodontol*.1967;38:271-279.

[34] Hove KA, Stallard RE. Diabetes and the periodontal patient. *J Periodontol*. 1970;41:713-718.

[35] Bay I, Ainamo J, Gad T. The response of young diabetics to periodontal treatment. *J Periodontol* 1974:45:806-808.

[36] Barnett ML, Baker RL, Yancey JM, MacMillan DR & Kotoyan M. Absence of periodontitis in a population of insulin-dependent diabetes mellitus (IDDM) patients. *J Periodontol* 1984:55:402-405.

[37] Carranza FA, Newman MG. Clinical periodontology. 8th ed. Philadelphia: WB Saunders Co; 1996. Irving Glickman's *Clinical Periodontology* Glickman; pp.281-297.

[38] Oliver RC, Brown LJ, Loe H. Periodontal diseases in the United States population. *J Periodontol* 1998:69:269-278.

[39] Katz PP, Wirthlin MR, Szpunar SM, Selby JV, Sepe SJ, Showstack JA. Epidemiology and prevention of periodontal disease in individuals with Diabetes.*Diabetes Care* 1991:14:375-385.

[40] Frantzis TG, Reeve CM, Brown AL. The ultrastructure of capillary basement mambranesin the attached gingiva of diabetics and nondiabetics patients with periodontal disease. *J Periodontol*. 1971;42:406-411.

[41] Ervasti T, Knuuttila M, Pohjamo L, Haukipuro K. Relation between control of diabetes and gingival bleeding. J Periodontol. 1985;56:154-157.

[42] Lopez R, Fernandez O, Jara G, Baelum   V. Epidemiology of necrotizing ulcerative gingival lesions in adolescents. *J Periodontal Research* 2002:6:439-444.

[43] Taylor GW, Burt BA, Becker MP, Genco RJ, Shlossman M, Knowler WC, Pettitt DJ: Severe periodontitis and risk for poor glicemic control in patients with non-insulin-dependent diabetes mellitus. *J Periodontol.* 1996;67:1085-1093

[44] Thorstensson H, Kuylenstierna J, Hugoson A: Medical status and complications in relation to periodontal disease experince in insulin-dependent diabetics. *J Clin Periodontol* 1996;23:194-202.

[45] Thorstensson H. Periodontal disease in adult insulin-dependent diabetics. *Swed Dent J Suppl.* 1995;107:1-68.

[46] Nelson RG. Periodontal disease and diabetes. *Oral Dis.* 2008;14:204-5.

[47] Mansour AA, Abd-Al-Sada N. Periodontal disease among diabetics in Iraq. *MedGenMed.* 2005;7:2.

[48] Arrieta-Blanco JJ, Bartolomé-Villar B, Jiménez-Martinez E, Saavedra-Vallejo P, Arrieta-Blanco FJ. Bucco-dental problems in patients with Diabetes Mellitus (I): Index of plaque and dental caries. *Med Oral.* 2003;8:97-109.

[49] van Adrichem LN, Hovius SE, van Strick R, van der Meulen JC. Acute effects of cigarette smoking on the microcirculation of the thumb. *Br J Plast Surg.* 1992;45:9-11.

[50] R. Genco, S.G. Grossi, A. Ho, F. Nishimura, Y. Murayama. A proposed model linking inflammation to obesity, diabetes and periodontal infections. J Periodontol. 2005;76:2075-2084.

[51] King GL. The role of inflammatory cytokines in diabetes and its complications. *J Periodontol*2008; 79: 1527– 1534.

[52] Serino M, Luche E, Chabo C, Amar J, Burcelin R. Intestinal microflora and metabolic diseases.*Diabetes Metab* 2009; 35: 262– 272.

[53] Darré L, Vergnes JN, Gourdy P, Sixou M. Efficacy of periodontal treatment on glycaemic control in diabetic patients: A meta-analysis of interventional studies. *Diabetes Metab.* 2008;34(5):497-506.

[54] Clarke NG, Shephard BC, Hirsch RS. The effects of intra-arterial epinephrine and nicotine on gingival circulation. *Oral Surg Oral Med Oral Pathol.* 1981;52:577-582.

[55] D'Aiuto F, Parkar M, Andreou G, Suvan J,   Brett PM, Ready D, Tonetti MS. Periodontitis and systemic inflammation: control of the local infection is associated with a reduction in serum inflammatory markers. *J Dent Res.* 2004;83:156-160.

[56] Mealey B, Oates T. Diabetes mellitus and periodontal diseases. *J Periodontol.* 2006;77:1289-1303.

[57] Petitti DB, Associations are not effects, *Am J Epidemiol.* 1991;133:101-102.

[58] Lalla E, Cheng B, Lal S, Tucker S, Greenberg E, Goland R, Lamster IB. Periodontal changes in children and adolescents with diabetes: a case-control study. *Diabetes Care.* 2006;29(2):295-9.

[59] Cutler CW,Machen RL, Jotwani R, Iacopino AM. Heightened gingival imflammation and attachment loss in type 2 diabetics with hyperlipidemia. *Journal of Periodontology.* 1999;70:1313-21.

[60] Salvi GE, Collins JG, Yalda B, Arnold RR, Lang N, Offenbacher S. Monocytic TNF secretion patterns in IDDM patients with periodontal diseases. *J Clin Periodontol.* 1997;248-16.

[61] Firatly E, Unal T, Saka N, Onan U,Oz H. serum fructosamine correlates with gingival index in children with insulin-dependent diabetes mellitus (IDDM). *J Clin Periodontol.* 1994;21:565-8.

[62] De Pommerau V, Dargent-Paré C, Robert JJ, Brion M. Periodontal status in insulin dependent diabetic adolescents. *J Clin Periodontol*. 1992;19:628-32.

[63] Raylander H, Ramberg P,Blomhé G,Lindhe J. Prevalence of periodontal disease in young diabetics. *Journal of Clinical Periodontology*. 1986;14:38-43.

[64] Sastrowuijoto SH, Hillemans P, Steenbergen TJN, Abraham-Inpijn L, Graaff J. Periodontal condition ond microbiology of healthy and diseased periodontal pockets in type 1 diabetes mellitus patients. *J Clin Periodontol*. 1989;16:316-22.

[65] Firatli E. The relationship between clinical periodontal status and insulin-dependent diabetes mellitus, Results after 5 years. *J Periodontol* 1997:68:136-140.

[66] Sahafian S, Mikó S, Albrecht M. 2010

[67] http://www.mondofacto.com/facts/dictionary?Russell's%20Periodontal%20Index

[68] MedlinePlus Encyclopedia *Dental Cavities*

[69] Twetman S, Aronsson S, Bjorkman S. Mutans streptococci and lactobacilli in saliva from children with insulin dependent diabetes mellitus. *Oral Microbiol Inmunol*.1989;4:165-8.

[70] Collin HL, Uusitupa M, Niskanen L, Koivisto AM, Markanen H, Meurman JH. Caries in patients with non insulin dependent diabetes mellitus. *Oral Surg Oral Med Oral Pathol Oral Radiol Endod*. 1998;85:680-5.

[71] Holloway PJ; Moore, W.J. The role of sugar in the etiology of dental caries. *J Dent*. 1983;11(3): 189–213.

[72] Silverstone LM. Remineralization and enamel caries: new concepts. *Dent Update*. 1983;10 (4): 261–73.

[73] Moore PA, Weyant RJ, Etzel KR, Guggenheimer J, Mongelluzzo MB, Myers DE *et al*. Type 1 diabetes mellitus and oral health: assessment of coronal and root caries. *Community Dent Oral Epidemiol* 2001; 29: 183–194.

[74] Lin B P, Taylor G W, Allen D J, Ship J A. Dental caries in older adults with diabetes mellitus. *Spec Care Dentist* 1999 19: 8–14.

[75] do Amaral F M, Ramos P G, Ferreira S R. Study on the frequency of caries and associated factors in type 1 diabetes mellitus. *Arg Bras Endocinol Metabol* 2006; 50: 515–522.

[76] Arrieta-Blanco J J, Bartolomé-Villar B, Jiménez- Martinez E, Saavedra-Vallejo P, Arrieta-Blanco F J. Bucco-dental problems in patients with Diabetes Mellitus(I): Index of plaque and dental caries. *Med Oral* 2003; 8: 97–109.

[77] Miralles L, Silvestre F J, Hernández-Mijares A, Bautista D, Liambes F, Grau D. Dental caries in type 1 diabetics: infl uence of systemic factors of the disease upon the development of dental caries. *Med Oral Patol Oral Cir Bucal* 2006; 11: 256–260.

[78] Siudikiene J, Machiulskiene V, Nyvad B, Tenovuo J, Nedzeiskiene I. Dental caries and salivary status in children with type 1 diabetes mellitus related to the metabolic control of the disease. *Eur J Oral Sci* 2006; 114: 8–14.

[79] Miralles L, Silvestre FJ, Hernández-Mijares A, Bautista D, Llambés F, Grau D. Dental caries in type 1 diabetics: influence of systemic factors of the disease upon the development of dental caries. *Med Oral Patol Oral cir Bucal*.2006;11:256-60.

[80] Sterky G O, Kjellman O, Högberg O, Löfroth A L. Dietary composition and dental disease in adolescent diabetics. A pilot study. *Acta Paediatr Scand* 1971; 60: 461–464.

[81] Iugetti L, Marino R, Bertolani M F, Bernasconi S. Oral health in children and adolescents with IDDM: A review. *J Pediatr Endocrinol Metab* 1999; 12: 603–610.

[82] Wegner H. Dental caries in young diabetics. *Caries Res* 1971; 5: 188–192.

[83] Wegner H. Increment of caries in young diabetics. *Caries Res* 1975; 9: 90–91.

[84] Twetman S, Nederfors T, Ståhl B, Aronson S. Two-year longitudinal observations of salivary status and dental caries in children with insulindependent diabetes mellitus. *Pediatr Dent* 1992;14: 184–188.

[85] Twetman S, Johansson I, Birkhed D, Nederfors T. Caries Incidence in young Type 1 diabetes mellitus patients in relation to metabolic control and cariesassociated risk factors. *Caries Res* 2002; 36: 31–35.

[86] Ben-Aryeh H, Serouya R, Kanter Y, Szargel R, Laufer D. Oral health and salivary composition in diabetic patients. *J Diabetes Complications*.1993;7:57-62.

[87] Got I, Fontaine A. Teeth and diabetes. *Diabete Metab*.1993;19:467-471.

[88] Kneckt M C, Syrjälä A M H S, Knuuttila M L E. Attributions to dental and diabetes health outcomes. *J Clin Periodontol*; 27: 205–211.

[89] Moore PA, Orchard T, Guggenheimer J, Weyant RJ. Diabetes and oral health promotion: a survey of disease prevention behaviors. *JADA*. 2000;131:1333-1341.

[90] Alves C, Márcia B, Andion J, Menezes R. Oral health knowledge and habits in children with type 1 diabetes mellitus. *Braz Dent*. 2009;20:70-73.

[91] Miko S, Ambrus S J, Sahafian S, Dinya E, Tamas G, Albrecht M G. Dental caries and adolescents with type 1 diabetes. *British Dental Journal* 2010;208:(6) p. E12.

[92] Ash, Major M, Stanley J. Nelson. Wheeler's Dental Anatomy, Physiology and Occlusion. 8th edition. 2003.P.41.

[93] American Academy of Pediatric Dentistry Clinical Affairs Comittee, Developing Dentition Subcommittee; American Academy of Pediatric Dentistry Council on Clinical Affairs. Guideline on management of the developing dentition and occlusion in pediatric dentistry. Pediatr Dent. 2005;27:143-155.

[94] Ziskin DE, Siegel EH, Loughlin WC, Diabetes in relation to certain oral and systemic problems. Part I: clinical study of dental caries, tooth eruption, gingival changes, growth phenomena and related observations in juveniles. *J Dent Res*. 1944;23:317-331.

[95] Bohatka L, Wegner H, Adler P. Parameters of the mixed dentition in diabetic children. *J Dent Res*. 1973;52:131-135.

[96] Adler P, Wegner H, Bohatka L. Influence of age and duration of diabetes an diabetes on dental development in diabetic children. *J Dent Res*. 1973;52:535-537.

[97] Lal S, Cheng B, Kaplan S, Softness B, Greenberg E, Goland RS, Lalla E, Lamster IB. Accelerated Tooth Eruption in Children With Diabetes Mellitus. *Pediatrics*. 2008;121:1139-1143

[98] Hastreiter RJ, Bakdash B, Roesch MH, Walseth J. Use of tobacco prevention and cessation strategies and techniques int he dental office. *JADA*. 1994;125(11):1475-84.

[99] Christen AG, Klein JA,Christen JA, McDonald JL Jr, Guba CJ. How-to-do-it quit-smoking strategies for the dental office team: an eight-step program. *JADA*. 1990;(suppl)S20-S7.

[100] Gerbert B, Coates T, Zahnd E, Richard RJ, Cummings SR. Dentists as smoking cessation counselors. *JADA*. 1989;118(1):29-32.

[101] Curriculum guidelines for predoctoral preventive dentistry. *J Dent Educ*. 1991;55(11):746-50.

9

The Effect of Type 1 Diabetes Mellitus on the Craniofacial Complex

Mona Abbassy[1,2,3], Ippei Watari[1] and Takashi Ono[1]
[1]*Orthodontic Science, Department of Orofacial Development and Function,*
Division of Oral Health Sciences, Tokyo Medical and Dental University,
[2]*Preventive Dental Sciences Department, Orthodontic Department Devision,*
King AbdulAziz University,
[3]*Alexandria University*
[1]*Japan*
[2]*Saudia Arabia*
[3]*Egypt*

1. Introduction

Diabetes mellitus (DM) is one of the systemic diseases affecting a considerable number of patients (Bensch *et al.*, 2003). Numerous experimental and clinical studies on the complications of diabetes mellitus have demonstrated extensive alterations in bone and mineral metabolism, linear growth, and body composition (Giglio and Lama, 2001). DM is a metabolic disorder characterized by disturbed glucose metabolism, manifesting primarily as chronic hyperglycemia.

Bone metabolism is impaired in Type 1 Diabetes Mellitus (T1DM), either through the direct effect of insulin deficiency or hyperglycaemia or via the more long-term effects of vascular disease. Previous data suggested that osteoblast function can be corrected by restoration of glycaemic control, indicating that hyperglycaemia produces direct impairment of bone metabolism (Shyng *et al.*, 2001).

Growth is a highly complex mechanism resulting not only in a major change in size, but also in minor changes in shape. The changes in shape of the craniofacial skeleton are of particular interest because pathological growth of certain anatomical regions may lead to functional and esthetic problems. In the craniofacial skeleton, it has been well known that growth involves a mosaic of growth sites that grow at different rates and mature at different times (Vandeberg *et al.*, 2004a; VandeBerg *et al.*, 2004b), its growth and by analogy, the response to growth disruption is much more complex than that of the appendicular skeleton (Vandeberg *et al.*, 2004a). Different parts of the craniofacial complex might be expected to respond differently to the same hormonal or biomechanical stimulus (VandeBerg *et al.*, 2004b). T1DM has been shown to affect the general growth of patients due to insulin deficiency and consequently leads to delayed skeletal maturation (Schwartz, 2003).

2. Types of bone formation in craniofacial complex

Bone forms in two ways, resulting in two types of mature bone – intramembranous and cartilage. Cartilage bone forms in a replacement process within the cartilage models of the embryo and infant. Intramembranous bone forms through the activation of the osteoblast cell or specialized bone forming cells in one of the layers of fetal connective tissue. The bones of the cranial vault, the face, and the clavicle are intramembranous in origin. All other bones of the body form from cartilage. Intramembranous bone include the mandible, the maxilla, the premaxilla, the frontal bone, the palatine bone, the squamous part of temporal bone, the zygomatic bone, the medial plate of the pterygoid process, the vomer, the tympanic part of the temporal bone, the nasal bone, the lacrimal bone, and the parietal bone. The original pattern of intramembranous bone changes with progressive maturative growth when these bones begin to adapt to environmental influences. This accounts for deformities due to malfunction, disease and other environmental factors (Salzmann, 1979).

3. Causes of growth problems

Growth disturbances can be associated with specific anatomic or functional defects. They may be of endocrine or non endocrine origin and may result from genetic, nutritional or environmental factors. Disturbances in somatic growth show themselves in retardation or acceleration of the skeletal system, including the facial and cranial bones. Causes for growth problems usually fall into the following categories (Kumar, 2009):

- **Familial short stature**
  Familial short stature is a tendency to follow the family's inherited short stature (shortness).
- **Constitutional growth delay with delayed adolescence or delayed maturation**
  A child who tends to be shorter than average and who enters puberty later than average, but is growing at a normal rate. Most of these children tend to eventually grow to approximately the same height as their parents.
- **Illnesses that affect the whole body (Also called systemic diseases)**
  Constant malnutrition, digestive tract diseases, kidney disease, heart disease, lung disease, hepatic disease, diabetes, and severe stress can cause growth problems.
- **Endocrine (hormone) diseases**
  Adequate production of the thyroid hormone is necessary for normal bone growth. Cushing's syndrome can be caused by a myriad of abnormalities that are the result of hypersecretion of corticosteroids by the adrenal gland. Growth hormone deficiency involves a problem with the pituitary gland (small gland at the base of the brain) that secretes several hormones, including growth hormone.
- **Congenital (present at birth) problems in the tissues where growth occurs**
  A condition called intrauterine growth restriction (IUGR), slow growth within the uterus occurs during a pregnancy. The baby is born smaller in weight and length than normal, in proportion to his/her short stature.

4. Outline of studying the effect of diabetes mellitus on craniofacial growth

Approximately 60% of adult bone mass including craniofacial bone is gained during the peak of the growth period which coincides with the onset of T1DM condition affecting the bone formation process (Eastell and Lambert, 2002). It is worth mentioning here that although T1DM condition exact etiological factors are totally unknown however; understanding the course of T1DM condition and its impact on craniofacial development may lead to improving the oral health for a large sector of the population worldwide.

Numerous experimental and clinical studies on the complications of DM have demonstrated extensive alterations in bone and mineral metabolism, linear growth, and body composition. Investigators in the fields of bone biology including orthodontics have long been interested in the general causes that affect the normal growth of the craniofacial region. T1DM has been shown to affect the general growth of patients with earlier onset of the disease, especially onset before or around the circumpubertal growth spurts (Chew, 1991).

In general, growth of the craniofacial complex is controlled by genetic and environmental factors (Giglio and Lama, 2001; Yonemitsu *et al.*, 2007). Regulatory mechanisms responsible for normal morphogenesis of the face and head involve hormones, nutrients, mechanical forces, and various local growth factors. The poor growth and alterations in bone metabolism have been associated with T1DM in both humans and experimental animals (Giglio and Lama, 2001). It is of prime importance investigating the changes in craniofacial bone structure and dynamic bone formation in DM condition to explore the impact of the diabetic condition on various mandibular growth elements and bone quality.

The following parts of this chapter are going to focus on these points:

- Investigating the effects of juvenile diabetes on general craniofacial growth and skeletal maturation.
- Analyzing the pattern of association between craniofacial morphology and skeletal maturation.
- Determination of the changes in bone morphology in diabetic rat mandible using micro-C.T.
- Determination of the mineral apposition rate and the bone formation rate in diabetic rat mandible using histomorphometric analysis.

5. Animal and experimental diabetic model

The animal studies using diabetic model presents various advantages when compared to studies carried out on human diabetic cases. Human studies can be limited by small sample sizes, cross-sectional designs, uncontrolled variables, and often retrospective nature, animal models have been used to yield more rigorous analyses (Singleton *et al.*, 2006).

5.1 Diabetic model

Experimental diabetic models include the streptozotocin-induced diabetic rat and the spontaneously diabetic BioBreeding rat. The occurrence of different abnormalities indicating altered bone formation after inducing DM with streptozotocin (STZ) is well documented (Giglio and Lama, 2001; Hough *et al.*, 1981; Tein *et al.*, 1998). Streptozotocin-induced diabetes mellitus (STZ-DM), caused by the destruction of pancreatic β-cells and is similar to T1DM in human, is characterized by mild to moderate hyperglycemia, glucosuria, polyphagia, hypoinsulinemia, hyperlipidemia, and weight loss. STZ-DM also exhibits many of the complications observed in human DM including enhanced susceptibility to infection and cardiovascular disease, retinopathy, alterations in angiogenesis, delayed wound healing, diminished growth factor expression, and reduced bone formation (Lu *et al.*, 2003).

5.2 Importance of testing the uncontrolled diabetic condition

In the usual clinical situation, although T1DM patient is treated with insulin, patient may still suffer from an overall poor diabetic metabolic state with an uncontrollable blood glucose level and a high and sometimes changing insulin requirement (Follak *et al.*, 2004).

5.3 Inducing diabetic condition

All the experimental protocols followed had been approved by the Institutional Animal Care and Use Committee of Tokyo Medical and Dental University, and the experiments were carried out under the control of the University's Guidelines for Animal Experimentation. In our investigation we explored the various effects of DM using the streptozotocin DM model. Twelve 3-week old male Wistar rats were used for this study. They were randomly divided into two groups, the control group and the diabetes group (DM group), each group consists of 6 rats. The rats in the control group were injected intra-peritoneal with a single dose of 0.1M sodium citrate buffer (pH 4.5), while the rats in the DM group were injected intra-peritoneal with a single dose of citrate buffer containing 60mg/kg body weight of streptozotocin (Sigma Chemical Co., St. Louis, MO, USA).(Alkan *et al.*, 2002; McCracken *et al.*, 2006; Shyng *et al.*, 2001; Tein *et al.*, 1998) All animals were fed on standard Rodent diet (Rodent Diet CE-2; Japan Clea Inc., Shizuoka, Japan) with free access to water. Body weights, the presence of glucose in urine and blood glucose levels were recorded on day 0, 2, 7, 14, 21 and 28 after STZ injection.

Diabetes condition was determined by the presence of glucose in urine and blood. The urine of the rats was tested using reagent strips (Uriace Ga; TERUMO). (Abdus Salam *et al.*, 2004; Matin *et al.*, 2002) Blood samples of the rats were obtained via vein puncture of a tail vein, and blood glucose levels were determined using a glucometer (Ascensia Brio. Bayer Medical). Positive urine test and a blood glucose level greater than 200 mg/dl was considered DM.(Giglio and Lama, 2001).

Fig. 1. shows the weights of the rats (mean±SD) in both groups. DM group showed a significant decrease in weight. After STZ injection by 48 hours the urine test showed that the entire DM group had a high glucose level and this was confirmed by the high blood glucose measurements as shown in Fig. 2. A Student's t-test was used to compare the mean of weights and blood glucose levels in both groups.

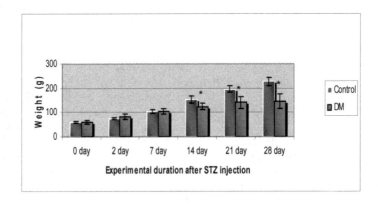

Fig. 1. Comparison between the changes of the rat's weight in the control and DM group. The weights of the DM group are significantly decreased as compared to the weights of the control group (*:$p<0.05$).

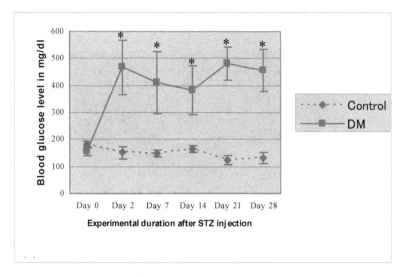

Fig. 2. Line graph represents the blood glucose levels for the control and DM group. The blood glucose level in DM group increased significantly 48h post-STZ injection and during the entire experimental period. Values are mean±SD. Significant differences between the two groups are marked with asterisks ($p< 0.05$).

6. Analytic studies conducted to test the effect of diabetic condition on craniofacial growth

6.1 Cephalometric analysis

Cephalometric measurements are still one of the most widely spread diagnostic aids crucial for the diagnosis of various abnormalities in the craniofacial complex (Chidiac *et al.*, 2002).

The protocol for examining the cephalometric measurements in DM rats involves the following steps:

- Prior to each radiographic session, the rats are anaesthetized with diethyl ether and intraperitoneal injection of 8% chloral hydrate using 0.5ml/100g of body weight.
- Each animal is then placed in this specially-designed apparatus (Fig. 3) to maintain standardized head posture and contact with the film (SGP-3, Mitsutoy, Tokyo, Japan) where the head of each rat is fixed firmly with a pair of ear rods oriented vertically to the sagittal plane and the incisors are fixed into a plastic ring.
- The settings of lateral and dorsoventral cephalometric radiographs are 50/55kVp, 15/10mA, and 20/60-sec impulses respectively (Singleton *et al.*, 2006; Vandeberg *et al.*, 2004a; VandeBerg *et al.*, 2004b).
- A 10 mm steel calibration rod is incorporated into the clear acrylic table on which the animals are positioned for the radiographs.
- All the radiographs are developed and scanned at high resolution by the same operator (Singleton *et al.*, 2006).

The cephalometric landmarks (Table 1; Fig. 4) were derived from previous studies on rodents (Engstrom *et al.*, 1988; Kiliaridis and Thilander, 1985; Singleton *et al.*, 2006; Vandeberg *et al.*, 2004a; VandeBerg *et al.*, 2004b). Selected linear measurements were then obtained (Table 2). To ensure reliability and replicability of each measurement, each distance was digitized twice and the two values were averaged.

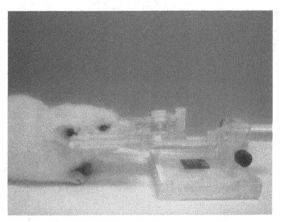

Fig. 3. Apparatus for roentgenographic cephalometry

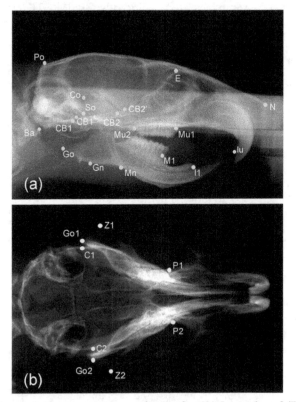

Fig. 4. Location of cephalometric points on radiographs: (A) Sagittal and (B) transverse.

On the sagittal radiograph

N: The most anterior point on the nasal bone

E: The intersection of the frontal bone and floor of anterior cranial fossa

Po: The most posterior and superior point on the skull

Ba: The most posterior and inferior point on the occipital condyle

Co: The most posterior and superior point on the mandibular condyle

Go: The most posterior point on the mandibular ramus

Mn: The most concave portion of the concavity on the inferior border of the mandibular corpus

Gn: The most inferior point on the ramus that lies on a perpendicular bisector of the line Go-Mn

Il: The most anterior and superior point on the alveolar bone of the mandibular incisor

So: The intersection of the most anterior tympanic bulla and the superior border of the sphenoid bone

CB1: The most anterior point on the occipital bone at the spheno-occipital synchondrosis

CB1′ : The most posterior point on the sphenoid bone at the spheno-occipital synchondrosis

CB2: The most anterior point on the sphenoid bone at the spheno-basispheno synchondrosis

CB2′ : The most posterior point on the basisphenoid bone at the spheno-basispheno-synchondrosis

Ml: The junction of the alveolar bone and the mesial surface of the first mandibular molar

Mu1: The junction of the alveolar bone and the mesial surface of the first maxillary molar

Mu2: The junction of the alveolar bone and the distal surface of the third maxillary molar

Iu: The most anterior-inferior point on the maxilla posterior to the maxillary incisors

On the transverse radiograph

Z1 & Z2: The points on the lateral portion of the zygomatic arch that produce the widest width

Go1 & Go2: The points on the angle of the mandible that produce the widest width

P1 & P2: The most anterior and medial points within the temporal fossae that produce the most narrow palatal width

C1 & C2: The points on the cranium that produce the widest cranial width

Table 1. Definition of radiographic points

Neurocranium
Po-N: total skull length
Po-E: cranial vault length
Ba-E: total cranial base length
So-E: anterior cranial base length
Ba-CB1: occipital bone length
CB1′ -CB2: sphenoid bone length
Ba-So: posterior cranial base length
Po-Ba: posterior neurocranium height
Viscerocranium
E-N: nasal length
Mu2-Iu: palate length
CB2-Iu: midface length
E-Mu1: viscerocranial height
Mandible
Go-Mn: posterior corpus length
Ml-Il: anterior corpus length
Co-Il: total mandibular length
Co-Gn: ramus height
Transverse X-ray
Go1-Go2: Bigonial width
C1-C2: Maximum cranial width
P1-P2: Palatal width
Z1-Z2: Bizygomatic width

Table 2. Measurements of craniofacial skeleton

In our studies, evaluation of the craniofacial growth of diabetic rats at the age of 7 weeks was done using lateral and dorsoventral cephalometric radiographs. All of the data in each experiment were confirmed the normal distribution, so a Student's t-test was used to compare the mean of each data recorded in the control group and in the DM group. All statistical analyses were performed at a 5% significance level using statistic software (v. 10; SPSS, Chicago, IL, USA).

6.1.1 Changes in the total skull
The size of total skull, denoted by Po-N, was significantly smaller in the DM group than in the control group.

6.1.2 Changes in the neurocranium
Cranial vault length (Po-E), total cranial base length (Ba-E), anterior cranial base length (So-E), Occipital bone length (Ba-CB1), and posterior cranial base length (Ba-So) showed statistically significant decrease in DM group (Table 3, Figs. 5, 6), while other dimensions exhibited no significant differences.

Po-N	total skull length
Po-E	cranial vault length
Ba-E	total cranial base length
So-E	anterior cranial base length
Ba-CB1	occipital bone length
Ba-So	posterior cranial base length

Table 3. Significant changes in the total skull and neurocranium

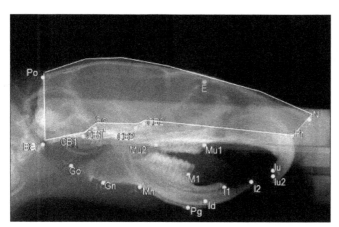

Fig. 5. Neurocranium

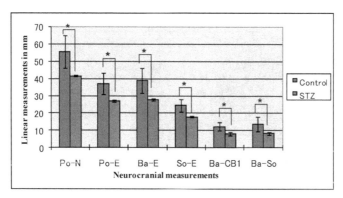

Fig. 6. Changes in the neurocranial measurements of the control and DM group. All the significant measurements are shown in this figure. Values are mean±S.D. Significant differences between the two groups are marked with asterisks ($p<0.05$).

6.1.3 Changes in the viscerocranium

All measurements of the viscerocranium, including the nasal length (E-N), palatal length (Mu2-Iu), midface length (CB2-Iu), and viscerocranial height (E-Mu1) showed a statistically significant decrease in DM group (Table 4, Figs. 7,8)

E-N	Nasal length
Mu2-Iu	Palate length
Cb2-Iu	midface length
E-Mu1	Posterior viscerocranial height

Table 4. Significant changes in the viscerocranium

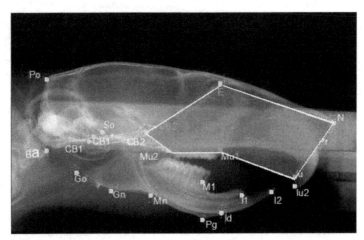

Fig. 7. Viscerocranium

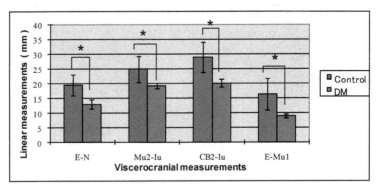

Fig. 8. Changes in the viscerocranial measurements of the control and DM group. All the viscerocranial measurements are significant. Values are mean±S.D. Significant differences between the two groups are marked with asterisks ($p<0.05$).

6.1.4 Changes in the mandible

In the DM group, the posterior corpus length (Go-Mn), total mandibular length (Co-Il) and the ramus height (Co-Gn) were significantly shorter than in the control group (Table 5, Figs. 9, 10), whereas no remarkable differences were found in the remaining dimensions.

Go-Mn	Posterior corpus length
Co-Il	Total mandibular length
Co-Gn	Ramus height

Table 5. Significant changes in the mandible

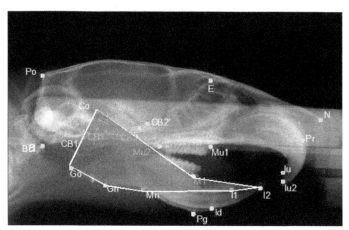

Fig. 9. Mandible

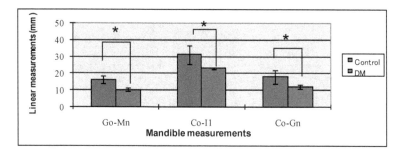

Fig. 10. Changes in the mandible measurements of the control and DM group. Values are mean ± S.D. Significant differences between the two groups are marked with asterisks ($p<0.05$).

6.1.5 Changes in the transverse X-ray

In transverse X-ray only the maximum cranial width (C1-C2) and the bizygomatic width (Z1-Z2) were statistically decreased in DM group (Table 6, Figs. 11, 12).
All other linear measurements showed no significant differences between both groups

C1-C2	Maximum cranial width
Z1-Z2	Bizygomatic width

Table 6. Significant changes in the transverse X-ray

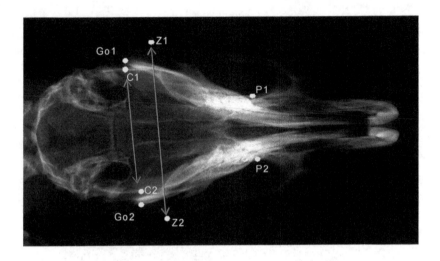

Fig. 11. Transverse X-ray measurements

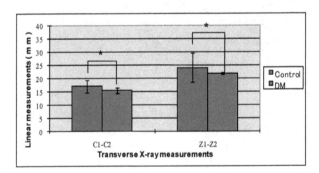

Fig. 12. Changes in the transverse X-ray measurements of the control and DM group. Two measurements in the transverse X-ray were significant. Values are mean±S.D. Significant differences between the two groups are marked with asterisks ($p < 0.05$).

Linear measurements	DM		C	
	Mean	SD	Mean	SD
Neurocranium				
Po-N	41.67	0.59*	55.61	9.48
Po-E	26.86	0.6*	37.12	6.35
Ba-E	27.74	0.64*	38.87	7.19
So-E	17.91	0.31*	24.41	3.72
Ba-CB1	8.23	1.08*	12.3	2.34
CB1' -CB2	4.78	0.74	5.93	1.18
Ba-So	8.44	0.7*	13.61	4.23
Po-Ba	10.03	0.83	13.14	2.81
Viscerocranium				
E-N	13.07	1.56*	19.57	3.48
Mu2-Iu	19.34	0.95*	25.01	4.5
CB2-Iu	20.16	1.29*	29	5.07
E-Mu1	8.93	0.69*	16.43	5.36
Mandible				
Go-Mn	10.27	1.04*	16	2.39
M1-I1	5.4	0.88	6.97	1.54
Co-I1	22.95	0.34*	31.13	5.51
Co-Gn	12.22	1.2*	17.9	4.04
Transverse X-ray				
Go1-Go2	18.42	0.42	19.77	1.32
C1-C2	15.43	0.67*	17.03	1.16
P1-P2	8.5	0.41	9.19	0.52
Z1-Z2	21.9	0.33*	24	1.4

*$p<0.05$ as compared to control values

Table 7. Comparision of skeletal cephalometric measurements for Type 1 Diabetes mellitus (DM) and controls (C)

6.2 Histomorphometric analysis
6.2.1 Fluorescent dyes used for double labeling in histomorphometric analysis
Fluorochromes are calcium binding substances that are preferentially taken up at the site of active mineralization of bone known as the calcification front, thus labeling sites of new bone formation. They are detected using fluorescent microscopy on undecalcified sections. Labeling bones with fluorochrome markers provides a means to study the dynamics of bone formation. The rate and extent of bone deposition and resorption can be determined using double and triple fluorochrome labeling sequences. The sequential use of fluorochromes of clearly contrasting colors permits a more detailed record of events relating to calcification. Flurochromes commonly used in mammals include tetracycline, calcein green, xylenol orange, alirazin red, and hematoporphyrin. Calcein is a fluoresces bright green when combined with calcium (Stuart and Smith, 1992).

6.2.2 Calcein administrations and sections preparation

The steps needed for detecting the double labeling involves the following:

- Rats are subcutaneously injected with 50 mg/kg body weight calcein fluorescent marker on day 21 and day 28 after STZ injection. The time difference between the 2 injections is one week to be able to compare the amount of bone formed during this period (Fig. 14).
- Sacrifice of all animals by transcardiac perfusion under deep anesthesia using 4% paraformaldehyde in 0.1 M phosphate buffer (pH 7.4).
- Mandibles are dissected and fixed in the same solution for 24 hours.
- All specimens are embedded in polystyrene resin (Rigolac, Nisshin EM Co. Ltd., Tokyo, Japan).
- Undemineralized ground frontal sections are processed to show the crown and both apices of buccal and lingual roots of the lower second molar (Shimomoto *et al.*, 2007).

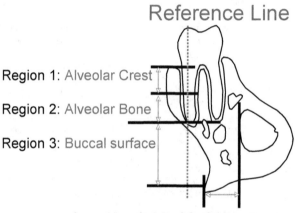

Fig. 13. Schematic drawing of observation regions for dynamic bone histomorphometry. The periosteal surfaces were delimited into 4 areas as alveolar crest (region 1), alveolar bone (region 2), buccal surface of the jaw bone (region 3), and inferior border of the jaw bone (region 4).

6.2.3 Method of analysis

The bone around the lower second molar is centrally located within the mandibular arch, and because of the parallel alignment of the buccal and lingual roots this made a precise reference when frontal sections are produced (Shimomoto *et al.*, 2005). To conduct the histomorphometric analysis it is essential to use a digitizing morphometry system to measure bone formation indices. The system consists of a confocal laser scanning microscope (LSM510, Carl Zeiss Co. Ltd., Jena, Germany), and a morphometry program (LSM Image Browser, Carl Zeiss Co. Ltd., Jena, Germany). Bone formation indices of the periosteal surfaces of the alveolar/jaw bone include mineral apposition rate ($\mu m/day$) and bone formation rate ($\mu m^3/\mu m^2/day$), according to the standard nomenclature described by (Parfitt *et al.*, 1987). The calcein-labeled surface (CLS, in mm) is calculated as the sum of the length of double labels (dL) plus one half of the length of single labels (sL) along the entire endosteal or periosteal bone surfaces; that is, CLS = dL + 0.5sL (Keshawarz and Recker, 1986). The mineral apposition rate (MAR, in μ/day) is determined by dividing the mean of the width of the double labels by the interlabel time (7 days). The bone formation rate (BFR) is calculated by multiplying MAR by CLS (Sheng *et al.*, 1999). Based on the reference line along the long axis of the buccal root, the area superior to the root apex was considered alveolar bone, while the area inferior to the root apex was considered the jaw bone. The lingual side of the bone is excluded, because the existence of the incisor root may influence bone formation.

The periosteal surfaces of the mandible are divided into four regions for analysis (Fig. 13):
Region 1: alveolar crest (upper 1/2 of the tooth root, near the tooth crown)
Region 2: alveolar bone (lower 1/2 of the tooth root, near the root apex)
Region 3: buccal surface of the jaw bone
Region 4: inferior border of the jaw bone

6.2.4 Histomorphometric indices

The obtained results in our study showed that in the alveolar bone (region 2), there was a significant decrease in the MAR (Fig. 15A) BFR (Fig. 15B) recorded in the DM group compared to the control group. However, in the alveolar crest (region 1), the MAR and the BFR in the control and the DM groups were not significantly different. ($p<0.05$). In the buccal surface (region 3) and inferior borders (region 4) of the jaw bone the MAR (Fig. 15A) and BFR (Fig. 15B) were significantly suppressed compared with those in the control group ($p<0.05$). Most of the periosteal surfaces in the mandibular regions of the control group showed significantly higher values recorded for the mineral apposition rate and the bone formation rate when compared to the DM group. These results agree with previous studies that recorded diminished lamellar bone formation in DM rats' femur and may suggest an association between the DM condition and the decreased number and function of osteoblasts (Follak *et al.*, 2004; Shyng *et al.*, 2001). The alveolar crest region was the only region that did not show a significant difference in the mineral apposition rate and the bone formation rate parameters among the two groups; this may be attributed to the unique nature of this region exhibiting a highly intensive bone remodeling process especially during the teeth eruption that decreases toward the base of the socket (Gerlach *et al.*, 2002), however further studies are needed to elaborate the detailed pattern of bone growth at the alveolar crest region.

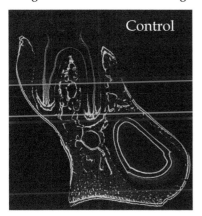 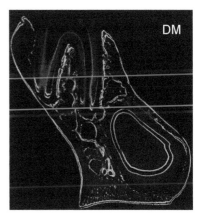

Fig. 14. Frontal sections of the mandibular second molar area. (A) Control; (B) DM. Fluorescent labeling on the periosteal surface indicates new bone formation.

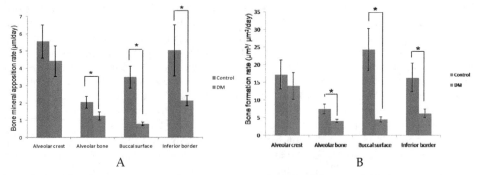

Fig. 15. (A) The changes in mineral apposition rate (MAR) of the mandible between the control group and the DM group. Alveolar crest (region 1, upper 1/2 of the tooth root, near the tooth crown). Alveolar bone (region 2, lower 1/2 of the tooth root, near the root apex). Buccal surface of the jaw bone (region 3). Inferior border of the jaw bone (region 4). The data are expressed as means ± SD. n = 5 for each group. *:$p<0.05$. (B) The changes in the bone formation rate (BFR/BS) of the mandible between the control group and the DM group. Alveolar crest (region 1, upper 1/2 of the tooth root, near the tooth crown). Alveolar bone (region 2, lower 1/2 of the tooth root, near the root apex). Buccal surface of the jaw bone (region 3). Inferior border of the jaw bone (region 4). The data are expressed as means ± S.D. n = 5 for each group. *:$p<0.05$.

6.3 Microtomography of the mandible (micro-CT)

Micro-computed tomography (micro-CT) has rapidly become a standard technique for the visualization and quantification of the 3D structure of trabecular bone. Bone architecture and mineralization are generally considered to be important components of bone quality, and determine bone strength in conjunction with bone mineral density.

6.3.1 Protocol adopted to examine the mandible using micro-CT

In our study all specimens were imaged by micro-CT (inspeXio SMX-90CT; Shimadzu Science East Corporation, Tokyo, Japan)

- After removing only the soft tissue, the mandibular plane is set orthogonal to the sample stage.
- Three dimensional images of each hemi mandible are acquired with a resolution voxel size of 15 μm / pixel.
- Raw data are obtained by rotating the sample stage 360 degrees. Then, slice images are prepared using multi-tomographic image reconstruction software (MultiBP; Imagescript, Tokyo, Japan).
- The resulting gray-scale images are segmented using a low-pass filter to remove noise and a fixed threshold to extract the mineralized bone phase.
- The volume of interest is drawn on a slice-based method starting from the first slice containing the crown of the first molar and moving dorsally 100 slices (Laib and Ruegsegger, 1999; Zhang *et al.*, 2008), in the area of the alveolar crest (Between the buccal and lingual roots of the second molar at the cervical region); and the buccal surface of the jaw bone (Shimomoto *et al.*, 2007). Trabecular bone was carefully contoured on the first and the last slice, while the intermediate slices were first interpolated by morphing.

- For observation and analysis of reconstructed 3D images, 3D trabecular structure analysis software (TRI/3D-BON; RATOC System Engineering, Tokyo, Japan) is used (Takada *et al.*, 2006). Reconstructed 3D images were prepared from slice images using the volume rendering method, to analyze the microstructure of the bone (Fig. 16).
- The following parameters are measured: tissue volume (TV), bone volume (BV), bone surface (BS), bone surface / bone volume (BS/BV), bone-volume fraction (BV/TV).
- Four properties of the trabeculae are evaluated: trabecular thickness (Tb.Th), trabecular number (Tb.N), trabecular separation (Tb.Sp), and Trabecular space (Tb.S) (Nakano *et al.*, 2004; Takada *et al.*, 2006).

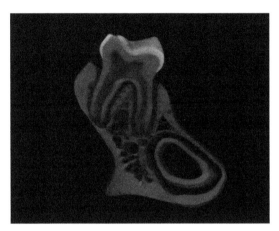

Fig. 16. The left mandible was imaged by micro-CT

6.3.2 Microtomography of the DM mandible

The quantification of micro-CT trabecular bone changes (mean±SD) is shown for the DM and the control groups in (Table 4). All trabecular parameters in both alveolar bone and buccal surface of jaw bone showed significant changes. Compared with the control group, bone volume fraction (BV/TV) was significantly decreased only in the alveolar bone; however, trabecular thickness (Tb.Th) and trabecular numbers (Tb.N) were significantly decreased both in alveolar and buccal surface of jaw bone, in the DM group. Correspondingly, significantly higher trabecular separation (Tb.Sp) and trabecular space (Tb.S) were revealed both in alveolar and buccal surface of jaw bone for the DM group when compared with that of the control group. Also, the bone surface / bone volume (BS/BV) was significantly increased only in alveolar bone ($p<0.05$). These findings indicate deterioration of the bone quality in the DM group. These results agree with other research work suggesting that the glycaemic levels play an important role in modulating the trabecular architecture especially in mandibular bone (Thrailkill *et al.*, 2005).

The DM condition resulted in alteration of the trabecular distance and thickness as compared to the control group indicating profound impact on the histological integrity of the bone. The reduction in trabecular bone volume accompanied by the expansion of the bone marrow space is in agreement with another investigation (Duarte *et al.*, 2005). In this context, these results may describe a state of osteopenia in experimental diabetic rats, which might be the result of an imbalance between bone formation and resorption

	Alveolar Bone		Buccal Surface Of The Jaw Bone	
	DM	Control	DM	Control
Bone Surface/Bone Volume (1/mm)	36.8±9.5*	63.93±15.3	87.8±5.6	70.0±15.5
Bone Volume/Tissue Volume (%)	22.1±11.6*	46.2±10.2	37.3±4.2	55.2±16.4
Trabecular Thickness (μm)	23.2±2.1*	34.3±4.5	21.5±2.9*	26.1±2.1
Trabecular Number (1/mm)	10.8±1.2*	14.4±2.6	15.2±1.7*	18.9±0.7
Trabecular Separation (μm)	37.5±1.0*	25.5±2.4	38.1±9.1*	25.9±2.4
Trabecular Space (μm)	87.6±4.3*	71.2±11.5	67.7±7.9*	53.1±2.0

*$p<0.05$ as compared to control values

Table 8. Microarchitectural properties in the mandible as measured by micro-CT

6.4 Histological analysis
6.4.1 Procedure for preparing mandibles for histological analysis
- Mandibles for all groups were decalcified in 10% EDTA solution pH 7.4 for 5 weeks at 4°C (Yokoyama *et al.*, 2009).
- Specimens are then dehydrated in an ascending ethanol series and embedded in paraffin (Figs. 9, 10, 11).
- Serial horizontal sections (5 μm thick parallel to the occlusal plane) are prepared using a microtome (Leica RM 2155, Nussloch, Germany) (Figs. 12, 13)

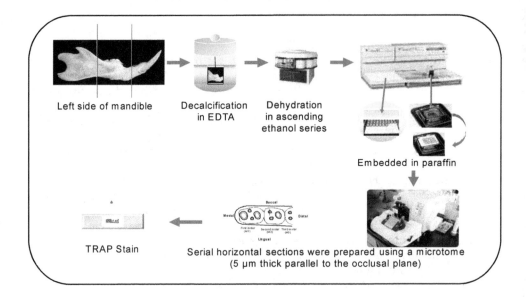

Fig. 17. Experimental procedure for histological section preparation

6.4.2 TRAP staining

Histological sections are incubated for 30–60 min at 37°C in a mixture of 0.8% naphthol AS-BI phosphate (Sigma, St Louis, MO, USA), 0.7% fast red violet salt (Sigma, St Louis, MO, USA) and 50mM sodium tartate diluted in 0.2M sodium acetate buffer (pH 5.4) (Tsuchiya and Kurihara, 1995). Sections were examined under a light microscope. For the histomorphometric assessment of resorption, the number of tartrate-resistant acid phosphatase-positive multinucleated cells (osteoclasts) on the distal surface of the alveolar bone adjacent to the mesio-buccal root of the second molar were counted in each 540 µm x 120 µm area in five consecutive sections, at the middle third of the root selected at least 25µm apart from each specimen (n = 5) of each group (Misawa *et al.*, 2007; Mishima *et al.*, 2002).

6.4.3 Histological analysis

Bone-resorption activity was assessed by counting the number of tartrate-resistant acid phosphatase-positive multinucleate cells (osteoclasts) on the distal surface of the alveolar bone adjacent to the mesio-buccal root of the second molar (Fig. 18A-D). Statistical analysis

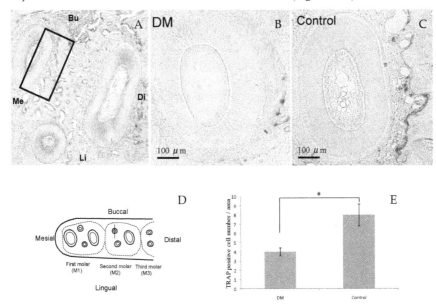

Fig. 18. Osteoclast counts in a horizontal section of the mandibular second molar region stained with Tartarate-resistant acid phosphatase (TRAP). (A) Low magnification photograph of the three roots of the second molar stained with TRAP stain. The black rectangle (540 X 120 µm) indicates the area on the distal surface of the alveolar bone adjacent to the middle third of the mesio-buccal root of the second molar in which the osteoclast cells were counted. Bu, buccal; Li, lingual; Me, mesial; Di, distal. (B) The mesio-buccal root of the control rat (original magnification 100X). (C) The mesio-buccal root of the DM rat (original magnification 100X). (D) A schematic drawing showing the observation area on the distal surface of the alveolar bone adjacent to the mesio-buccal root of the second molar in which the osteoclast cells were counted. (E) The number of TRAP-positive cells on the distal surface of the mesio-buccal root of the mandibular second molar. Values are mean ± SD. *:(p<0.05), bars = 100 µm.

demonstrated a significantly higher number of osteoclast cells in the control group when compared with the DM group ($p<0.05$) (Fig. 18). Results revealed that the number of osteoclasts was significantly lower in the DM rats than in the controls, in line with previous studies on DM rats' mandible (Mishima *et al.*, 2002) and long bones (Glajchen *et al.*, 1988; Shires *et al.*, 1981). These results confirm that the decreased rate of bone turnover may be associated with the DM condition.

7. Suggested mechanisms for the effect of diabetic condition on craniofacial complex

Growth of the craniofacial complex is controlled by genetic and environmental factors (Giglio and Lama, 2001; Yonemitsu *et al.*, 2007). Regulatory mechanisms responsible for normal morphogenesis of the face and head involve hormones, nutrients, mechanical forces, and various local growth factors. The poor growth and alterations in bone metabolism have been associated with T1DM in both humans and experimental animals (Giglio and Lama, 2001). Because human studies can be limited by small sample sizes, cross-sectional designs, uncontrolled variables, and often retrospective nature, animal models have been used to yield more rigorous analyses (Singleton *et al.*, 2006). In our studies we observed the rat growth from the age of 3 weeks old till 7 weeks old. This time period is corresponding to early growth stage in human according to previous craniofacial growth studies (Losken *et al.*, 1994; Siegel and Mooney, 1990). Consequently, in the current study STZ-DM model was used to investigate the effect of T1DM on craniofacial growth.

The studied STZ-DM rats showed significantly reduced growth in most of the craniofacial skeletal units but no significant differences were observed between controls and DM group as regards the remaining craniofacial skeletal units (Sphenoid bone length, posterior neurocranium height, anterior corpus length, bigonial width and palatal width). Craniofacial growth as a whole was also significantly lower in DM group compared to controls in all three dimensions. Previous study investigated the DM effect exclusively on the growth of the mandible and suggested that the diabetic condition had a differential effect on the osseous components and / or its associated non-skeletal tissues. They found that the disharmonious growth of the mandible was due to DM condition and might not be associated with diabetic condition complications such as renal failure, anemia, body weight change or alteration in the food intake qualities (Giglio and Lama, 2001). Thus we hypothesize that the deficiency in the craniofacial growth in our experiment might be attributed to the diabetic condition in the DM group as it was reported that specific alterations in bone metabolism are associated with DM. Moreover, several pathogenic possibilities have been proposed, such as insulinopenia, bone microangiopathy, impaired regulation of mineral metabolism, alterations in local factors that regulate bone remodeling, and even an intrinsic disorder associated with T1DM (Duarte *et al.*, 2005; Ward *et al.*, 2001). The aforementioned insulin hormone deficiency that is associated with T1DM cases may have direct effect on bone metabolism. It was mentioned in literature that normal insulin hormone level exerts direct anabolic effects on bone cells (Duarte *et al.*, 2005). Multiple osteoblast-like cell lines express insulin receptors on the cell surface and have a high capacity for insulin binding (Pun *et al.*, 1989). Moreover, osteoclasts exhibit reduced bone resorption in response to insulin stimulation (Thomas *et al.*, 1998). These findings support the idea that the actions of insulin in bone could be mediated directly via stimulation of osteoblasts in combination with inhibition of osteoclasts, (Thomas *et al.*, 1998; Thrailkill *et al.*,

2005) and this mechanism of action may explain the retardation of craniofacial growth in STZ-DM.

Diabetes has a deleterious effect on osseous turnover due to decreased osteoblast and osteoclast activities and numbers and, a lower percentage of osteoid surface and osteocalcin synthesis, as well as increased time for mineralization of osteoid (Duarte *et al.*, 2005). It was reported that the influence of diabetes on discrete stages of matrix-induced endochondral bone formation could have profound effects on the biomechanical behavior of bone. Also, chondrogenesis and calcification of bone were reduced by 50% in diabetic animals (Reddy *et al.*, 2001). This was evident in the current study results that showed a significant decrease in the craniofacial linear measurements of the DM group.

In addition to this, insulin may exert synergistic effects with other anabolic agents in bone, such as parathyroid hormone (PTH) (Thomas *et al.*, 1998; Thrailkill *et al.*, 2005). An animal model of T1DM has frequently demonstrated alteration in bone turnover, retarded growth, increased concentration of PTH, and reduced concentration of 1,25-dihydroxivitamin D (Duarte *et al.*, 2005; Tsuchida *et al.*, 2000). The effects of PTH on the bones are complex; it stimulates resorption or bone formation depending on the concentration used, the duration of the exhibition, and the administration method (Duarte *et al.*, 2005; Toromanoff *et al.*, 1997; Tsuchida *et al.*, 2000). Also, 1,25-dihydroxivitamin D, like PTH, belongs to the most important group of bone regulatory hormones. It regulates osteoclastic differentiation from hematopoietic mononuclear cells, and osteoblastic functions and activity (Collins *et al.*, 1998; Duarte *et al.*, 2005).

Moreover, Insulin may indirectly regulate the enhancement of growth hormone serum concentration by direct regulation of the hepatic growth hormone receptor, this results in abnormalities in the insulin growth factor-1 in T1DM (Chiarelli *et al.*, 2004) which consequently may have lead to the retarded growth in uncontrolled DM in the current study.

In the present study most of the periosteal surfaces in the mandibular regions of the control group showed significantly higher values recorded for the mineral apposition rate and the bone formation rate when compared to the DM group. These results agree with previous studies that recorded diminished lamellar bone formation in DM rats' femur and may suggest an association between the DM condition and the decreased number and function of osteoblasts (Follak *et al.*, 2004; Shyng *et al.*, 2001). The alveolar crest region was the only region that did not show a significant difference in the mineral apposition rate and the bone formation rate parameters among the two groups; this may be attributed to the unique nature of this region exhibiting a highly intensive bone remodeling process especially during the teeth eruption that decreases toward the base of the socket (Gerlach *et al.*, 2002).

Micro CT analysis showed a significant decrease of bone volume fraction, trabecular thickness, and trabecular number. Also, it showed a significant increase of the trabecular separation and the trabecular space in the DM group when compared with the control group. This finding indicates deterioration of the bone quality in the DM group. These results agree with other research work suggesting that the glycaemic levels play an important role in modulating the trabecular architecture especially in mandibular bone (Thrailkill *et al.*, 2005). In this context, these results may describe a state of osteopenia in experimental diabetic rats, which might be the result of an imbalance between bone formation and resorption.

A histometric evaluation of bone resorption was performed by counting the number of osteoclast cells on the distal surface of the alveolar bone adjacent to the mesio-buccal root of the second molar.   These evaluations revealed that the number of osteoclasts was significantly lower in the DM rats than in the controls, in line with previous studies on DM rats' mandible (Mishima *et al.*, 2002) and long bones (Glajchen *et al.*, 1988; Shires *et al.*, 1981). These studies confirm that the decreased rate of bone turnover may be associated with the DM condition.

This deteriorating effect on mandibular bone structure and dynamic bone formation might be be attributed to several pathogenic possibilities, such as insulinopenia, bone microangiopathy, impaired regulation of mineral metabolism, alterations in local factors that regulate bone remodeling, and even an intrinsic disorder associated with DM (Abbassy *et al.*, 2008; Duarte *et al.*, 2005).   However, the detrimental effects observed may not be associated with the significant loss of rats` weights observed in the diabetic group starting from day 14 because previous research (Abbassy *et al.*, 2008; Giglio and Lama, 2001; Shires *et al.*, 1981; Thrailkill *et al.*, 2005) showed that the mandibular growth was not affected in normal rats supplied with restricted diet and having same pattern of weight loss resembling weight loss pattern observed in DM rats.

8. Conclusions

It is obvious that the T1DM condition significantly affects craniofacial growth, bone formation mechanism and the quality of the bone formed which may alter many aspects of planning and treatment of orthodontic patients affected by this globally increasing hormonal disturbance.

There should be a new strategy for treating orthodontic patients suffering from metabolic disorders specially those disorders having direct and indirect effects on bone growth as the diabetic condition.   The orthodontic craniofacial linear measurements were significantly decreased in the T1DM cases when compared to normal cases.   These facts should be considered when orthodontic problems are diagnosed and treated in T1DM, because this may alter the orthodontic treatment period and the final treatment outcome. In this chapter it was suggested that a better understanding of how diabetes affects bone will improve our ability to protect bone health in diabetic patients.   Also, it was recommended to conduct further studies in order to elucidate the exact mechanism by which diabetes produces alterations in most of the craniofacial units.

Thus, T1DM condition had detrimental effects on the different bone regions of the mandible, that shed the light on the complexity of the craniofacial structure which is affected by many hormonal disorders suggesting further examination for the overlying soft tissues which are directly affected by any underlying boney changes.   Diabetes condition had detrimental effect on bone architecture, as shown by micro-CT, and impaired the rate of the mandibular bone formation, as examined by the dynamic histomorphometric analysis.   All of these results were verified on the cellular level by a histological study that showed the diminished number of osteoclasts on the alveolar wall, suggesting that the early stage of T1DM resulted in low bone turnover.   These results may suggest that more care is needed during the consideration of the force needed for treatment of orthodontic patients affected by T1DM, also, the retention period and rate of success in these patients may be affected.

These comprehensive studies done on bone and craniofacial growth suggest that planning the treatment in craniofacial region for patients affected with hormonal disorders is a more complex procedure when compared to the treatment of normal patients, moreover it is suggested that it is of prime importance to keep close attention to the general systemic condition of these patients and administer the proper hormonal therapy for these patients when needed to avoid any detrimental effects on bone resulting from any hormonal imbalance.

Within the limitations of this *in vitro* study, it was concluded that:

1. T1DM reduces craniofacial growth, resulting in retardation of skeletal development.
2. DM in the rat affects the bone architecture, as shown by micro-CT, and impairs the rate of the mandibular bone formation, as examined by the dynamic histomorphometric analysis.
3. All of these results were verified on the cellular level by a histological study that showed the diminished number of osteoclasts on the alveolar wall, suggesting that the early stage of DM resulted in low bone turnover.
4. These findings should be considered when conducting any treatment in the craniofacial region in T1DM since the better understanding of how diabetes affects bone will improve our ability to protect bone health in diabetic patients.
5. Good control of diabetes mellitus should be considered before orthodontic treatment by a long time inorder to obtain the best outcome.

9. References

Abbassy MA, Watari I, Soma K (2008). Effect of experimental diabetes on craniofacial growth in rats. *Archives of Oral Biology,* Vol.53, No.9, (September 2008), pp. 819-825

Abbassy MA, Watari I, Soma K (2010). The effect of diabetes mellitus on rat mandibular bone formation and microarchitecture *European Journal of Oral Sciences,* Vol.118, No.4, (August 2010), pp. 364-369

Abdus Salam M, Matsumoto N, Matin K, Tsuha Y, Nakao R, Hanada N, Senpuku H (2004). Establishment of an animal model using recombinant NOD.B10.D2 mice to study initial adhesion of oral streptococci. *Clinical and Diagnostic Laboratory Immunology,* Vol.11, No.2, (March 2004), pp. 379-386

Alkan A, Erdem E, Gunhan O, Karasu C (2002). Histomorphometric evaluation of the effect of doxycycline on the healing of bone defects in experimental diabetes mellitus: a pilot study. *Journal of Oral and Maxillofacial Surgery,* Vol. 60, No.8, (August 2002), pp.898-904

Bensch L, Braem M, Van Acker K, Willems G (2003). Orthodontic treatment considerations in patients with diabetes mellitus. *American Journal of Orthodontics and Dentofacial Orthopedics,* Vol.123, No.1, (January 2003), pp. 74-78

Chew FS (1991). Radiologic manifestations in the musculoskeletal system of miscellaneous endocrine disorders. *Radiologic Clinics of North America,* Vol.29, No.1, (January1991), pp. 135-147, ISSN 0033-8389

Chiarelli F, Giannini C, Mohn A (2004). Growth, growth factors and diabetes. *European Journal of Endocrinology,* Vol.151, Suppl 3, (November 2004), pp.U109-117

Chidiac JJ, Shofer FS, Al-Kutoub A, Laster LL, Ghafari J (2002). Comparison of CT scanograms and cephalometric radiographs in craniofacial imaging. *Orthodontics and Craniofacial Research,* Vol.5, No.2, (May 2002), pp.104-113

Collins D, Jasani C, Fogelman I, Swaminathan R (1998). Vitamin D and bone mineral density. *Osteoporosis International,* Vol.8, No.2, (March 1998), pp. 110-114, ISSN 0937-941X

Duarte VM, Ramos AM, Rezende LA, Macedo UB, Brandao-Neto J, Almeida MG, Rezende
        AA (2005). Osteopenia: a bone disorder associated with diabetes mellitus. *Journal of
        Bone and Mineral Metabolism*, Vol.23, No.1, (January 2005), pp. 58-68

Eastell R, Lambert H (2002). Diet and healthy bones. *Calcified Tissue International*, Vol.70,
        No.5, (May 2002), pp. 400-404

Engstrom C, Jennings J, Lundy M, Baylink DJ (1988). Effect of bone matrix-derived growth
        factors on skull and tibia in the growing rat. *Journal of Oral Pathology*, Vol.17, No.7,
        (August 1988), pp. 334-340, ISSN 0300-9777

Follak N, Kloting I, Wolf E, Merk H (2004). Histomorphometric evaluation of the influence
        of the diabetic metabolic state on bone defect healing depending on the defect size
        in spontaneously diabetic BB/OK rats. *Bone*, Vol.35, No.1, (July 2004), pp. 144-152

Gerlach RF, Toledo DB, Fonseca RB, Novaes PD, Line SR, Merzel J (2002). Alveolar bone
        remodelling pattern of the rat incisor under different functional conditions as
        shown by minocycline administration. *Archives of Oral Biology*, Vol.47, No.3,
        (March 2002), pp. 203-209

Giglio MJ, Lama MA (2001). Effect of experimental diabetes on mandible growth in rats.
        European Journal of Oral Sciences, Vol.109, No.3, (June 2001), pp. 193-197

Glajchen N, Epstein S, Ismail F, Thomas S, Fallon M, Chakrabarti S (1988). Bone mineral
        metabolism in experimental diabetes mellitus: osteocalcin as a measure of bone
        remodeling. *Endocrinology*, Vol.123, No.1, (July 1988), pp. 290-295, ISSN 0013-7227

Hough S, Avioli LV, Bergfeld MA, Fallon MD, Slatopolsky E, Teitelbaum SL (1981).
        Correction of abnormal bone and mineral metabolism in chronic streptozotocin-
        induced diabetes mellitus in the rat by insulin therapy. *Endocrinology*, Vol. 108,
        No.6, (June 1981), pp. 2228-2234, ISSN 0013-7227

Keshawarz NM, Recker RR (1986). The label escape error: comparison of measured and
        theoretical fraction of total bone-trabecular surface covered by single label in normals
        and patients with osteoporosis. *Bone*, Vol. 7, No.2, (February 1986), pp. 83-87

Kiliaridis S EC, Thilander B. (1985). The relationship between masticatory function and
        craniofacial morphology. I. A cephalometric longitudinal analysis in the growing
        rat fed a soft diet. *European Journal of Orthodontics*, Vol.7, pp. 273-283

Kitabchi AE UG, Murphy MB, Barrett EJ, Kreisberg, RA, Malone JI, et al. (2001).
        Management of hyper-glycemic crises in patients with diabetes. *Diabetes Care*,
        Vol.24, pp. 131-153

Kumar P, Clark, M. (2009). *Kumar and Clark's Clinical Medicine* (7th edition), Elsevier, ISBN
        10: 0-7020-2993-9, ISBN 13: 978-0-7020-2993-6, London, UK

Laib A, Ruegsegger P (1999). Calibration of trabecular bone structure measurements of in vivo
        three-dimensional peripheral quantitative computed tomography with 28-microm-
        resolution microcomputed tomography. *Bone*, Vol.24, No.1, (January 1999), pp. 35-39

Losken A, Mooney MP, Siegel MI (1994). Comparative cephalometric study of nasal cavity
        growth patterns in seven animal models. *Cleft Palate Craniofacial Journal*, Vol.31,
        No.1, (January 1994), pp.17-23

Lu H, Kraut D, Gerstenfeld LC, Graves DT (2003). Diabetes interferes with the bone
        formation by affecting the expression of transcription factors that regulate
        osteoblast differentiation. *Endocrinology*, Vol.144, No.1, (January 2003), pp.346-352,
        ISSN 0013-7227

Matin K, Salam MA, Akhter J, Hanada N, Senpuku H (2002). Role of stromal-cell derived
        factor-1 in the development of autoimmune diseases in non-obese diabetic mice.
        Immunology, Vol.107, No.2, (October 2002), pp.222-232, ISSN 0019-2805

McCracken MS, Aponte-Wesson R, Chavali R, Lemons JE (2006). Bone associated with implants in diabetic and insulin-treated rats. *Clinical Oral Implants Research,* Vol.17, No.5, (October 2006), pp. 495-500

Misawa Y, Kageyama T, Moriyama K, Kurihara S, Yagasaki H, Deguchi T, Ozawa H, Sahara N (2007). Effect of age on alveolar bone turnover adjacent to maxillary molar roots in male rats: A histomorphometric study. *Archives of Oral Biology,* Vol.52, No.1, (January 2007), pp. 44-50

Mishima N, Sahara N, Shirakawa M, Ozawa H (2002). Effect of streptozotocin-induced diabetes mellitus on alveolar bone deposition in the rat. *Archives of Oral Biology,* Vol.47, No.12, (December 2002), pp. 843-849, ISSN 0003-9969

Nakano H, Maki K, Shibasaki Y, Miller AJ (2004). Three-dimensional changes in the condyle during development of an asymmetrical mandible in a rat: a microcomputed tomography study. *American Journal of Orthodontics and Dentofacial Orthopedics,* Vol.126, No.4, (October 2004), pp. 410-420

Parfitt AM, Drezner MK, Glorieux FH, Kanis JA, Malluche H, Meunier PJ, Ott SM, Recker RR (1987). Bone histomorphometry: standardization of nomenclature, symbols, and units. Report of the ASBMR Histomorphometry Nomenclature Committee. *Journal of Bone and Mineral Research,* Vol.2, No.6, (December 1987), pp. 595-610

Pun KK, Lau P, Ho PW (1989). The characterization, regulation, and function of insulin receptors on osteoblast-like clonal osteosarcoma cell line. *Journal of Bone and Mineral Research,* Vol.4, No.6, (December 1989), pp. 853-862

Reddy GK, Stehno-Bittel L, Hamade S, Enwemeka CS (2001). The biomechanical integrity of bone in experimental diabetes. *Diabetes Research and Clinical Practice,* Vol.54, No.1, pp. 1-8, ISSN 0168-8227

Salzmann JA (1966). Practice of orthodontics. *American Journal of Orthodontics,* Vol. 76, No.1, (July 1979), pp. 103-104

Schwartz AV (2003). Diabetes Mellitus: Does it Affect Bone? *Calcified Tissue International,* Vol.73, No.6, (December 2003), pp. 515-519

Sheng MH, Baylink DJ, Beamer WG, Donahue LR, Rosen CJ, Lau KH, Wergedal JE (1999). Histomorphometric studies show that bone formation and bone mineral apposition rates are greater in C3H/HeJ (high-density) than C57BL/6J (low-density) mice during growth. *Bone,* Vol.25, No.4, (October 1999), pp. 421-429

Shimomoto Y, Chung CJ, Iwasaki-Hayashi Y, Muramoto T, Soma K (2007). Effects of occlusal stimuli on alveolar/jaw bone formation. *Journal of Dental Research,* Vol.86, No.1, (January 2007), pp. 47-51

Shimomoto Y IY, Chung C-R, Muramoto T, Soma K. (2005). Occlusal stimuli affects alveolar and jaw bone formation during the growth period. . *Journal of Japanese Society of Bone Morphometry,* Vol.15, No.1, pp. 29–34, ISSN 0917-4648

Shires R, Teitelbaum SL, Bergfeld MA, Fallon MD, Slatopolsky E, Avioli LV (1981). The effect of streptozotocin-induced chronic diabetes mellitus on bone and mineral homeostasis in the rat. *Journal of Laboratory Clinical Medicine,* Vol.97, No.2, (February 1981), pp. 231-240, ISSN 0022-2143

Shyng YC, Devlin H, Sloan P (2001). The effect of streptozotocin-induced experimental diabetes mellitus on calvarial defect healing and bone turnover in the rat. *International Journal of Oral and Maxillofacial Surgery,* Vol.30, No.1, (February 2001), pp. 70-74

Siegel MI, Mooney MP (1990). Appropriate animal models for craniofacial biology. *Cleft Palate Journal,* Vol.27, No.1, (January 1990), pp. 18-25

Singleton DA, Buschang PH, Behrents RG, Hinton RJ (2006). Craniofacial growth in growth hormone-deficient rats after growth hormone supplementation. *American Journal of Orthodontics and Dentofacial Orthopedics*, Vol.130, No.1, (July 2006), pp. 69-82

Stuart A, Smith D (1992). Use of the Fluorochromes xylenol orange, calcein green, and tetracycline to document bone deposition and remodeling in healing fractures in chickens. *Avian diseases*, Vol.36, (July 1992), pp. 447-449

Takada H, Abe S, Tamatsu Y, Mitarashi S, Saka H, Ide Y (2006). Three-dimensional bone microstructures of the mandibular angle using micro-CT and finite element analysis: relationship between partially impacted mandibular third molars and angle fractures. *Dent Traumatol*, Vol.22, No.1, (February 2006), pp. 18-24

Tein MS, Breen SA, Loveday BE, Devlin H, Balment RJ, Boyd RD, Sibley CP, Garland HO (1998). Bone mineral density and composition in rat pregnancy: effects of streptozotocin-induced diabetes mellitus and insulin replacement. *Experimental Physiology*, Vol.83, No.2, (March 1998), pp. 165-174

Thomas DM, Udagawa N, Hards DK, Quinn JM, Moseley JM, Findlay DM, Best JD (1998). Insulin receptor expression in primary and cultured osteoclast-like cells. *Bone*, Vol.23, No.3, (September 1998), pp. 181-186

Thrailkill KM, Liu L, Wahl EC, Bunn RC, Perrien DS, Cockrell GE, Skinner RA, Hogue WR, Carver AA, Fowlkes JL, Aronson J, Lumpkin CK, Jr. (2005). Bone formation is impaired in a model of type 1 diabetes. *Diabetes*, Vol.54, No.10, (October 2005), pp. 2875-2881

Toromanoff A, Ammann P, Mosekilde L, Thomsen JS, Riond JL (1997). Parathyroid hormone increases bone formation and improves mineral balance in vitamin D-deficient female rats. *Endocrinology*, Vol.138, No.6, (June 1997), pp. 2449-2457, ISSN 0013-7227

Tsuchida T, Sato K, Miyakoshi N, Abe T, Kudo T, Tamura Y, Kasukawa Y, Suzuki K (2000). Histomorphometric evaluation of the recovering effect of human parathyroid hormone (1-34) on bone structure and turnover in streptozotocin-induced diabetic rats. *Calcified Tissue International*, Vol.66, No.3, (March 2000), pp. 229-233

Tsuchiya T MY, Kurihara S. (1995). The fluorescent simultaneous azo dye technique for demonstration of tartarate -resistant acid phosphatase (TRAP) activity in osteoclast-like multinucleate cells. *Journal of Bone and Mineral Metabolism*, Vol.13, pp. 71-76

Vandeberg JR, Buschang PH, Hinton RJ (2004a). Craniofacial growth in growth hormone-deficient rats. *The Anatomical Record. Part A, Discoveries in Molecular, Cellular and Evolutionary Biology*, Vol.278, No.2, (June 2004), pp. 561-570, ISSN 1552-4884

VandeBerg JR, Buschang PH, Hinton RJ (2004b). Absolute and relative growth of the rat craniofacial skeleton. *Archives of Oral Biology*, Vol.49, No.6, (June 2004), pp. 477-484, ISSN 0003-9969Ward DT, Yau SK, Mee AP, Mawer EB, Miller CA, Garland HO, Riccardi D (2001). Functional, molecular, and biochemical characterization of streptozotocin-induced diabetes. *Journal of the American Society of Nephrology*, Vol.12, No.4, pp. 779-790, ISSN 1046-6673

Yokoyama M, Atsumi T, Tsuchiya M, Koyama S, Sasaki K (2009). Dynamic changes in bone metabolism in the rat temporomandibular joint after molar extraction using bone scintigraphy. *Europen Journal of Oral Sciences*, Vol.117, No. 4, (August 2009), pp. 374-379, ISSN 1600-0722

Yonemitsu I, Muramoto T, Soma K (2007). The influence of masseter activity on rat mandibular growth. *Archives of Oral Biology*, Vol.52, No.5, (May 2007), pp. 487-493, ISSN 0003-9969

Zhang X, Fei Y, Zhang M, Wei D, Li M, Ding W, Yang J (2008). Reversal of osteoporotic changes of mineral composition in femurs of diabetic rats by insulin. *Biological Trace Element Research*, Vol.121, No.3, (March 2008), pp. 233-242

10

The Role of Genetic Predisposition in Diagnosis and Therapy of Periodontal Diseases in Type 1 Diabetes Mellitus

M.G.K. Albrecht

Department of Conservative Dentistry Semmelweis University, Budapest, Hungary

1. Introduction

The prevalence of diabetes mellitus (DM) and its probable influence on periodontal disease suggests that DM patients will very likely probably become an increasing proportion of the patient population seen by both general dentists and periodontists. Many investigators have studied the oral manifestations involving periodontitis as a complicating factor in the periodontal therapy of DM patients, whose disease may be more prevalent and more severe and progress rapidly.[1][2][3] Periodontal disease makes chewing difficult or painful, thereby leading to an improper diet. On the other hand, uncontrolled periodontal disease may upset metabolic control of DM.[2]

Until the past 15 years, the management was based on the periodontology model of care, and the aim of these methods was to diagnose the problem and resolve it via treatment. Consequently, repairs were made, but the periodontitis generally recurred or progressed unabated. Disease prevention was not practised. It is clear that the risk of periodontal disease varies greatly from one patient to another.[4-8]

Today many practitioners are providing better and more complete service to their patients because they are beginning to incorporate the principles of the information-intense medical model.[9] Changes in our political and social structure have affected how health care is being managed. With increasing evidence of the influence of periodontal disease on systemic health, dentist and hygienists are taking a more intensive look at the risk factors associated with its onset and progression. Bacteriology, immunology, genetics, and systemic cofactors are often used to determine what is wrong with the patients. Genetic knowledge is an important part of the medical model because it allows for a complete and comprehensive picture of all of the factors contributing to the patient's past, current, and future status.

2. Classification and characterization of periodontal diseases

2.1 Gingivitis

Gingivitis is an inflammatory pathologic alteration affecting the gingival epithelium and connective tissue (Fig.1). Clinical symptoms comprise reddness and swelling of the gingiva, bleeding on probing, and a periodontal pocket deph ≥1mm.

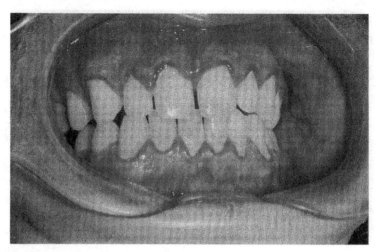

Fig. 1. Gingivitis

Gigivitis is characterized by a subgingival microflora that is slightly shifted in favor of gramm-negativ, anaerobic bacteria without any periodontopathogenic microorganisms. ANUG is the acronym of the acute necrotic ulcerative gingivitis.

2.2 Chronic Adult Periodontitis (AP)

The slowly progressing AP is clinically characterized by persistent loss of attachment, a positive bleeding on probing (BOP), periodontal pockets depths of 1-3 mm, and slight loss of alveolar bone tissue (Fig.2). This is the most common type of periodontitis and generally occurs at the age of 30 years or later. It may be either generalized or limited to molars and/or incisors. The subgingival microbial panel is slightly shifted in favor of gram-negative, anaerobic bacteria with an increased amount of periopathogenic microorganizms.

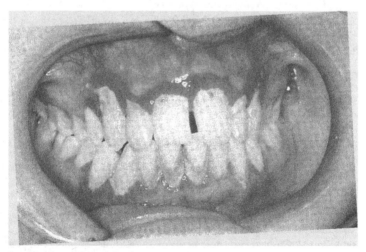

Fig. 2. Periodontitis (loss of alveolar bone tissue)

2.3 Refractory marginal periodontitis

Refractory or therapy-resistant AP shows a progressive loss of attachment even with diligent mechanical therapy and positive compliance of the patients. This type of periodontitis is characterized by a progressive loss of supporting tissue even if treated thoroughly. In most cases the lesions compromise more than one tooth and are infected by high concentration s of periodontal pathogens. After a massive degradation of supporting tissue the affected teeth are often lost (Fig.3).

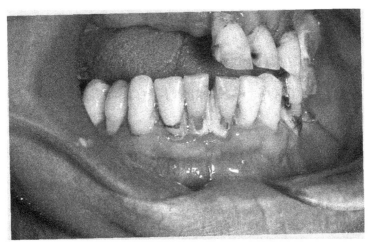

Fig. 3. Periodontitis (degradation of supporting tissue the affected teeth are often lost)

2.4 Localised Juvenile Periodontitis (LJP)

This type usually affects healthy adolescents at the age of 10 to 20 years. It is distinguished by a severe, but localized loss of bone tissue combined with the development of deep pockets at the first molars and/or the incisors. *Actinobacillus actinomycetemcomitans* is considered to be the marker pathogen for LJP.

2.5 Rapidly Progressive Periodontitis (RP)

RPP is mostly seen in patient's at the age of 20 to 35 years. The patients medical history frequently shows a prior LJP. This form of periodontitis is generalized and progresses intermittently with severe loss of bone tissue, gingival bleeding and acute inflammation.The subgingival oral microflora is characterized by a high concentration of periodontal pathogens.

3. The oral cavity ecosystem

The human oral cavity accomodates about 50 billion bacteria belonging to about 400 different species.[10] The various habitats are occupied by microbial populations specifically adapted to their enviroments.

The deep periodontal lesion is a unique eco-system within the oral cavity providing particular living conditions. It is the only place within the oral cavity not being flushed by saliva. Instead is filled with crevicular fluid. Moreover, the acigen concentration decreases progressively with pocket depth creating optimal growth conditions for anaerobic bacteria.[1]

These bacteria lack the enzymes necessary to detoxify oxigen radicals resulting in a severely reduced growth or even death in the presence of oxigen. Dispite the great variety of the microbial flora only a fraction of the bacterial species is etiologically connected to the development of periodontitis. The flora of a healthy sulcus usually consists of aerobic grampositive cocci and rods. These bacteria known as „beneficial flora" show no pathogenic potential but, by their presence, are able to prevent the colonization is progressing the microbial spectrum is shifted in favor of anaerobic gram-negative rods.

The marker pathogens of periodontitis belong to the group of obligatory anaerobic, black pigmented Bacteroides species as *Porphyromonas gingivalis* and *Prevotella intermedia* as well as *Bacteroides forsythus, Treponema denticola, and Actinobacillus actinomycetemcomitans*.[11,12] A strict correlation of the alveolar pocket depth and presence of periodontopathogens could be proven by several clinical studies.[13,14,15]

Several metabolites produced by the periodontitis-associated pathogens either destroy the sorrounding periodontal tissue or inactivate the humoral host defense system. The most important virulence factors produced by the three marker pathogens *P. gingivalis*, *P. intermedia* and *A. actinomycetemcomitans*.[14]

4. Aetiology of periodontitis

The development of plaque is considered to be the primary cause of periodontitis. Especially at the gingival margin plaque hardens to tartar resulting in a mechanical irritation. Exotoxins produced by the plaque bacteria diffuse into adjacent tissue and give rise to reddening and swelling -the typical clinical characteritics- of gingivitis. After professional removal of plaque and dental calculus a healthy periodontium is quickly restored indicating that gingivitis is a reversible condition. In case no professional removal of the dental calculus is performed the infection will progress and a periodontitis becomes established showing the typical clinical characteristics like bleeding on probing (BOP), increasing pocket deph and loss of alveolare bone tissue.[11]

At the age play a roule development of periodontitis[16], and the age of 40 far more teeth are lost by periodontitis than by caries.

Periodontitis associated bacteria are found in low concentration even in the healthy sulcus. Therefore, additional factors must exist that determine the onset and the progress of disease. In case of an impaired immune system e.g. by stress, medication, hormonal imbalances, diabetes or smoking the pathogens utilize the selective advantages for prompt proliferation leading to the establishment of an manifest infection of the periodontium.[17-20]

5. Genetic component to periodontitis

For approximately the past 15 years, dental researchers have been focusing on dental plaque. Clinicians have made treatment decisions as though the plaque-disease interrelationship was quantitative: the more plaque, the more bacteria, the more inflammation, the more disease. However, clinical experience demonstrates that not all people respond the same way to similar accumulations of plaque. There are patients with a lot of plaque who have moderate and advanced disease. Some types of plaque simply are more virulent than others. However, clinical experience demonstrates that not all people respond the same way to plaque accumulations. Because so much variability respond to plaque, and respond to treatment. Some type of plaque symply are more virulent than others. In adults, these bacteria routinely colonize the teeth when tooth cleaning is not performed on a regular basis. Although bacteria are essential for the initiation of periodontitis, there is currently no mechanism for determing the clinical trajectory of the disease for individual patients, i.e., differentiating those patients who will have a mild to moderate form of disease and respond well to simple professional care from those who are likely to develop a more severe periodontitis that demands extensive therapy and results in tooth mobility. Individual differences in disease progression are dramatic and are often not predictable by currently known mechanisms.

Identification of a risk factors may explain why individual patients do not respond uniformly to standard treatment. For example, a patient who is a heavy smoker may not heal as soon or as well as expected after treatment. Patients react differently to bacterial stimulation. This is a result not only of the type and amount of bacteria but also of the underlying genetic characteristics of the patient's immune system.The cytokines tumor necrosis factor alpha(TNFά) and interleukin 1 (IL-1) are key mediators of the inflammatory process and modulate the extracellular matrix components and bone which comprise the periodontal tissues.The genes encode pro-inflammatory proteins (IL 1A and IL-1B producing IL-1 ά and IL-1β). Several genetic polimorphisms have been described in the genes of the IL-1 cluster and, in case control studies, associations have been reported with increased severity of several chronic inflammatory diseases.

The genetic risk of developing periodontitis has been investigated by studying families and populations as well as twin.[21-26] The studies conducted on twins have reported a significant genetic component explaining the variation in clinical attachment loss, probing depth and gingivitis. An association between the severe chronic form of the disease and a composite genotype in the interleukin IL-1ά and IL-1β genes has been reported.[21] However, this association was found only in non-smokers. Other authors have subsequently investigated the IL-1ά - IL-1β genotypes with a chronic form of periodontitis with different results.[27,28]

The genetics influence resistance on periodontal disease has been determined from a wide variety of sources.[29-32] Genotype positive patients had significantly more clinical expression of inflammation, as determined by bleeding on probing. In healthy patients 46.7 % of genotype positive patients had bleeding as compared with only 8.6% of genotype-negative patients.[32,33] Their results from genetic susceptibility testing have the real potential to improve patient management. Many of the genetic markers for common disease involve polymorphisms in gene sequences involved in cytokine biological activity. Researchers know that in healthy subject IL-1 plays a very important role in inflammation and the expression of periodontitis. Patients with this genotype progress more rapidly toward severe periodontitis and have statistically significant increased inflammation.[32] It has been established that this genotype occurs in approximately 30% of most of the populations that have been tested for this genotype.

Cells from people with a positive genotype produced up to four times more IL-1 in response to the same bacterial challenge.[34] Because IL-1 in high concentrations is involved with destruction of tissues, this increased IL-1 response may explain the more rapid progression of periodontal disease in genotype-positive patients when faced with a bacterial challenge in their plaque. For patients with this genetic susceptibility to periodontitis, tooth loss was be minimized by good plaque control and definitive periodontal therapy.[35]

6. Genetic test for susceptibility to periodontal disease

Two polymorphisms within the IL-1 gene cluster show a close association with periodontitis. One polymorphism is located at position -899 of the Interleukin 1ά gene, the other at position +3953 of the Interleukin 1β gene.[32,36] Within both polymorphisms allele 1 harbors a cytidin c, whereas allele 2 carries a thymidin (T) at the respective position. Allele 2 of the +3953 polymorphism of the IL-1β gene leads to an alteration of the corresponding protein resulting in an overproduction of IL-1β.[37] This overproduction of IL-1 seems to override the feedback mechanisms which normally limit inflammation resulting in the development of massive gingival pockets and degradation of periodontal tissue. These data allow a risk assessment, defining a patients as PRT-positive or PRT negative, the presence of periodontitis risk alleles at positions IL-1ά-889 and IL-1β +3953.

6.1 Genotyp[R] PRT test

With the Genotyp[R] PRT test (Hain Lifescience) the base composition and allelic combination of the two IL1 loci can be analysed. The test is a molecular biological assay based on the identification of gene loci associated with an elevated risk in developing periodontitis by means of highly specific DNA probes. It is based on the analysis of nucleic acids, there is no need for viable bacteria to perform the test and no special precautions are required during transport. A detailed sequence analysis has to be performed by additional examinations. The Genotyp[R] PRT test is not a diagnostic test for periodontal disease. It is rather a test determing the patient's genetic susceptibility to developing severe, generalized periodontitis in the future and helps to plan a comprehensive therapy. Processing and interpretation of the test is performed in clinical laboratories from a buccal swab containing cells of the mucous membrane of the patient's cheek.

7. Indications for microbiological testing of the subgingival flora

It is generally accepted that periodontitis is initiated by the establishment of a specific subgingival bacterial flora. Some of the marker pathogens belong to the group of obligatory anaerobic, black pigmented *Bacteroides species* such as *Porphyromonas gingivalis* and *Prevotella intermedia*. In addition, the bacterial species *Actinobacillus actinomycetemcomitans* (*Haemophilus a.*), *Bacteroidea forsythus*, and *Treponema denticola* play a pivotal role in the initiation of periodontal disease (Table 1).

Strong evidence for etiology	Moderate evidence for etiology
Actinobacillus actinomycetemcomitans	Campylobacter rectus
Porphyromonas gingivalis	Eubacterium nodatum
Bacteroides forsytus	Fusobacterium nucleatum
	Prevotella intermedia
	Peptostreptococcus micros
	Streptococcus intermedius-complex
	Treponema denticola

Table 1. Specific Bacteria Associated with Periodontal Disease (Annals of Periodontology 1:928,1996)

7.1 MicroDent^R test

Like Genotyp^R PRT the microDent^R test is a molecular biological diagnostic device. Since it is based on the analysis of nucleic acids, there is no need for viable bacteria to perform the test and no special precautions are requireed during transport. The microDent^R test a highly sensitive and highly specific molecular bological PCR-DNA-probe method. Due to the high specificity of the PCR, any potential contamination of the probe by concomitant flora has no influence on the test results.

A defined cut-off ensures that every positive test result is of clinical relevance and that bacterial concentrations present in a healthy sulcus lead to a negative result. Sampling is performed from the gingival pocket with strile paper points. These marker species can be detected with the microDent^R test: *Actinobacillus actinomycetemcomitans, Porphyromonas gingivalis, Prevotella intermedia, Bacteroides forsythus, Treponema denticola.*

Periodontopathogenic bacteria activate inflammatory mechanisms within the local periodontal tissue throught the production of toxins and other metabolites. The degree of this response depens on the general health and immunologic state of the patients. Besides that, exogenic risk factors such as haevy smoking, stress and medication can negatively influence the progression of periodontal disease. Patients who in addition are PRT-positive suffer from an overproduction of IL-1 leading to a significantly increased immunologic response to the presence of periodontopathogenic bacteria. This individuals therefore are at an even higher risk for developing severe disease and losing teeth. Knowledge of the IL−1 genotype, the bacterial load, and possible additional risk factors allow for the prediction of the patient's future periodontal status including the risk of further tooth loss.

8. Risk factor influence on periodontitis in type 1 DM

A number of studies have demonstrated a relationship between DM and periodontal diseases, which are among the most prevalent complications of DM.[38-57] Individuals with DM tend to have a higher prevalence of periodontal diseases and more severe and rapidly progressing forms than those who do not have DM.[41,48] DM is a known risk factor for periodontitis in adults. Seppälä et al.[49] demonstrated that patients with type 1 DM exhibit a higher degree of attachment loss and bone loss than control subjects under similar dental plaque conditions. This finding was confirmed in a follow-up site-by-site study by the same authors.[50]

The changes in the periodontal conditions are mostly expressed in the first year of the disease, and the damage to the periodontium which develops at this time is not greatly influeced in the further course of the disease (Fig 4).

It is an interesting result that younger DM subjects display more periodontal destruction than do non-DM subjects at a later age. In the all-age groups, the periodontal status varied according to the age of the patient at the onset of DM. This suggests that the early onset of DM (before 14) is a much greater risk factor for periodontal diseases than mere disease duration (Fig 5).

Earlier investigators[51,52] noted that the duration of DM was greater in groups with severe periodontal disease. Our results[53] indicated that DM is associated with an increased risk of the development of periodontal disease in the event of an increased duration of the DM, and the level of oral hygiene is considered to be a contributory factor rather than the primary etiologic factor in the initiation of gingivitis and periodontitis in those with DM. In agreement with Gusberti et al.[57] the findings of our study[53] demonstrate that poorly controlled type 1 DM patients with elevated blood glucose and HbA$_{1c}$ levels have a greater prevalence to more severe periodontal diseases. The severity of periodontal disease was observed to decrease as the control of the DM improved, in agreement with Tervonen and Knuuttila[55], Rylander et al.[58]

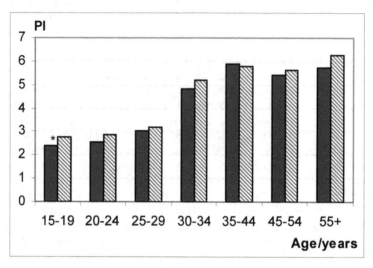

Duration of DM: < 1year / > 1year: *P<0.001

Duration of DM: ■ <1 year, □ >1 year

Fig. 4. Periodontal conditions (PI) in patients with short and long histories of DM.

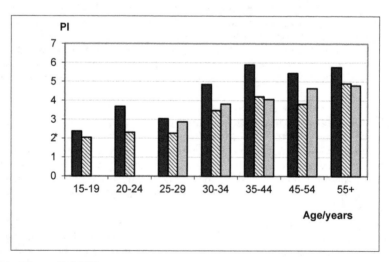

< 14 year / > 14 year: P<0.0001

■ < 14 year, ▨ 15-25 year, □ > 25 year

Fig. 5. Age of the patient at the onset of DM

Type 1 DM to increase the prevalence and severity of periodontitis independent of the effects of oral hygiene, and duration time of DM.[42] However the severity of periodontal disease increased with the duration of DM only among those with an adequate level of oral hygiene (OHI-S = 0) The association between periodontal disease and the duration of diabetes mellitus is consistent with trends seen in other complications of DM whereas the longer duration of diabetes mellitus is in direct proportion of the prevalence and severity of periodontal disease. The development of systemic complications of diabetes such as retinopathy, nephropathy, is also is relationship with the duration of diabetes mellitus agreement with Rylander[58], Galea et al.[59], Rosenthal et al.[60] and Lopez.[52]

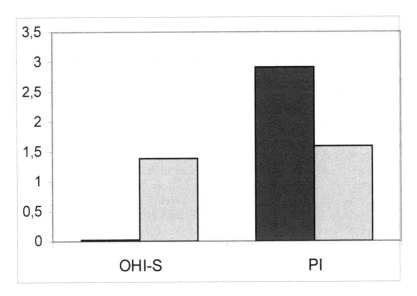

PI = The intensity of gingivitis and periodontitis
OHI-S = oral hygiene
OHI-S= 0 / PI: p<0.0001
Duration time: ■ < 1 year □ > 5 year

Fig. 6. The intensity of gingivitis and periodontitis(PI) according to the level of oral hygiene (OHI-S) and the duration of DM

On the other hand, the presence of severe periodontal infection may also increase the risk for microvascular and macrovascular complications. DM patients with severe periodontal disease demonstrate a significantly higher prevalence of proteinuria and a greater number of cardiovascular complications.[31,54,55] Karjalainen et al.[56], Genco,[31] Lopez et al.[52], Albrecht[59] examined the association between the severity of periodontal disease and organ complications (retinopathy) and found that advanced periodontal disease was associated with severe ophthalmic complications in type 1 DM.

A more pronounced incidence of poor glycemic control in subjects with a shorter duration of DM would be consistent with the hypothesis that hyperglycemia increases linearly with time, but at different rates in different people. This hypothesis suggests that patients with rapidly increasing hyperglycemia would have more severe periodontal disease at the onset of DM, resulting in damage to the periodontium.

A positive correlation between the level of control of the disease and the intensity of gingivitis and periodontitis. In the well-controlled type 1 DM patients the intensity of gingivitis and periodontitis was lower than in those with poor glycemic control agreement with Gusberti et al.[57], Albrecht et al.[41] Good metabolic control of DM reduces the susceptibility to infection and is therefore also important for the prevention of periodontal disease in people with type 1 DM. In patients with poorly controlled DM, an improvement of the metabolic control may improve the periodontal condition.[61-64] Conversely, periodontal disease can interfere with the control of DM and can increase the insulin requirements in previously stable patients.[65-67,56,68,2,69]

Smoking is associated with an increased intensity of periodontitis. Very light or occasional smokers did not show statistically significant differences compared to non-smokers respect to the prevalence and intensity of gingivitis or periodontitis. No periodontally healthy subjects who has been, or who use to be heavy smokers. Tobacco contains cytotoxic substances such as nicotine which may also have a negative effect on the cellular turnover and repair of the periodontium.[68,70,53]

9. Genetic predisposition and periodontal disease in type 1 DM

Recently several study demonstrates that specific genetic markers, that have been associated with increased IL-1 production, are a strong indicator of susceptibility to severe periodontitis in healthy adults. [22,29,31] The study presented here was to explore a possible association between IL-1A and IL-1-B genotypes in patient with type 1 DM and controls with periodontitis. The frequency -in type 1 DM and controls- of the composite genotype that comprises allele 2 of the IL-1A plus IL-1B is shown in Fig.7. All subject were non-smokers.

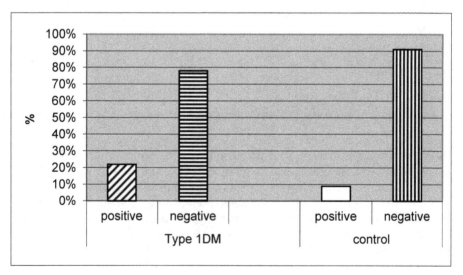

Fig. 7. Frequency of the Genotype[R] PRT positive and negative type 1 DM adult patients and control with periodontitis.

To control the effect of age on disease severity, data were analyzed separately for type 1 DM adolescents aged 14-19 years. In this age range, the composite genotype was present in 22,7 % of DM adolescents and 8,57% of healthy individuals were estimated to carry the IL-1 risk genotype. Distribution of the PAG (Periodontitis Associated Genotype)[21] positive and negative subjects in type 1 DM adolescents shows the Fig. 8.

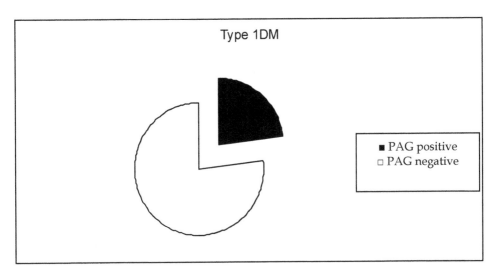

Fig. 8. Frequency of PAG positive and negative adolescents with type 1 DM

Gingivitis was more severe in those adolescents with positive GenoType[R]PRT test (Fig.9).

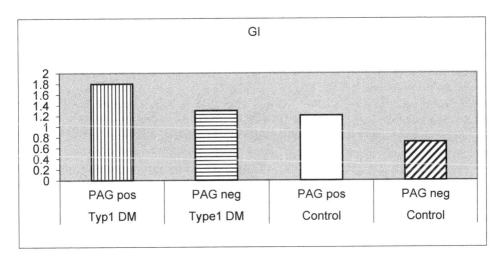

PAG positive/PAG negative: p<0.001

Fig. 9. The intensity of gingivitis (GI) of PAG positiv and in negative adolescents with type 1 DM.

In type 1 DM there was significant more extracted teeth in Genotype[R] PRT positive subjects than in negative group or non-diabetic people (p< 0.001) (Fig.10).

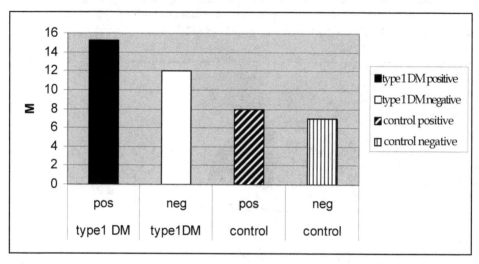

P< 0.001

Fig. 10. The mean value of extracted teeth (M) in DM patients and metabolically healthy individuals with positive Genotype.

Periodontitis involves multiple clinical patterns including various severities of periodontitis, uncommon early onset forms that affect children and young adults with type 1 DM, and patients who do not respond predictably to conventional therapy refractory periodontitis.

Guzman et al.[71] have shown a possible interactions between genetic an enviromental factors that there is interplay between genetic an environmental factors that results in periodontal disease.

The finding that a specific genotype in the IL-1 gene cluster correlates with severe periodontitis suggest a genetic mechanism by which some individuals, if challenged by bacterial accumulations, may have a more vigorous immuno-inflammatory response leading to more severe periodontitis in type 1 DM. The lack of reliable markers for type 1 DM patient susceptibility to severe periodontitis has prevented the early identification of those at most risk and has prevented delivery of therapy appropriate for the degree of the risk.

10. The modification of the subgingival microflora in patients with type 1 DM

Periodontopathogenic bacteria activate inflammatory mechanisms within the local periodontal tissue throught the production of toxins and other metabolites. The degree of this response depends on the general health and immunologic state of the patients. Besides that, exogenic risk factors such as heavy smoking, stress, and medication can negatively influence the progression of periodontal disease. Of all of the various microorganism that colonize the mouth in healthy subjects, there are three, Porphyromonas gingivalis, Actinobacillus actinomycetemcomitans, and Bacteroides forsythus have been implicated as etiologic agents in periodontitis. The presence of periodontal pathogen, though necessary to cause disease, is not sufficient. According our findings there were a significant difference between the severity of the gingivitis, parodontitis and the bacteria identified from the gingival pocket of patients with type 1 DM (Fig.11, Table 2). In case of gingivitis alone, the most prevalent bacterium was *Bacteroides forsythus* (11.11%), whereas in parodontitis it was *Treponema denticola* (75.92%). In type 1 DM the presence of *Treponema denticola* no additional risk of developing agressive periodontitis, despite the fact its presence is necessary for the disease to develop. The *Bacteriodes forsythus, Prevotella intermedia, Porphyromonas gingivalis, Actinobacillus actinomicetemcomitans* may be risk indicators for periodontal disease in population with type 1DM though they are not risk factors.

Patients who in addition are PRT positive suffer from an overproduction of IL-1 leading to a significantly increased immunologic response to the presence of periodontopathogenic bacteria. These individuals therefore are at an even higher risk for developing severe disease and losing teeth.

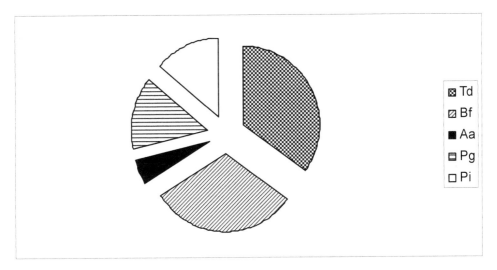

Td: *Treponema denticola*
Bf: *Bacteroides forsythus*
Aa: *Actinobacillus actinomycetemcomitans*
Pg: *Porphyromonas gingivalis*

Fig. 11. The distribution of the subgingival microflora in adult patient with type 1 DM.

Subgingival bacterial flora in type 1 DM

Actinobacillus actinomycetemcomitans(Aa)	Porphyromonas gingivalis (Pg)	Prevotella inermedia(Pi)	Bacteroides forsythus (Bf)	Treponema denticola (Td)
5%	15%	14%	31%	35%

Table 2. Distribution of the Subgingival Microflora in Type 1 DM with Periodontal Disease

11. Diagnosis and therapy of periodontal disease in type 1 DM

A considerable fraction of periodontal diseases can be stabilized for years using classical mechanical treatments as root planing or deep scaling. However, this treatment often is not sufficient for elimination of the tissue invading periodontal pathogens. Subsequently, progressive loss of attachment and bone tissue might occur in spite of diligent treatment. In these cases a specific concomitant therapy with antibiotics promises to be more efficient -of course only after careful microbiological testing-.

The choice of medication and mode of application depends on the composition of the subgingival flora and the clinical manifestation of the periodontitis. Where tissue-invasive, periopathogenic bacteria such as *Treponema denticola* are present, mechanical methods like root-planing or deep-scaling are often ineffective in eliminating the pathogen. Despite careful treatment, the result is progressive attachment loss and bone resorption. In such cases, a one-of antimicrobial concomittal therapy – only undertaken after microbiological diagnostics, of course – is much more effective while causing less side effects.

In the main, both local and systemic antibiotic applications are available. In the case of a generalized periodontal disease, an adjuvant systemic therapy is indicated. If the infection focus is limited to individual sites, a local treatment is a sensible alternative.

Antibiotic therapies should in any case only be implemented after microbiological diagnostics (e.g.microDent^R test) have been completed, in order to avoid both excessive and under treatment.

In most cases a negative bacterium test result can be equated with periodontal stability. However, the presence of periodontal marker organisms indicates an increased risk for progressive destruction of the periodontium. It is obvious that a therapy with antibiotics should be initiated only after thorough microbiological test.

A sustained success of the therapy depends on an optimal compliance of the patients and regular recall sessions. Regular control examinations of the subgingival flora are rather helpful in early diagnosis of potential rezidives.

Genetics factors should also be determined because they play a key role in providing information to make better treatment decisions. A genotype result is always important to consider when making treatment decisions, even if the patient is genotype-negative. A negative result does not mean that a patient will be periodontal-disease-free. Genotype negative individuals must still be cautious about other risk factors, such as stress, smoking, bad oral hygiene-, and diabetes control.

The genetic predictive test for periodontitis complements the dentist's full scope of services by providing additional wanted and useful information. Indications for the genetic predictive test may be of value to the following patients groups:

- DM patients exhibiting refractory, therapy-resistent periodontitis. A positive test result might explain previous treatment failures and is an indicator for planing an alternative therapy.
- DM patients exhibiting progressive periodontitis. A positive test result might indicate the necessity for a more agressive therapy and shortes recall intervals.
- Type 1 DM adolescens -under 14 years- exhibiting early clinical sign of periodontitis. Before starting treatment, the test helps to plan an individual therapy maching the patient's t.i. a therapy stopping progress of the disease without risking over-treatment.
- Haewy smokers patients with type 1 DM.

Treatment decisions will be affected if a patient has risk factors, for example, haevy smokers. Haevy smokers are counseled that the treatment outcome from regenerative therapy will not be as good as outcomes for those who do not smoke.

In all cases where patient motivation and compliance are major obstacles to efficient prophylactic measures the situation can be dramatically improved when high risk patients are informed about their condition.

Knowledge of the IL-1 genotype, the bacterial load, and possible additional risk factors allow for the prediction of the patient's future periodontal status including the risk of further tooth loss. For the first time, these data enable the dentist to plan an individual therapy matching the patient's needs. Knowledge of the IL-1 genotype also allows a more efficient therapy from an economic point of view because over- and under-treatment can be minimized.

12. Conclusion

Periodontitis is a complex multifactorial disease. Similarly, Type 1 DM is a complex metabolic syndrome. Periodontal disease can be especially problematic for individuals with type 1 DM, in whom the disease may have an early onset or may progress more rapidly. Many characteristics and local factors such as dental calculus, the smoking habits and general factors (the duration of DM, the age, the degree of metabolic control, and the complications of DM) have been identified as factors that put people et an enhanced risk.

The initial dental therapy for patients with type 1 DM, as for all patients, must be directed toward the control of acute oral infections at the onset of DM. It is important to advise the phisician of the periodontal status, since the presence of infections including advanced periodontal disease may increase the insulin resistance and cotribute to a worsening of the DM state. Regular dental care may help maintain good oral health and it is especially important at the onset of the disease. Patients should also be checked regularly for bleeding gums or inflammation. Educating the patient in proper home oral care is a standard routine of periodontal treatment and prevention. Plaque control and scaling procedures frequently resolve gingivitis. However, where more tissue destruction has occurred, it may still be difficult or impossible for the patient to remove plaque deposits from the periodontal pockets.

Periodontitis is a disease leading to destruction of connective tissue and bone that support the teeth. Due to the multifunctional etiology of the disease its clinical appearence and progression greatly vary resulting in difficulties in planing an effective therapy. Smoking should be avoided because it is associated with an increased intensity of periodontitis.

Patients who are genotype positive do not lose all of their teeth to periodontitis because, for the most part, it is a treatable and preventable disease. If patients are identified as having the genetic susceptibility factor and begin a treatment or prevention plan, there are high expectations for favorable outcomes and there is no known risk from being tested. Determining the patient's genetic susceptibility in the future helps to plan a comprehensiv therapy and regular dental control to improve patients care prevent to developing severe, generalized periodontitis and toothlos. This IL-1 genotype does not cause periodontal disease directly, this marker is not a causative factor, instead it is a severity risk factor for susceptibility or predisposition to periodontitis. Optimal prophylaxis and efficient therapy of the polymorphisms defining the periodontitis risk genotype (PRT-positive) patients a careful microbiological testing of the subgingival bacterial flora for allows for the timely application of appropriate therapeutic measures. In case of positive test results proving the presence of specific periodontopathogenic bacterial species antibiotics should be applied. Choice of medication and mode of application depend on the composition of the subgingival flora and the clinical manifestation of the periodontal disease.

13. References

[1] Rutledge, CE. Oral and roentgenographic aspects of the teeth and jaws of juvenile diabetics. J Am Dent Assoc 27:1740-1750,1941.

[2] Thorstensson H, Kuylenstierna J, Hugoson A: Medical status and complications in relation to periodontal disease experience in insulin-dependent diabetics. J Clin Periodontol 23:194-202,1996.

[3] Taylor GW. Bidirectional interrelationships between diabetes and periodontal diseases: an epidemiological perspectiv. Ann Periodontol 6:99-112,2001.

[4] Ismail AI, Morrison CE, Burt BA, Affese RG, Kavanagh MT. Natural history of periodontal disease in adult: findings from the Tecumseh Periodontal Disease Study, 1959-87. J Dent Res 69:430-435,1990.

[5] Page RC, Beck JD. Risk assessment for periodontal disease. Int Dent J 47:61-87,1997.

[6] Hart TC, Kornman KS. Genetic factors in the pathogenesis of periodontitis. Periodontol 14: 202-215, 2000.

[7] Salvi GE, Lawrence HP, Offenbacher S, Beck JD. Influence of risk factors on the pathogenesis of periodontitis. Periodontol 14:173-201,2000.

[8] Page RC, Krall EA, Martin J, Mancl L, Garcia RI. Validity and accuracy of a risk calculator in predicting periodontal disease. JADA 133:569-576,2002.

[9] Cooper M. Contending for the Future. Vol.4. Seattle, MBC Consultants, Inc, 1998.

[10] Haffajee AD, Socransky SS. Microbial etiological agents of destructive periodontal diseases. Periodontol 5:78-11,2000.

[11] Joshi VM, Vandana KL. The detection of eight putative periodontal pathogens in adult and rapidly progressive periodontitis patients: an institutional study. Indian J Dent Res. 18:6-10,2007.

[12] Faveri M, Figueiredo LC, Duarte PM, Mestnik MJ, Mayer MP, Feres M. Microbiological profile of untreated subjects with localized aggressive periodontitis. J Clin Periodontol 36:739-49,2009.

[13] Petsios A, Nakou M, Manti F. Microflora in adult periodontitis. J Periodontol Res 30: 325-331, 1995.

[14] Guentsch A, Puklo M, Preshaw PM, Giockmann E, Pfister W, Potempa J, Eick S. Neutrophils in chronic and aggressive periodontitis in interaction with Porphyromonas gingivalis and Aggregatibacter actinomycetemcomitans. J Periodontol Res 44:368-77,2009.

[15] Meng S, Zhao L, Yang H, Wu Y, Ouyang Y. Prevalence of Actinobacillus actinomycetemcomitans in Chinese chronic periodontitis patients and periodontally healthy adults. Quintessence Int. 40:53-60,2009.

[16] Avlund K, Schultz-Larsen K, Krustrup U, Christiansen N, Holm-Pedersen P. Effect of inflammation in the periodontium in early old age on mortality at 21-year follow-up. J Am Geriatr Soc 57:1206-12,2009.

[17] Haffajee AD, Socransky SS. Relationship of cigarette smoking to attachment level profiles. J Clin Periodontol 28:283-295,2001.

[18] Bergstrom J, Eliasson S. Cigarette smoking and alveolar bone height in subjects with high standard of oral hygiene. J Clin Periodontol 14:466-468,1987.

[19] Bergstrom J. Influence of tobacco smoking on periodontal bone height. Long- term observations and a hypothesis. J Clin Periodontol 31:260-266,2004.

[20] Jervøe-Storm PM, Alahdab H, Koltzscher M, Fimmers R, Jepsen S. Quantification of periodontal pathogens by paper point sampling from the coronal and apical aspect of periodontal lesions by real-time PCR. Clin Oral Investig 14:533-41,2010.

[21] Kornman KS and di Giovine FS. Genetic variations in the cytokine expression: a risk factor for severity of adult periodontitis. Ann Periodontol 3:327-338,1998.

[22] Michalowitz BS, Aeppli D, Virag JG, Klump DG, Hinric Michalovitz BS. Genetic and hereditable risk factors in periodontal disease. J Periodontol 65:479-488,1994.

[23] Michalovitz BS, Diehl SR, Gubsolley JC, Sparks BS, Schenkein HA. Evidence of substantial genetic basis for risk of adult periodontitis. J periodontol 71:1699-1701,2000.

[24] Page RC, Offenbacher S, Schroeder HE, Seymour GJ, Kornman KG: Advances in the pathogenesis of periodontitis: summary of developments. Periodontol 14:216-248,2000.

[25] Hart TC, Kornman KS. Genetic factors in the pathogenesis of periodontitis. Periodontol 14:202-215,2000.

[26] Gonzales JR, Michel J, Rodriguez EL, Hermann JM, Bödeker RH, Meyle J. Comparison of interleukin-1 genotypes in two populations with agressive periodontitis. Eur J Oral Sci. 111:395-399,2003.

[27] Armitage GC, Wu Y, Wang HY, Sorrell J, Di Giovine FS, Duff GW. Low prevalence of a periodontitis-associated interleukin-1 composite genotype in individuals of Chinese heritage. J Periodontol 71:164-171, 2000.

[28] Walker SJ, van Dyke TE, Rich S, Kornman KS, di Giovine FS, Hart T. Genetic polymorphisms of the IL-1ά and IL-1β genes in African-American control population. J Periodontol 71: 723-728, 2000.

[29] Loe H, Anerud A, Boysen H, et al. Natural history of periodontal disease in man. Rapid, moderate and no loss of attachment in Sri Lankan laborers 14-to 16 years of age. J Clin Periodontol 13:431-440, 1986.

[30] Michalovicz BS, Aeppli D, Virag JG et al. Periodontal findings in adult twins. J Periodontol 62:293-299,1991.

[31] Genco RJ. Periodontal disease and risk for myocardial infarction and cardiovascular disease. Cardiovasc Rev Rep March:34-40,1998.

[32] Kornman KS, Crane A, Wang HY et al. The interleukin-1 genotype as a severity factor in adult periodontal disease. J Clin Periodontol 24:72-77,1997.

[33] Jotwani R, Avila R, Kim BO, et al. The effects of an antiseptic moutrinse on subclinical gingivitis in IL-1 genotype positive ad negative humans. IADR Abstract, 1998.

[34] DiGiovine FS, Cork MJ, Crane A, et al. Novel genetic association of an IL-1β gene variation a +3953 with IL-1β protein production and psoriasis. Cytokine 7:606. Abstract, 1995.

[35] Nunn M, Mc Guire M. Relationship of clinical parameters and interleukin-1 genotype to tooth survival. J Dent Res 77:647. Abstract 125. 1998.

[36] Gore EA, Sanders JJ, Pandey JP, Palesch Y, Galbraith GM. Interleukin 1-β+3953 allele 2 association with disease status in adult periodontitis. J Clin Periodontol 25:781-785.1998.

[37] Pociot F, Mølvig J, Wogensen L, Worsaae H, Nerup J. A Taql polymorphism in the human interleukin-1 beta (IL 1 b) gene correlates with secretion in vitro. Eur J Clin Invest 22:396-402,1992.

[38] Golub L, Nicoll G, Jacono V, Ramamurthy N. In vivo cervicular leukocyte response to a chemotactic challenge. Inhibition by experimental diabetes. Infect Immun 37:1013-1020,1982.

[39] Albrecht M., Bánóczy J., Baranyi É., Tamás Gy. jr., Szalay J., Egyed J., Simon G., Ember Gy. Studies of dental and oral changes of pregnant diabetic women. Acta Diab. Lat. 24:1-7,1987.

[40] Hayden P and Buckley LA. Diabetes mellitus and periodontal disease in an Irish population. J Periodontol Res. 24:398-402,1989.

[41] Albrecht M., Bánóczy J., Tamás Gy.: Dental and Oral symptoms of Diabetes Mellitus. Comm. Dent. Oral Epidemiol. 16:378-380,1988.

[42] Albrecht M., Bánóczy J., Dinya E., Tamás Gy. :Occurrence of oral leukoplakia and lichen planus in diabetes mellitus. J Oral Patol Med 21:364-366,1992.

[43] Pinson M, Hoffman WH, Garnick JJ and Litaker MS: Periodontal disease and type 1 diabetes mellitus in children and adolescents. J Clin Periodontol 22:118-123,1995.

[44] Takahashi K, Nishimura F, Kurihara M, Iwamoto Y, Takashiba S, Miyata T, Murayama Y. Subgingival microflora and antibody responses against periodontal bacteria of young Japanese patients with type 1 diabetes mellitus. J Int Academy Periodontol 3:104-111,2001.

[45] Oh Tae-Ju, Eber R, Wang HL. Periodontal diseases in the child and adolescent. J Clin Periodontol 29:400-403,2002.

[46] Pavez V, Araya V, Rubio A, Rios L, Meza P, Martinez B. Periodontal health status in patients with diabetes mellitus type 1, from 18 to 30 years-old, from Santiago de Chile. Revista Medica de Chie 130:402-408,2002.

[47] Cutress TW. Periodontal health in South Pacific populaions: a rewiew. Pac Health Dialog 10:68-75,2003.

[48] Oliver RC, Tervonen T: Diabetes: a risk factor for periodontitis in adults. J Periodontol 65:530-538,1994.

[49] Seppälä B, Seppälä M and Ainamo J: A longitudinal study on insulindependent diabetes mellitus and periodontal disease. J Clin Periodontol 20:161-165,1993.

[50] Seppälä B, and J Ainamo: A site-by-site follow-up on the effect of controlled versus poorly controlled insulin-dependent diabetes mellitus. J Clin Periodontol 21:161-1651994.

[51] Rosenthal IM, Abrams H, Kopczyk A: Relationship of inflammatory periodontal disease to diabetic status in insulin-dependent diabetes mellitus patients. J Clin Periodontol 15:425-429,1988.

[52] Lopez R, Fernandez O, Jara G, Baelum V: Epidemiology of necrotizing ulcerative gingival lesions in adolescents. J Periodontal Research 6:439-444,2002.

[53] Albrecht Mária. Fog- és szájbetegségek diabetes mellitusban. Medicina Könyvkiadó Rt. Pg. 43. 2001.

[54] Ervasti T, Knuuttila M, Pohjamo L, Haukipuro K. Relation betweeen control of diabetes and gingival bleeding. J Periodontol 56:154-157,1985.

[55] Tervonen T, Knuuttila M. Relation of diabetes control to periodontal pocketing and alveolar bone level. Oral Surg 61:346-349,1986.

[56] Karjalainen KM, Knuuttila MLE, von Dickhoff KJ. Assotiation of the severity of periodontal disease with organ complications in Type 1 diabetic patients. J Periodontol 65:1067-1072,1994.

[57] Gusberti FA, Grossman N and Loesche WJ. Puberty gigivitis in insulin-dependent diabetic children. I. Cross-sectional observation. J Periodontol 54:714-720, 1983.

[58] Rylander H, Ramberg P, Blohme G, Lindhe J. Prevalence of periodontal disease in young diabetics. J Clin Periodontol 14:38-43,1986.

[59] Galea H, Aganovic I, Aganovic M: Dental caries and periodontal disease experience of patients with early onset insulin dependent diabetes. Int Dent J 36:219-224,1986.

[60] Rosenthal IM, Abrams H and Kopczyk A. The relationship of inflammatory periodontal disease to diabetic status in insulin dependent diabetes mellitus patients. J Clin Periodontol 15:425-429,1988.

[61] Yki-Jarvien H, Sammalkorpi K, Koivisto VA, Nikkilä EA. Severity, duration, and mechanisms of insulin resistance during acute infections. J Clin Endocrinol Metab 69:317-323,1989.

[62] Miller LS, Manwell MA, Newbold D, Reding ME, Rasheed A, Blodgett J: The relationship between reduction in periodontal inflammation and diabetes control: A report of 9 cases. J Periodontol 63.843-848,1992.

[63] Harris MI. Summary. In: National Diabetes Data Group. Diabetes in America. 2 nd. Ed. NIH Publication No. 95-1468. Washington DC. Government Pronting Office; p.11-113,1995.

[64] Committee on Research, Science and Therapy of the American Academy of Periodontology. Diabetes and Periodontal Diseases. J Periodontol 70:935-949,1999.

[65] Sammalkorpi K. Glucose intolerance in acute infections. J. Intern Med 225:15-19,1989.

[66] Sastrowijoto SH, van Steenbergen TJM, Hillemans P, Hart AAM, de Graff J, and Abraham –Inpijn L. Improved metabolic control, clinical periodontal status and subgingival microbiology in insulin-dependent diabetes mellitus. J Clin Periodontol 17:233-242,1990.

[67] American Diabetes Association (ADA). Self-monitoring of blood glucose (consensus statement).Diabetes Care 16:60-65,1993.

[68] Taylor GW and Arbor A: Periodontal treatment and its effects on glycemic control. J Pathol Oral Radiol Endod 98:311-316,1999.

[69] Grossi SG, Skrepcinski FB, DeCaro T, Robertson DC, Ho AW. Treatment of periodontal disease in diabetics reduces glycated hemoglobin. J Periodontol 68:713-719,1997.

[70] Grossi SG, Skrepcinski FB, DeCaro T, Zambon JJ, Cummins D, Genco RJ. Response to periodontal therapy in diabetics and smokers. The relation of periodontal infections to systemic diseases. J Periodontol 67:1094-1102,1996.

[71] Guzman S, Karima M, Wang HY, Van Dyke TE. Association between interleukin-1 genotype and periodontal disease in a diabetic population. J Periodontol 74:1183-1190,2003.

Permissions

The contributors of this book come from diverse backgrounds, making this book a truly international effort. This book will bring forth new frontiers with its revolutionizing research information and detailed analysis of the nascent developments around the world.

We would like to thank David Wagner, for lending his expertise to make the book truly unique. He has played a crucial role in the development of this book. Without his invaluable contribution this book wouldn't have been possible. He has made vital efforts to compile up to date information on the varied aspects of this subject to make this book a valuable addition to the collection of many professionals and students.

This book was conceptualized with the vision of imparting up-to-date information and advanced data in this field. To ensure the same, a matchless editorial board was set up. Every individual on the board went through rigorous rounds of assessment to prove their worth. After which they invested a large part of their time researching and compiling the most relevant data for our readers. Conferences and sessions were held from time to time between the editorial board and the contributing authors to present the data in the most comprehensible form. The editorial team has worked tirelessly to provide valuable and valid information to help people across the globe.

Every chapter published in this book has been scrutinized by our experts. Their significance has been extensively debated. The topics covered herein carry significant findings which will fuel the growth of the discipline. They may even be implemented as practical applications or may be referred to as a beginning point for another development. Chapters in this book were first published by InTech; hereby published with permission under the Creative Commons Attribution License or equivalent.

The editorial board has been involved in producing this book since its inception. They have spent rigorous hours researching and exploring the diverse topics which have resulted in the successful publishing of this book. They have passed on their knowledge of decades through this book. To expedite this challenging task, the publisher supported the team at every step. A small team of assistant editors was also appointed to further simplify the editing procedure and attain best results for the readers.

Our editorial team has been hand-picked from every corner of the world. Their multi-ethnicity adds dynamic inputs to the discussions which result in innovative outcomes. These outcomes are then further discussed with the researchers and contributors who give their valuable feedback and opinion regarding the same. The feedback is then collaborated with the researches and they are edited in a comprehensive manner to aid the understanding of the subject.

Apart from the editorial board, the designing team has also invested a significant amount of their time in understanding the subject and creating the most relevant covers. They scrutinized every image to scout for the most suitable representation of the subject and create an appropriate cover for the book.

The publishing team has been involved in this book since its early stages. They were actively engaged in every process, be it collecting the data, connecting with the contributors or procuring relevant information. The team has been an ardent support to the editorial, designing and production team. Their endless efforts to recruit the best for this project, has resulted in the accomplishment of this book. They are a veteran in the field of academics and their pool of knowledge is as vast as their experience in printing. Their expertise and guidance has proved useful at every step. Their uncompromising quality standards have made this book an exceptional effort. Their encouragement from time to time has been an inspiration for everyone.

The publisher and the editorial board hope that this book will prove to be a valuable piece of knowledge for researchers, students, practitioners and scholars across the globe.

List of Contributors

Daniel Rappoport, Yoel Greenwald, Ayala Pollack and Guy Kleinmann
Ophthalmology Department, Kaplan Medical Center, POB 1, Rehovot, Israel

Pedro Romero-Aroca, Nuria Soler, Marc Baget-Bernaldiz and Isabel Mendez-Marin
Department of Ophthalmology, University Hospital Sant Joan, Institut de Investigació Sanitaria Pere Virgili (IISPV), Reus, Spain

Juan Fernández-Ballart
Epidemiology, Department of Basic Sciences, University Rovira i Virgili (Tarragona), Spain

Nepton Soltani
Molecular Medicine Research Center, Hormozgan University of Medical Science, Iran

Maria M. Zanone, Vincenzo Cantaluppi, Enrica Favaro, Elisa Camussi, Maria Chiara Deregibus and Giovanni Camussi
Renal and Vascular Physiopathology Laboratory, Department of Internal Medicine, Molecular Biotechnology Centre and Research Centre for Molecular Medicine, University of Torino, Italy

A. Criscimanna
Division of Immunogenetics, Department of Pediatrics, Children's Hospital of Pittsburgh, University of Pittsburgh, USA
Division of Endocrinology, DOSAC, Universita' degli Studi di Palermo, Italy
Department of Surgery, Children's Hospital of Pittsburgh, University of Pittsburgh, USA

S. Bertera, M. Trucco and R. Bottino
Division of Immunogenetics, Department of Pediatrics, Children's Hospital of Pittsburgh, University of Pittsburgh, USA

F. Esni
Department of Surgery, Children's Hospital of Pittsburgh, University of Pittsburgh, USA

Stephen J. M. Skinner, Paul L. J. Tan, Olga Garkavenko, Marija Muzina, Livia Escobar and Robert B. Elliott
Living Cell Technologies (NZ) Ltd, New Zealand

Ivana Maria Saes Busato, Maria Ângela Naval Machado, João Armando Brancher, Antônio Adilson Soares de Lima, Carlos Cesar Deantoni, Rosângela Réa and Luciana Reis Azevedo-Alanis
Pontifical Catholic University of Paraná, Brazil

S. Mikó and M. G. Albrecht
Semmelweis University, Department of Conservative Dentistry, Hungary

Mona Abbassy
Orthodontic Science, Department of Orofacial Development and Function, Division of Oral
Health Sciences, Tokyo Medical and Dental University, Japan
Preventive Dental Sciences Department, Orthodontic Department Devision, King AbdulAziz
University, Saudia Arabia
Alexandria University, Egypt

Ippei Watari and Takashi Ono
Orthodontic Science, Department of Orofacial Development and Function, Division of Oral
Health Sciences, Tokyo Medical and Dental University, Japan

M.G.K. Albrecht
Department of Conservative Dentistry Semmelweis University, Budapest, Hungary

Printed in the USA
CPSIA information can be obtained
at www.ICGtesting.com
JSHW011408221024
72173JS00003B/463

9 781632 411532